Beautiful Skin

Beautiful Skin

The Eight Basic Steps to a Lifetime of Glowing Health

Gail M. Gross
Honora M. Finkelstein, Ph.D.

FAWCETT COLUMBINE   NEW YORK

A Fawcett Columbine Book
Published by Ballantine Books
Copyright © 1985 by Gail Gross and Honora Finkelstein
Illustrations copyright © 1985 by Elaine Yabroudy
All rights reserved under International and Pan-American Copyright
Conventions. Published in the United States by Ballantine Books,
a division of Random House, Inc., New York, and simultaneously in
Canada by Random House of Canada Limited, Toronto.

Library of Congress Catalog Card Number: 85-90857

ISBN: 0-449-90108-4

Cover design by Georgia Morrissey
Cover photo by Don Banks
Text design by Ann Gold
Manufactured in the United States of America
First Edition: November 1985
10 9 8 7 6 5 4 3 2 1

This book is dedicated to my beloved husband, Jenard, who taught me the best of what I know and gave me the courage to blossom and grow. —G.G.

To my husband, Jay, who loves me unconditionally and reminds me to take my own advice; and to my cheering section—Aileen, Kathleen, Bridget, and Michael—without whose cooperation this book would never have been written. —H.F.

Contents

Acknowledgments

To my wonderful children, Dawn and Shawn Gross, whose loving and supportive ways make me so proud to be their mother.

To my mother, Ida Clawans, for all of her love and guidance along the way.

To Eileen Eastham who gave me the idea for this book.

To Lynn Wyatt who not only gave me the idea for the chapter "Secrets of Internationally Recognized Beauties" but also helped to develop it.

To Nina Brown who helped with the illustrations.

To Lois Stark who encouraged me to explore the psychological ramifications of dermatological problems.

To Gayle Bentsen, Marie Curran, and Ann Fluor for helping proofread this manuscript.

To Barbara Hines, Adriana Banks, Brenda Duncan, Laura Sakowitz, Lauren McCollum, and Paula Douglas for all of their creative ideas.

To Warner Roberts for having faith in me and making me a regular on her show.

To Gail Adler, Barbara Hurwitz, and Cynthia Colt for listening chapter by chapter.

To all of my dearest friends for all of their support, understanding and love.

To all of the doctors and famous women who gave of their time and energy to help make this book possible. . . . Dr. Milton Altshuler, Dr. Thomas E. Biggs Jr., Dr. William Boylston, Dr. Alan J. Garber, Dr. Roy Knowles, Dr. Alfred Leiser, Dr. Doyle Rogers, Dr. Melvin Spira, and Dr. John E. Wolf Jr., B. A. Bentsen, Winifred Hirsch, Rosemarie Stack, Marjorie Reed, Warner Roberts, Nellie Connally, Carolyn Hunt Schoellkopf, Neile McQueen, Joan Schnitzer, Maxine Mesinger, Debra Paget, Mary Ann Mobley, Jane Dudley, Joan Benny, Margaret, Duchess of Argyle, Gene Tierney, C. Z. Guest, Princess Mary Obolensky, Margie McConn, Eva Gabor, Louise Cooley, Alexandra Marshall, Paula Douglass, JoAnne Herring, Lollie Lowe, Laurie Sands, Betsy Bloomingdale, Joanna Carson, Victoria McMahon, Diane Von Fürstenberg, Mary Greenwood, Paige Rense, Eileen Eastham, Nina Brown, Madelyn Renée, Viscountess Harriet de Rosière, Louise Shepard, and Margaret Love.

To Roland Patino and Sandra Colter for their expert advice.

To Marilyn Sike for her fabulous secretarial skills, which have helped me on every level, and her uncanny ability to get the job done.

To Anne Lippman for all of her time and talent in both word processing and editing.

To Peggy Cayan for helping me reach those out-of-reach people.

To Hal Foster and Sarah Turner for not giving up.

To Leon Davis for sharing his incredible knowledge on Interferon.

To Eleanor Cruikshank Moore for her dedication and help always above and beyond the call of duty.

A special thank you to Dr. Creigton Edwards and Dr. Taylor Wharton for extra help along the way. —G.G.

I wish to thank our editor at Ballantine, Elizabeth Sacksteder, for invaluable advice and recommendations during all revisions of this book; my husband for making me buy a personal computer and word processor, without which large portions of manuscript might never have been generated; Patrick McGowan for legal advice and friendship; Tricia McGowan and Fran Herbst for friendship, hugs, and leads on an assortment of good research sources on nutrition, avoidance of common poisons, and stress relief; my friends in various Edgar Cayce A.R.E. study groups and the Church of Unity for many years' worth of advice in "beautiful thinking"; the staff of the Library of Congress for research assistance on the relationship of sex, sun, nutrition, and exercise to skin health; and, of course, my co-author, Gail Gross, for inviting me on the ride. —H.F.

Beautiful Skin

The Bottom Line First....

With so many books about overall body beauty and health on the market today, you may ask, "Why do I need a book addressed only to skin care?" The answer is that skin is not just one of many concerns of the woman who would be beautiful. It is, or should be, *the* most important concern.

The first impression you offer the world is your face. It gives a clue to your age, health, and outlook on life. And the skin, the largest organ in the body, is a barometer of your general well-being—both physical and mental. Both the blemishes of youth and the wrinkles of age are signs that the body isn't functioning in a balanced way.

"Wait!" we hear you say. "I can understand how acne might be the result of body disorders, but don't try to tell me that wrinkles aren't normal. Isn't everyone (at least everyone who lives long enough) going to get wrinkles eventually?"

The answer to this objection is only a partial "yes." The key words here are *normal* and *eventually*.

It's true that eventually the skin will begin to wrinkle as the body ages. But recent breakthroughs in understanding of the body's functions indicate that what we consider a normal aging process may in fact be premature aging. As evidenced by the Hunzans in the Himalayas, the Vilcabambams of the Andes, and the Abkhasians in Russia, who live in good health up to ages of between 100 and 140 years, the human body is capable of staying in good working order and operating at an optimal level for much longer than we usually assume, perhaps even twice as long.

3

Even in our own society, some people really do seem to age more slowly than others; as a result, they wrinkle less rapidly. What are their secrets? How do they slow down what for most of us seems to be inevitable deterioration?

Longevity researchers are daily turning up new evidence on the factors involved in the relationship between life-style and the rate at which we age. It would seem that it really is possible to slow down the process of aging and retard the development of the furrows resulting from this process. So a concern for the health, maintenance, and good looks of the skin has a multitude of ramifications, not the least of which is that healthy, young-looking skin is proof of a young, healthy body.

Would you like to look younger? Would you like, in fact, to *be* younger, to slow down the aging process, to retain the glow of youth longer? Would you like, in effect, to postpone "middle age" until your seventies? Or, if you've already accumulated the signs of aging, would you like to begin erasing them? Would you like to take ten to fifteen years of the ravages of age off your face? You *can*. That's what the Figure-8 program can teach you to do.

In other words, you can look better longer. And you can do it naturally.

How the Figure-8 Program Was Developed

The authors of this book are two ordinary women who, for personal reasons, became interested in the subjects of skin care, aging, and the importance of taking responsibility for their own health. They share their stories below.

GAIL: My interest in skin care developed as a direct result of a nearly fatal accident. In 1971, my father suffered a massive heart attack, and the entire family returned home to rally around his bedside. He was placed in an intensive care unit, and the all-night vigils kept everyone in a constant state of exhaustion.

We divided our time with Dad into day and night shifts, so that he was never alone, and so that we each received periods of rest. Mother, however, never seemed to eat or sleep, and my mounting concern for her well-being led me to take matters into my own hands. Although unfamiliar with Mother's kitchen, I proceeded to prepare a simple dinner for her. Assuming, incorrectly, that Mother's oven operated electrically, I turned it on and set the timer for one hour. At the sound of the buzzer, I opened the oven door and immediately realized my mistake. Without thinking, I struck a match to light the gas pilot, and the oven, by now entirely filled with gas, blew up in my face. All my senses, except that of pain, seemed to heighten, and as an overwhelming flood of fear washed over my entire body, I somehow managed to reach the phone and call for help.

THE BOTTOM LINE FIRST. . . .

As I lay in my hospital bed, I felt five years old again, dependent and hurt, desperately searching the eyes of my elders for reassurance, as the masked doctors packed my face, first in ice and then in antibiotic creams applied with tongue depressors. The memories of my recuperation are a total blur, except for the gentleness of the nurses who cared for me. When the shock and trauma had subsided, my doctors braved the moment to clarify my prognosis. I had damaged the deepest layer of skin, altering its elasticity and pigmentation. Skin damage has a cumulative effect, and I had, in a sense, gone through an accelerated time warp; my skin would age more quickly as a result of the injury it had already received. I would have to change my lifestyle just to keep things at a status quo, for my now fragile skin was, in effect, more vulnerable to assault.

Being a goal-oriented and tenacious person, I found myself reassuring the doctors that I would be fine, and that I would, somehow, find a way to make everything all right again. This is how my concern for skin care began. I became obsessed with aging, digging deeply into the research for concrete answers and solutions. Before I knew it, I had come upon a great deal of information about possible ways of slowing down aging in the future based on present knowledge. I began to experiment on myself, adding one thing and then subtracting another. Ultimately, the results became too dramatic to ignore: not only was I not aging at an accelerated rate, I was actually appearing to grow younger. The startling changes in the skin all over my body became apparent to friends and family alike, and I began to share my newfound perceptions with them. Finally, my dear friend, Eileen Eastham, suggested that I gather up the information I had accumulated and write a book so that others could benefit from these findings. By this time I had been teaching school for several years, and I was working on a master's degree in Psychology and English. A book seemed a natural extension of all of my interests, and that is how *Beautiful Skin* was born.

HONORA: As a university teacher for ten years, I needed to face my classes with an appearance that was reasonably attractive, or at least not frightening to the freshmen, and on a minimal budget, since teachers are notoriously underpaid. Since I didn't have time for much fuss, my beauty regimen for years consisted of soap and water cleansing, occasional moisturizing with a nonoily lotion, and application of inexpensive base, blush, lipstick, and eyeshadow. I passed the magic number thirty, which anyone associated with journalism knows means "the end," without a thought about being over the proverbial hill. In fact, I was so busy earning higher degress, supporting and raising a family, teaching, and working as a professional writer and editor that by the time I realized that thirty-five was supposed to be middle-aged, I'd already passed it!

Fortunately, I had for years been doing a few things that were beneficial to my skin without really thinking about them. The first was a change in diet—

moving away from the heavy use of prepared foods, sugar, salt, white-flour products, and beef and pork, and toward a diet of fresh fruits and vegetables, light meats like fish and chicken, and occasional vitamins and other potent nutritional supplements. The reason for my interest in diet was that both my parents had died in their early sixties of serious degenerative diseases—my mother of multiple types of cancer, and my father of cardiovascular disease. Because I wanted to improve my chances of living a longer and healthier life, I began to gather information as early as 1968 on the relationship of disease to dietary habits.

The second thing I had incorporated into my life-style that seemed to help me retain a more youthful outlook was positive mental attitude as a means of relieving stress. Both optimism and meditation are effective stress—and wrinkle—relievers.

On the other hand, I had been doing a good many things that were not positive—smoking for twelve years, using alcohol, caffeine, and other common poisons, and overtaxing my body as a whole by trying to get by on four to six hours of sleep a night, especially when I had an editorial deadline to meet. I never seemed to have time for a regular exercise program, so physical fitness was a matter of catch-as-catch-can. But probably worst of all, I managed to get sunburned every couple of years. Unfortunately, by the time I learned how to handle sun exposure, it was too late to prevent some permanent damage.

Then, at the age of forty, I married a second time and started a new family with another baby. Not wanting to be the only mommy on the block to be mistaken for her child's grandmother, I took a good look at my own middle-aged reflection, became vitally interested in the condition of my skin, and began a skin care program of my own devising. Apparently, it has had a beneficial effect.

A young mother of my acquaintance was recently telling me about her seven-year-old's science project. Referring to my four-year-old son, she said, "You still have all the thrills of school projects to look forward to." My reply was simply, "Again," since I have three nearly grown daughters. A startled look momentarily crossed my friend's face; then she said, "You know, you look so young, I completely forgot you've been through all these motherhood joys before!" So I was delighted when Gail invited me to join her on this project.

The Merlin Effect

The earlier you start our positive skin care program, the longer you can expect to reap benefits in terms of beauty, health, and longevity. Abuse has a cumulative effect; the damage you do at fifteen will emerge in middle age. The wrinkle or freckle or liver spot that then presents itself is the result of earlier damage, either to the skin itself or to the body's repair mechanisms. If young girls were warned against such damaging practices as excessive exposure to the sun, indulgence in improper diet, and the abuse of common poisons, and were given a few basic instructions about the benefits to the skin of exercise, proper cleansing, and certain foods, we'd see more women of forty who looked twenty-five—more women of seventy who looked forty.

But most of us have a mañana attitude toward our looks and our youth— as long as the bloom is with us, we blithely assume it will stay, no matter how we abuse it. So the majority of us don't begin to concern ourselves with the damage we do to our skin until the day we notice the telltale wrinkles, and realize we are indeed getting older.

The important thing to understand, however, is that no matter what your age or the condition of your skin, you can begin now to reverse the aging process, to improve your health, your vitality, and your looks. The famed magician Merlin was reputed to have lived backward; instead of aging, he "youthened." You can, too, if you're willing to follow the natural approach we outline for you. And you may do so in such a short time it will seem like magic, although the principles behind your youthening skin will mean sound good health for all the years ahead of you.

Meet Your Skin: The Ultimate Organ

The skin you live in is the hardest-working organ of your body and far more complex than its surface appearance suggests. It is truly the ultimate organ: it is sensitive and sensual; it breathes, it helps keep the body temperate, it eliminates wastes. Because you really should become better acquainted with its complexities and all the jobs it does for you, we hope you'll pardon us for becoming technical here while we explain some terms you'll be seeing throughout the rest of the book.

The skin is actually comprised of three primary layers: the *epidermis*, the *dermis*, and the *subdermis*. Like the walls of your house, each layer performs a special function, with the outermost layer providing protection from the elements, and the inner layers providing padding and insulation and containing a support network similar to the plumbing and electrical wiring system in your house.

1.   THE EPIDERMIS, the external protective covering of the body, is itself composed of multiple layers of protein called *keratin*. You probably know that snakes and some other animals seasonally shed their entire skins. Well, people shed their skins every day. The cells on the surface of the epidermis are dead and are continually

flaking off. As the very outer layer is removed, newer cells rise to the top and become the new surface. The lower layer of the epidermis is the "mother layer" where new cell growth takes place. The life span of a skin cell is quite short; it usually takes two to three weeks for new cells generated in this lower part of the epidermis to rise to the surface. (That's one reason why a change in body health takes only three weeks to make a real change in your skin's appearance.)

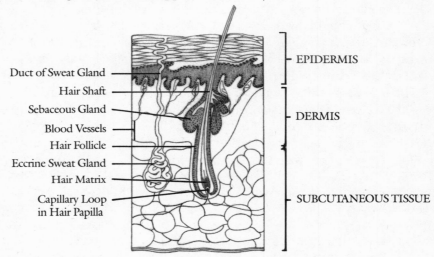

Duct of Sweat Gland — EPIDERMIS

Hair Shaft

Sebaceous Gland — DERMIS

Blood Vessels

Hair Follicle

Eccrine Sweat Gland

Hair Matrix

Capillary Loop
in Hair Papilla — SUBCUTANEOUS TISSUE

2.   THE DERMIS is the support system of the skin; its function in the body is comparable to your house's plumbing and electrical wiring. Part of the "plumbing" consists of glands that help keep the outer layer of skin soft and supple: the sebaceous glands which manufacture sebum, or body oil, and the sweat glands, which extend to the top layer of the skin, forming pores through which the glands release moisture. Perspiration and sebum are the skin's natural lubricants and the means by which it carries out the process of self-hydration. And moisture is, of course, absolutely essential to young-looking skin.

Another part of the plumbing system in the dermis is the network of blood vessels that give the skin its glow when the body is healthy and the circulation good. In addition, the dermis contains a portion of the body's "electrical wiring," in its complex network of nerve endings and nerve tissue. The dermis also contains hair follicles and two protein substances called *collagen* and *elastin*, which stretch and flex with every moment. Collagen is a basic part of the body's connective tissue and makes up about a third of the body's total proteins, while elastin is the chief ingredient of elastic fiber. Both collagen and elastin alter with exposure to the elements, illness, and age; wrinkles are the ultimate result of this damage.

3.   THE SUBCUTANEOUS TISSUE is the "insulation" layer of the skin, containing mostly fatty tissue; fat, of course, plumps up the skin as well as keeping the body warm.

Your skin is busy working for you on a twenty-four-hour basis in ways that you are usually not even conscious of. One is sensation, which a healthy person takes for granted. There are numerous nerve endings under the skin's outer layer that respond to stimuli such as heat, cold, pain, and pressure; some stimuli may cause positive, pleasurable responses, while others cause negative ones, eliciting self-protective reactions. Stroke a piece of fur and you'll get a positive response; touch a hot stove and you'll get a negative one. The numbing of sensation is usually a signal that something is amiss in the body, since numbness is a result of nerve dysfunction or damage.

Like the kidneys and bowel, the skin is also an organ of elimination, bringing waste products, toxins, and salts to the surface of the body in the sweat, where they remain until you wash them away. The process of perspiration also allows the skin to serve as a temperature regulator, helping to maintain the body's inside temperature at a constant level regardless of winter's chill or summer's heat. As an adjunct to the lungs, the skin "breathes," taking in oxygen and removing carbon dioxide from the body. Even more important is the skin's function as a shield against fluid loss; except for the moisture lost in the sweat, the skin keeps the cells of the inner body from losing water and dehydrating through contact with the external environment.[1] Indeed, the skin is the body's great protector, absorbing very few substances in the external environment, and then only on a selective basis, and keeping out harmful substances. One of the ways it does this is through the creation of an acid pH balance that develops when body perspiration, oil, and dead skin cells combine with carbon dioxide on the skin's surface. Known as the "acid mantle," this acid pH level combats bacteria and protects against infection.[2]

Considering everything the skin does for you, don't you think you ought to stop neglecting it and start giving it the respect, love, and care it deserves? If your answer is affirmative, then the Figure-8 Program can help.

The Figure-8 Program

When we began organizing the materials we had collected for this book, we realized our recommendations for healthier, younger-looking skin fell naturally into eight categories. In brief, these involved the following topics:

1. Nutrition and vitamin therapy
2. Elimination of common poisons

3. Sensible exercise
4. Regular enjoyment of sex
5. Proper cleansing, moisturizing, and use of makeup
6. Protection from the environment
7. Adequate rest, mental quieting, and stress relief
8. Positive imaging

These eight topics form the basis of our program. Any woman, young or mature, who wants to have healthier skin can achieve her goal by following our recommendations in these eight areas.

Nothing in nature stands alone. If the skin is to look young, fresh, and healthy, the body-mind complex must be in balance within itself and in harmony with its environment. Healthy skin requires that the major body systems—glands, circulation, digestion, respiration, elimination—be working well. The first key to the program we outline is therefore *balance*—of the inner and the outer selves, of body and mind, of the individual within her environment. The other two keys are *awareness*—of both what we do with our bodies and our minds and what it is possible for us to accomplish—and *attitude*, because a person's mental attitudes are of tremendous importance in maintaining both health and youth.

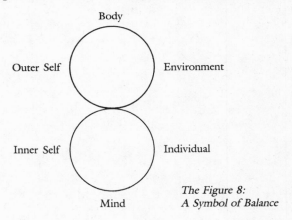

The Figure 8:
A Symbol of Balance

It seemed natural, given the above list and the idea of balance, that we adopt as a symbol of our approach the figure 8. It consists of two perfect circles, one balanced on the other. We'll use this symbol of balance and perfection in our chapter on positive imaging. But for the present, let's just note that there are eight steps to good health and youthful skin. Some of the steps apply to good care of the physical body; others involve mental health and discipline. We want to help our readers incorporate these eight steps into a routine that can be not only simple to accomplish but individually tailored. We want to approach any necessary life-style changes in such a way that inclusion of the new disciplines will be relatively painless. And we want those who try the program to get results that are so rapid they'll be encouraged to continue.

Of course, everyone who tries the program will need to become committed to the accomplishment of goals in all eight areas. But it's often easier to make the effort if you can see you're already doing some positive things in pursuit of your goals even if you may be doing them accidentally or without premeditation. You'll find a check list at the end of each chapter, which you can use to see at a glance what you may already be doing and what you may still want to incorporate into a daily routine. Try always to modify your present actions in the least stressful way and tailor your personal youthening program to your individual needs. If you need to revise your life-style drastically in all areas, then give yourself plenty of time, and work into the program slowly.

One More Thing Before We Start . . .

It's not just a truism that very often we're our own worst enemies—we think, for one reason or another, that we can't or don't deserve to attain the good things we see others enjoying. It is in fact true that some of us are predisposed, through our genetic makeup and what our parents and grandparents did with their bodies before we were born, toward a certain type of skin and indeed toward a certain degree of good or poor health. That's why we sometimes say it's best to "pick your parents wisely"! But it's *not* true that there's nothing we can do about it. And the first step in changing is to love ourselves enough to make the effort.

So, whether you believe in magic or not, there's an incantation we want you to try every morning. Go to the mirror and say to the person you see in it some variation of the following:

"Your body deserves to be beautiful. Your skin deserves to be youthful. You are entitled to live fully, vigorously, and in glorious health throughout the entire span for which you were created. I love you."

Saying these words with conviction will put you well on the road to making the skin you live in younger, healthier, and more beautiful—a suitable temple for the perfected, youthened you.

---

[1] John A. Parrish, Barbara A. Gilchrest, and Thomas B. Fitzpatrick, *Between You and Me* (Boston: Little, Brown and Co., 1978), p. 18.

[2] Irwin I. Lubowe, and Barbara Huss, *A Teen-Age Guide to Healthy Skin and Hair* (New York: E.P. Dutton, 1979), p. 5.

Step One:
Nutrition and Vitamin Therapy

The skin is the largest and most visible organ in the body. But, like any other organ, it can't function at optimal efficiency unless your body as a whole is functioning well. That's why the first step in the Figure-8 approach to younger, more beautiful skin is a younger, healthier body, nourished with fresh, high-quality, natural foods and vitamins. We've devised a diet plan for better skin, based on all we've been able to learn about present nutritional theories, longevity research, and our own personal experiences.

Within ten days of beginning the Figure-8 diet plan, you should begin to feel more energetic. In three weeks you'll start to see an improvement in your skin tone. Eventually, wrinkles should begin to fade. If you suffer from occasional breakouts or acne, the diet may help to clear your complexion. And, while this is not a weight-loss diet, you may find you'll lose weight. The reasons for this are twofold: by switching to high-quality, high-energy foods, you'll lose your taste for the empty-calorie foods you're probably used to; you'll also feel more energetic and become more active. So, while skin improvement may be your primary focus, your body as a whole is going to benefit from the Figure-8 diet plan.

No living thing is ever static. As a living organism, the body is in a constant state of flux, renewing itself out of the materials it takes in. Each body cell has a life span; when a cell dies it is superseded by a new cell, the blueprint for which was contained in the old cell. If the materials the body takes in are toxic, that blueprint may be damaged; then, new cells will be just a little bit weaker than the older cells they are replacing. But if the body is nourished on wholesome, natural food, fresh water, and clean air, the new cells have a better chance of remaining as strong and healthy as their predecessors.

It's known that the body needs more than forty nutrients if it is to grow and repair itself and have adequate energy to function properly. Among them are fats, proteins, carbohydrates, vitamins and minerals, and, of course, water, which comprises about 65 percent of the body's weight. It's very likely that there are other necessary nutrients which have not yet been identified.

Since science hasn't yet revealed all the secrets of nutrition, it's important to eat foods in as natural a state as possible, rather than foods that have been refined and "enriched." Artificial "enrichment" puts back some of the vitamins and minerals that a food loses in processing, but it doesn't put back the potentially important nutrients that researchers haven't yet isolated and given a name to. Enriched white rice, for example, contains synthetic B-complex vitamins to replace the vitamins stripped from the rice in the polishing process, but it doesn't contain the natural fiber of brown rice, and probably loses other healthful qualities as well. By eating natural foods, you insure that your body gets not only those nutrients that are known to be necessary for good health, but also any the importance of which hasn't yet been discovered.

The Figure-8 diet plan was devised to be well balanced and to include large amounts of those nutrients that have the most benefits to the skin. Balancing the body is the key to skin health and beauty. Whether your skin is dry, oily, showing signs of aging, or prone to acne, the nutritional benefits of the Figure-8 diet should get your system in better balance and thereby help eliminate your skin's problems, whatever they may be. Some of the foods we recommend are sure to be part of your diet already. Others may be unfamiliar to you. Liver, sardines, brewer's yeast, and wheat germ are high on the list because they're especially rich in such nutrients as vitamins A, B-complex, E and RNA, all of which will have an immediate effect on your energy and your skin's health. As we outline the plan, we'll explain to you what each food does for both your skin and your overall well-being, and give you some pointers on how to integrate the foods you're not now eating into your daily diet.

We hope you'll find eating the Figure-8 way an adventure in healthy eating, and a delight to you as you watch your body grow younger and stronger. For many years, both authors have had a lot of fun experimenting with the foods on this diet, collecting, testing, and creating recipes for themselves and their families. A lot of foods that used to be no-nos, such as nuts and complex carbohydrates, are really very nutritional. You can eat such a wide variety of delicious foods that you never feel deprived. (And, for those of you who have tried more restrictive eating plans, with this diet you may almost feel as if you're cheating!) Frankly, we *love* the way we eat, and we hope you'll come to value *your* new way of eating as you begin following the Figure-8 diet plan.

On the next few pages, you'll find a reference chart summing up the program, with some specific ways the foods listed can help your skin. Then, at the end of the chapter, you'll find menu suggestions and recipes to help you prepare your meals as you convert your present diet to the Figure-8 plan. Happy eating!

THE FIGURE-8 DIET PLAN

1. *Eat a 3- to 4-ounce serving of liver or other organ meat once a month.*

Most people think of meat as the best source of protein, and Americans have long had a love affair with beefsteak. However, red meats such as beef and pork are high in saturated fats, and not as rich in other nutrients as the organ meats. The functions that most Americans expect a thick steak to serve—lots of iron and protein—are fulfilled better and more efficiently by the so-called "variety meats," which offer a number of other benefits as well.

Organ meats contribute substantial amounts of many vitamins, especially *vitamin A* and *vitamin B$_{12}$*. Vitamin A is one of the most important substances for your skin's health—so much so that according to Dr. John Wolf, Houston proteins; hormones, which regulate all body functions; enzymes necessary for body processes, such as digestion; and antibodies which defend against disease.

Protein is especially important if you want good skin, because *collagen*, the elastic fibrous tissue which supports the dermis, is made up of protein. Collagen fibers, which bind together in strands underneath the skin, provide the mechanical strength of the skin and allow it to stretch and contract without damage.

Proteins are composed of amino acids. These are referred to as *nonessential*, meaning those which the body can synthesize, or *essential*, meaning those which the body can't synthesize and which therefore have to be supplied by food sources. Food sources are spoken of as being complete proteins if they contain all the essential amino acids in quantities sufficient to support life and growth. Meat, eggs, and dairy products are complete animal proteins, and all, in the proper forms, are part of the Figure-8 diet. Except for brewer's yeast, and according to some authorities soybeans and wheat germ, vegetable proteins are usually incomplete.

If you are a vegetarian, you can get enough essential amino acids by combining complementary types of vegetable protein to form complete proteins. Some good combinations include legumes with grains, or grains with nuts and seeds, or nuts and seeds with legumes, or any of these with dairy products.

However, Houston endocrinologist Dr. Alan Garber maintains that there is a qualitative difference in the amino acid content of animal proteins as compared to vegetable proteins; he believes that we require a certain amount of animal proteins in our diets in order to meet the essential amino acid dietary requirement for good health.

How much dietary protein is the right amount? In general, the recommended optimal daily protein allowance for adults is .8 grams for every kilogram of body weight, or .36 grams of protein per pound of body weight. For example, a 125-pound female would require 44 grams of dietary protein daily. This is quite a bit less than authorities used to think was healthful, and less than most Americans eat. To make the most of your daily protein allowance, you need to eat protein sources that are particularly high in other nutrients as well.

Organ meats, especially liver, also supply generous quantities of *iron*, which is a component of hemoglobin and a part of the enzyme systems in the body. A deficiency of iron causes anemia, the symptoms of which are pale skin and a lack of energy. Women, because they menstruate, pregnant women, because they must share their blood systems with developing babies, and children and teenagers, because of their growth spurts, are prone to iron deficiencies unless they add iron-rich foods to their diets.[1] Liver is probably the best source of iron in the human diet.

Organ meats contribute substantial amounts of many vitamins, especially *vitamin A* and *vitamin B_{12}*. Vitamin A is one of the most important substances for your skin's health—so much so that according to Dr. John Wolf, Houston dermatologist and present Chief of Staff of Dermatology at Baylor College of Medicine, it has become a significant part of serious acne treatment, administered both orally (as Accutane) and topically (as Retin-A). Also, a report at the Third International Symposium of Psoriasis, in 1981, showed that vitamin A administered orally has even been found effective in the treatment of psoriasis. What concerns us more is its role in the maintenance of normal skin.

When the diet isn't sufficient in vitamin A, cell development speeds up, but cells also die more quickly. As they deteriorate, these dying cells can plug pores and oil ducts, making the skin dry and rough, or attracting the bacterial growth that leads to acne.[2] Vitamin A taken orally can prevent or clear up many skin infections and encourage new cell growth because it's stored just beneath the surface of the skin. Because too much vitamin A can have serious toxic effects, however, it's preferable to get your supply of this vital nutrient from natural food sources, not from vitamin supplements, unless you have a serious skin ailment and are under a doctor's care. (*continued on page 20.*)

THE FIGURE-8 DIET AT A GLANCE
*A total of eight meals a week should include a selection from items 1 through 3 to insure a dietary sufficiency of both protein and RNA.

Food	How Much	How Often	Important Nutrients
1. *Liver or other organ meat*	3–4 oz.	Once a month	protein iron vitamin A vitamin B12 RNA
2. *Sardines*	3–4 oz.	2–4 times a week	RNA protein iodine calcium
3. *Other seafood or poultry dark meat*	3–4 oz.	2–4 times a week	iodine (in seafood) RNA protein
4. *Brewer's yeast*	2–4 tablespoons	daily	RNA B-complex vitamins choline inositol phosphorus
5. *Lecithin granules*	1–2 tablespoons	daily	choline inositol phosphorus essential fatty acids
6. *Skim milk and/or some no-fat cultured milk product*	16 oz.	daily	B12 calcium (vitamins A and D are usually added) protein "friendly" bacteria (in cultured milk products)
7. *Thin vegetable oils*	substitute for other fats in your food preparation	generally; use any fats *very* sparingly	essential fatty acids vitamin E
8. *Wheat germ*	1–2 tablespoons	daily	protein vitamin E vitamin A B-complex vitamins minerals

Benefits to skin

Helps sustain collagen in the dermis; prevents anemia; prevents wrinkling, dryness, skin infections; may help control acne. Rich source of B_{12}.

Reduces wrinkles, decreases age pigmentation, prevents dryness; may help control acne; helps balance the thyroid gland, which controls many skin afflictions.

Reduces wrinkles; helps balance skin oiliness and dryness.

Reduces wrinkles, dryness; helps balance skin oiliness; prevents skin disorders.

Prevents skin imbalances; improves skin texture; helps balance fat utilization, by emulsifying fat.

Prevents anemia; helps prevent cell damage; promotes body's production of vitamin K (through use of cultured milk products), which helps control some skin blemishes. Vitamin D in milk products prevents skin infections; assists in absorption of calcium for healthy cells; improves skin texture.

Improves skin texture; provides fat required by every body cell; prevents cellular oxidation; aids in absorption of fat soluble vitamins A, D, E, and K.

Helps sustain collagen in the dermis; prevents wrinkling and the depredations of aging; improves glandular activity; prevents cellular oxidation.

Food	How Much	How Often	Important Nutrients
9. *Whole grains and whole grain products*	substitute for your usual portions of refined grain products	generally	B-complex vitamins fiber protein magnesium rutin (a bioflavinoid found in large quantities in buckwheat)
10. *Bran*	1–2 tablespoons	daily	RNA fiber niacin
11. *Eggs*	2	weekly	protein unsaturated fatty acids vitamin A B-complex vitamins vitamin D iron and other minerals
12. *Legumes*	3–4 oz.	once or twice weekly	RNA protein (many legumes are high in various vitamins and minerals)
13. *Soy products*	substitute for red meat in your cooking	generally	B-complex vitamins vitamin E calcium protein
14. *Spinach, asparagus, onions, mushrooms, radishes, celery, beets*	1 or 2 3–4 oz. servings	daily (vary with selections from 16 and 17)	RNA various vitamins, minerals, and digestive enzymes (beets in particular contain an enzyme that promotes the body's own production of RNA)
15. *Peppers, broccoli, cauliflower, kale*	3–4 oz.	daily (see above)	vitamin A vitamin C various other vitamins, minerals, and digestive enzymes

Benefits to skin

Prevents skin disorders; improves digestive function, which helps control some blemishes; needed for healthy collagen maintenance; required for proper use of calcium by the cells; may help control spider veins.

Helps balance skin oiliness and dryness; helps prevent skin disorders; improves digestive function which helps control some skin blemishes.

Promotes healthy collagen; helps prevent skin disorders; aids in absorption of calcium for healthy cells; helps prevent anemia.

Helps sustain healthy collagen; helps prevent wrinkling, drying, and pigmentation due to age.

Helps prevent skin disorders; prevents wrinkling and the depredations of aging; helps promote healthy collagen.

Helps prevent the depredations of aging; promotes healthy digestion, which helps control some skin blemishes.

Helps prevent skin dryness and roughness; detoxifies; prevents cellular oxidation; promotes healthy digestion; acts as a cancer preventive.

Food	How Much	How Often	Important Nutrients
16. *Other vegetables*	3–4 oz.	daily (see above)	vitamins, minerals, and enzymes
17. *Sprouts*	1 oz.	daily	vitamin C B vitamins
18. *Citrus fruits*	3–4 oz.	daily	vitamin C other vitamins, minerals, and digestive enzymes
19. *Apricots or cantaloupe*	3–4 oz.	twice a week	vitamin A other vitamins, minerals, and digestive enzymes
20. *Other fruits*	3–4 oz.	daily	vitamins, minerals, and digestive enzymes
21. *Nuts and seeds*	1–2 oz.	as occasional replacement for other protein; use sparingly	zinc phosphorus vitamin E B-complex vitamins
22. *Blackstrap molasses, honey, fructose, or aspartame*	substitute wherever you now use table sugar	generally	B-complex vitamins (in molasses) aspartic acid, protein, vitamins, minerals, the gonadotropic hormone (in honey)
23. *Pure water*	6–8 8-oz. glasses	daily	

Vitamin B_{12} is important for healthy sexual functioning, and a deficiency of it can contribute to anemia. The B vitamins, all of which are found in liver, appear to affect a number of skin disorders; for example, one of the B-complex elements, PABA (para-aminobenzoic acid), is used both in sunscreen products and as a treatment for sunburn and vitiligo, an irregularity in which nonpigmented areas of skin develop. We'll discuss B vitamins in more detail shortly.

Finally, all organ meats are much richer than regular muscle meats in *nucleic acids*, of which more below.

Unfortunately, many Americans seldom eat organ meats, and therefore haven't learned to find them palatable. If you fall into this category, try starting with the milder-tasting organs, such as beef or calf hearts, which taste quite similar

Benefits to skin

Promotes healthy digestion.

Detoxifies; prevents cellular oxidation; helps prevent skin disorders.

Detoxifies; prevents cellular oxidation; promotes healthy digestion.

Helps prevent skin roughness and dryness; promotes healthy digestion.

Promotes healthy digestion.

Important to healthy hair, nails, and skin; prevents depredations of aging; prevents skin disorders.

Prevents skin disorders.

Prevents fatigue and may stimulate sexual interest.

Prevents skin dryness by moisturizing from within; detoxifies system directly and hence helps clear skin blemishes.

to regular beef. Chop some organ meat in a food grinder and mix it with an equal quantity of ground muscle meat. Then prepare it as you would a regular chopped meat recipe. Traditional spaghetti sauce is a good thing to start with, because the tomatoes and garlic will completely disguise the taste of the organ meat. Meat loaf and chili are other good ways to use this ground beef/chopped organ meat combo.

As you get used to eating organ meats in this way, gradually become more adventurous, reducing the amount of muscle meat in your recipe and trying new organs and new ways of preparing them. Two meats that are quite mild and delicate in flavor—easy to eat by themselves—are brains and sweetbreads. If you're interested in trying them, get a good French cookbook out of the library or at the bookstore and follow one of the classic recipes it will surely contain. One bite of *cerevelles au beurre noire* or creamed sweetbreads in puff pastry, and you'll be an instant convert!

One of the authors told her son that he'd live longer if he ate liver regularly. He quickly replied, with a gleam in his eye, "I think it would only *seem* longer." If this is your attitude toward liver, just bear in mind that it remains one of the richest foods you can eat, and even if you think you're not fond of it, it's worthwhile to experiment with it. One way of preparing liver that non-liver lovers sometimes like is traditional Jewish chopped chicken liver; the delicious flavor of garlic blends so delightfully with the liver that you may find you like it, after all. Most people also find they like liver in pâtés or as stuffing. Another favorite liver recipe is thin slices of veal liver sauteed with onions. The trick is to cook the liver very quickly, so that it's still pink and juicy inside. If you're used to leathery, dried-out liver, this dish is an eye-opener.

You may also find that you enjoy liver more if it's very fresh; our experience is that the fresher the liver, the less the unpleasant aftertaste. Try to buy it fresh from a local butcher and consume it the same day.

Both of the authors love liver, and one of them, who practiced vegetarianism for a while, found it to be the only meat she craved. We hope you'll learn to love it, too, and that you'll try to eat a serving of liver or other organ meat once a month, especially if you are premenopausal or pregnant. The benefits to your skin and general well-being will be tremendous.

2. *Eat a 3- to 4-ounce can of sardines two to four times a week.*

"Canned sardines?" you're thinking. "Why not fresh fish?" Yes, fresh seafood is an important part of your diet, as you'll learn below, and it usually is better to eat fresh rather than canned foods. Canned sardines, though, are an exception. This food is inexpensive and extremely high in *nucleic acids*, especially *RNA*, which are important in the life cycle of your body's cells.

The two main nucleic acids—RNA (ribonucleic acid) and DNA (deoxyribonucleic acid)—are responsible for the proper functioning and renewal of the cells. When we take in toxic materials, whether in the form of chemicals or other pollutants, common poisons (to be discussed in the next chapter), disease bacteria, viruses, or radiation, the nucleic acid in the cells becomes damaged and produces weaker cells in the next generation. If we bombard our bodies with toxins while feeding them lifeless foods, we will eventually develop degenerative diseases and begin to show signs of aging. If, however, we eat foods rich in high quality nucleic acids, the body's new cells will remain strong, young, and full of energy.[3]

A prominent physician, Dr. Benjamin S. Frank, has used nucleic acid therapy with great success to treat a variety of illnesses, including alcoholism and drug abuse, lung ailments, heart disease, arteriosclerosis, diabetes, osteoarthritis, and, believe it or not, acne! With respect to the health of the skin, Dr. Frank's research has shown that an increase in intake of RNA, especially when taken with B-complex vitamins, reduces wrinkles and decreases the brown spotting associated with aging, lightens senile keratoses (brownish, warty skin growths), decreases foot calluses, and lessens the dryness associated with aging skin. On the other hand, younger patients report decreases in skin oiliness, which may account in part for the decrease in acne. Ingestion of natural sources of RNA therefore seems to help alleviate abnormal skin conditions.[4]

A diet similar to Dr. Frank's was initiated several years ago at a famous cancer hospital for the purpose of raising the lowered antibody levels of cancer patients. It has been found that a diet high in good-quality foods which happen also to be high in RNA tends to raise the body's antibody levels and thus improves the immune system's ability to combat cancer. A more complete explanation of the beneficial effects of such diets still needs to be found, but the results of this research speak for themselves: in many cases, improved nutrition restored health and vigor to these patients. We can all benefit from adding this information about diet to our own knowledge.

The only precaution to take with a nucleic acid-rich diet is to maintain a good fluid intake so that the uric acid levels in your blood don't become too high.

Fish and shellfish are both extremely rich in RNA. Most seafood is best eaten fresh, since fresh seafood has more RNA than canned. The exception, as we indicated above, is sardines. Sardines have the highest RNA content of any fresh seafood, and for some reason, when they're canned, the RNA content of sardines is reputed to double.[5] Since canned sardines are cheap, readily available, and very tasty, they're an excellent way to boost the RNA levels in your diet. They also come packed in many different ways: in water, in safflower or soy oil, in mustard or tomato sauce, headless, skinless, or boneless. Just nosh them straight from the can, on crackers. You might think of them as the "good-skin convenience food."

A certain reporter interviewed the husband of one of the authors a few years ago, trying to determine whether or not his wife really did eat all the sardines she claimed to eat. Her husband mischievously replied, "Not only does my *wife* eat sardines, but we feed them regularly to our 11- and 15-year-olds, and neither one of *them* has any wrinkles so far! However," he continued with an impish wink, "we have begun to notice that their tails have started to wiggle when they walk."

Seafood, including sardines, is also a reliable natural source of *iodine*, a mineral that's essential for the proper functioning of the thyroid gland and for the production of thyroid hormones. Acne patients for years have been urged to avoid iodine-containing foods, which are believed to aggravate acne, but if you aren't an acne sufferer and haven't been so warned by your doctor, you should make sure your iodine intake is adequate. Since on the Figure-8 plan you'll be restricting your use of iodized salt, as explained in the next chapter, you should rely on seafood to supply an appropriate amount of this mineral. Even if you do have mild acne, you need small quantities of iodine to insure proper thyroid function. So, restrict your iodized salt intake, and ask your doctor how much seafood it's advisable for you to eat. It may be that avoidance of just shellfish (the biggest offender in the iodine-acne syndrome) will be sufficient.

If you find you don't care for the plain sardines, there are a number of simple, delicious ways to prepare them. Try one of the recipes below:

SARDINE HORS D'OEUVRES

1 3½-ounce can sardines
⅓ cup grated Swiss or Cheddar cheese
2 teaspoons finely chopped onion
2 teaspoons lemon juice
a dash of Worcestershire sauce
1 tablespoon low-fat mayonnaise (see recipe p. 55)
  freshly grated black pepper
  toasted rounds or large whole-wheat crackers or bread
  slices, trimmed and quartered

Drain the sardines and mash them. Mix in the grated cheese, onion, and lemon juice, Worcestershire sauce, and mayonnaise. Season with pepper to taste. Spread on bread, crackers, or melba toast and heat (approximately 350°F) until hot (about five or six minutes).

SARDINE LOAF

4 3½-ounce cans sardines
2 hard boiled eggs
1 large apple, cored and peeled
½ cup blanched almonds
  freshly grated black pepper
1 teaspoon honey
1 teaspoon vinegar
  fresh parsley (optional)

Drain the sardines and mash them. Put the apple, eggs, and almonds through a food chopper until mealy, then mix them with the sardines. Season with pepper to taste then add honey and vinegar. Place in a greased 1-quart mold; set mold in a pan half full of water and bake at 350°F for half an hour. Unmold and garnish with fresh parsley before serving.

You can also try canned oysters and canned mackerel—not as rich as sardines, but good sources of RNA nonetheless. Canned caviar, if you can afford it, is also high in RNA. On a trip to Iran, six years ago, when we roughed it by going into the hinterlands, we had the good fortune of finding huge tins of unprocessed, salt-free caviar available for six dollars each; tins this size would run several hundred dollars today. Iran was extremely dry, but we saved ourselves from wrinkling by regularly eating the caviar; because of its high nucleic-acid content, we stayed healthy, and our skins never looked better.

Just remember that with the single exception of sardines, no canned fish is ever as rich in RNA as its fresh equivalent.

We'd like to conclude with a disclaimer: People have charged the authors with having stock in a sardine company. We don't. (But look how long Charlie the Tuna has been around. And *he's* ageless!)

3. *Eat a 3- to 4-ounce serving of some other seafood or of poultry dark meat two to four times a week.*

Fresh seafood and poultry dark meat are high in complete *protein* and low in *saturated fats*, which can clog your arteries, and which may also cause blockage of the sebaceous glands in your skin. Both are also fairly high in *RNA*. Particularly recommended for their RNA content are fresh anchovies, fresh salmon, and fresh mackerel.[6] Of course, you can eat poultry light meat as well as the dark meat—both are low in fat and calories, especially if you don't eat the skin—but the dark meat is nutritionally richer and higher in RNA content. In many parts of the country, poultry packers have begun to market packages of chicken thighs, turkey drumsticks, and other formerly hard-to-find dark-meat parts in addition to the traditional breasts and quarters. Buying only the dark-meat parts may simplify your meal planning and help you to follow the diet.

4. *Include 2 to 4 heaping tablespoons of brewer's yeast and 1 to 2 tablespoons of lecithin in your diet every day.*

Two especially powerful foods at your health-food store that can work miracles on your skin, as well as on your energy level, your circulation, your sex drive, your nerves, your elimination processes, and your general body balance, are brewer's yeast and lecithin.

Brewer's yeast is a complete *protein*, that is, it has all the essential amino acids. It's also a rich source of the *B vitamins*, with the possible exception of B_{12}; nowadays, many nutritional yeasts are fortified with B_{12}.

What can the B vitamins do for your skin? So far, studies have shown that undersupplies of riboflavin, biotin, PABA, niacin, B6, and inositol, all of which are B vitamins, can cause skin disorders. PABA has been used topically as a remedy for sunburn and a sunscreen to prevent burns, and taken internally with pantothenic acid and fresh liver, has helped clear up vitiligo, an irregularity in which the skin develops white, nonpigmented spots. Pantothenic acid seems to be essential to proper adrenal function and is helpful in the treatment of the collagen disease, arthritis. And folic acid and choline, other B-complex elements, are necessary for the synthesis and production of nucleic acids in the cells.[7] Brewer's yeast provides more B vitamins per ounce than any other food source.

Yeast also contains over a dozen *minerals*. And it's a rich source of *RNA*; RNA extracts are generally made from brewer's yeast. It's useful both for people who want to lose weight and for people who want to gain weight because it helps to balance all the body's systems.

Don't mistake brewer's yeast for baker's yeast; the latter can absorb all the B vitamins in your system and create vitamin deficiencies. At one time, brewer's yeast was actually a by-product of the brewing industry, although today it's grown primarily as a food source and is sometimes referred to as "primary yeast," or "fortified nutritional yeast."[8]

Brewer's yeast comes in three forms: powders, flakes, and tablets. We recommend the powder because it has more concentrated vitamins by volume than the other types, although many people think that the flakes are sweeter in flavor. Some of the debittered brands of both powders and flakes are really quite tasty, so if you've never taken yeast before, you might buy only small quantities at first and shop around until you find a brand you like.

You should work up to a daily dosage of 2 to 4 tablespons of powdered yeast. However, you may have to approach this amount slowly; if your body is really deficient in both nutrients and the enzymes you need to digest the yeast, you'll have digestive disturbance, at first, from this much yeast. So start slowly, with ½ tablespoon, and work up to the full amount. Also, a very few people have demonstrated allergies to yeast, and in some rare cases it may actually cause skin breakouts, so starting slowly is wise from this standpoint, too. There is medical information to support the theory that consumption of excessive fat or antibiotics triggers yeast allergies, so be extra careful if you are in this risk group.

Lecithin, found naturally in a multitude of food sources, is an emulsifier, useful for dissolving fats. Among the well-touted benefits of lecithin are its ability to lower the cholesterol level in the blood and help dissolve hardened cholesterol deposits already laid down in the arteries; its aid to the entire endocrine (hormone) system; and its function in redistributing the body's weight, moving it from areas where it isn't wanted to areas where it is. Most important for our purposes, it is also supposed to help eliminate yellow fatty deposits on the skin; improve imbalances such as acne, eczema, and even psoriasis; and soften and plump up dry, aging skin, filling out wrinkles and improving the skin's texture.[9]

Most lecithin on the market today is made from soy and, considering all its benefits, is fairly inexpensive. Take one to two tablespoons of granular lecithin a day; you won't notice instant results, but stick with it and after a month or two, lecithin should begin to rebuild tissue and help prevent its further deterioration.

Both yeast and lecithin are very high in *phosphorus*, so *calcium* and *magnesium* must be added to the diet to prevent an imbalance and perhaps even a calcium deficiency. Some yeasts on the market have calcium and magnesium added, or, as Adelle Davis has suggested, you can add ¼ cup of calcium lactate and one tablespoon of magnesium oxide to every pound of brewer's yeast or lecithin you buy, if they aren't already listed as ingredients.[10]

There are several ways to take these two miracle foods: you can add them to soups, stews, breads, goulashes, and any strongly flavored sauces, or you can take them in juice or milk. One delicious way to include yeast in the diet is to sprinkle it on hot popcorn; it caramelizes, and *voila!* you have the healthful equivalent of caramel popcorn. Some brands of yeast are stronger in both potency and taste than others; you should read labels to compare nutritional potencies; buy small quantities and shop around until you find a brand that's palatable. Definitely the tastiest way to take yeast and lecithin that we've found is mixed with skim or low-fat milk and flavored with fruit, vanilla extract, or rum flavoring. The following recipe is a favorite:

BREWER'S YEAST SHAKE

> 2 cups very cold skim or lowfat milk
> 2 to 4 heaping tablespoons of brewer's yeast
> 1 to 2 heaping tablespoons of granular lecithin
> 2 packets of fructose or aspartame or 2 tablespoons of honey
> a small banana *or* 2 tablespoons of frozen orange juice concentrate *or* 1 teaspoon rum flavoring and nutmeg to taste (for a simulated egg nog flavor) *or* 1 teaspoon vanilla extract

Put all ingredients in a blender for about ten seconds; if you like it very cold, add a couple of ice cubes as you blend; then drink.

If you opt to take brewer's yeast and lecithin in this fashion, the milkshake is a meal; made with skim milk, it provides approximately 300 to 500 calories and 30 to 45 grams of protein, depending on how much yeast and lecithin you use. Drink it for breakfast and you'll need no other food until lunch. You'll also feel energetic all day. Or you can drink a cup for breakfast and the rest later in the day for quick pick-me-up.

We enjoy the tremendous energy boost that comes from taking yeast daily, and one of the authors lost nearly thirty pounds of unwanted weight simply by making the yeast milkshake her daily breakfast. Because yeast improves digestive functioning and peristalsis, we've found it virtually eliminates the need for laxatives. And some of our young friends have actually cleared their acne by eliminating sugar from their diets and drinking the yeast shake daily.

You can also add a tablespoon of wheat germ and two tablespoons of yogurt to this drink for added nutrition. We'll discuss their benefits below.

5. *Drink 2 cups of skim milk, plus 2 ounces of plain no-fat yogurt, acidophilus milk, or some other cultured-milk product every day.*

When you were growing up, your mother probably told you that milk was nature's perfect food. Well, mother was very nearly right. Milk is loaded with *protein* and *calcium*, and contains just about all the nutrients the body needs, except iron. It's an excellent source of *vitamin B$_{12}$*.

Calcium is the most plentiful mineral in the body because it's a basic component of bones and teeth. It's also essential in the clotting of the blood, and needed by the entire body for decreasing the permeability of the cell walls in order to keep toxic substances from entering the cells and damaging them. Calcium is also the great relaxer, often used to treat nervousness, mental confusion, insomnia, and muscular cramps; the mental symptoms of a severe calcium deficiency parallel those of anxiety neuroses.[11] Calcium assists in the absorption and functioning of vitamin C and is itself absorbed and used most efficiently in the presence of plenty of vitamins A, C, and especially D,[12] which is why most milk sold today is enriched with vitamin D.

Whole milk is high in saturated fat, so it's preferable to drink skim milk. If you're used to drinking whole milk, it's easy to learn to drink skim milk. The first step is to switch to lowfat milk. Buy some lowfat milk along with your whole milk the next time you go to the store. For a couple of days, whenever you drink milk, fill your glass halfway with whole milk and the rest of the way with lowfat milk. You won't notice any difference in taste. Gradually, over several days, increase the proportion of lowfat milk in the glass until you're drinking it straight.

By this time it will taste absolutely normal to you—the way whole milk used to taste. Then use the same method for switching from lowfat to skim milk.

If you can't drink milk for some medical reason, you'll need to get the calcium, viamin D, and vitamin B_{12} it provides from another source. Liver is a good source of B_{12}. Chewable calcium carbonate and calcium gluconate tablets are good calcium supplements. And cod liver oil is an excellent natural source of vitamin D. Just remember to use all oils sparingly.

When you buy milk, choose milk packaged in cardboard containers rather than plastic bottles, if possible. The opaque cardboard protects the milk from the flourescent lighting in the grocery store, helping it retain its nutrients longer.

If you are able to tolerate milk physically but you don't like the taste, you can substitute other nonfat dairy products. Nonfat yogurt and other nonfat cultured-milk products like buttermilk are preferable to cheeses, which tend to be high in fat. If you don't drink milk, start eating or drinking at least 16 ounces of yogurt or cultured milk each day. But remember to choose only nonfat dairy products, as there has been a lot of documented evidence linking high butterfat dairy products such as milk and cheese to breast cancer and heart disease.

Even if you do like sweet milk, add at least two ounces of yogurt or other cultured milk to your daily diet. In addition to all the benefits of milk, cultured-milk products such as yogurt and acidophilus milk contain bacteria that promote the body's production of *vitamin K*, which is necessary for normal blood clotting. These bacteria promote good digestion by encouraging the growth of "friendly" bacteria in the bowels,[13] and help prevent the skin eruptions caused by elimination irregularity.

Yogurt, in particular, creates bacteria in the bowel that produce B vitamins. The Balkan people, who often live to be well over a hundred in good health, use yogurt as a dietary staple, drinking a quart or so of it every day.

Use unflavored yogurt because the commercial fruit flavored brands usually contain large amounts of sugar and other additives. Add your own fresh fruit to the unflavored, live-culture type, and sweeten with honey for a delicious dessert. Or make a yogurt "shake" in your blender or food processor: blend one banana, 4 ounces of yogurt, a tablespoon of wheat germ, and a little honey, if desired, until the mixture is smooth and creamy. It makes a great breakfast or snack.

6. *Substitute thin, unrefined vegetable oils for other fats in your food preparation; use all oils sparingly.*

If you watch your weight or your cholesterol, you probably consider fat your Number One food enemy, although some fat is needed in the diet to insure supple skin, glossy hair, and healthy glands. The nerves and brain require fats for proper functioning. The adrenal glands and gonads secrete hormones composed of fats. Fat keeps the gall bladder functioning and prevents gallstone formation. It's essential for the production of vitamin D. It must be available in the intestines for the manufacture of friendly bacteria.[14] And fat is required in the formation of every body cell, so your skin can't renew itself without some fat in your diet.

When you eat fat, it's broken down into glycerine and fatty acids. Even without fat in the diet, the body can synthesize some fatty acids out of sugar. These acids are called "nonessential" because they aren't required in the diet. But there are some fatty acids the body can't manufacture on its own. These are termed "essential" because they *have* to be included in the diet. That's why you need small amounts of fat in your diet, in spite of the hazards of excessive fat consumption.

What's most important is the *kind* of fat you eat. Saturated fats like butter, lard, and suet are solid at room temperature and are usually of animal origin. Animal fats contain cholesterol, and often contribute to such ailments as heart disease and atherosclerosis, which is the clogging of the blood vessels with fat deposits. Saturated fats may also clog the sebaceous glands, thereby worsening skin blemishes. Monounsaturated fats, such as olive oil and peanut oil, and polyunsaturated fats, such as corn oil, safflower oil, and sunflower oil, are thin and liquid at room temperature and contain no cholesterol.

Although some evidence suggests that the polyunsaturated fats seem to be able to reduce cholesterol levels in the blood, helping to reverse arterial deterioration that has already taken place, their higher degree of unsaturation may also make them more susceptible to the unpleasant effects of "autoxidation," a term which simply means that they oxidize more readily and may therefore be more likely to contribute to premature aging. The more saturated the fat, the less likely it is to oxidize.[15] Both polyunsaturated and saturated fats are now related to cancer, diabetes, and heart disease. In addition, there is new evidence that while polyunsaturated and monounsaturated fats reduce the level of blood cholesterol, they may still contribute to the buildup of plaque in the arteries.

Since both saturated and polyunsaturated fats may have some negative effects, we suggest you take a middle of the road approach: avoid the saturated fats as much as possible because of their relationship to clogged arteries and sebaceous glands, and generally substitute thin vegetable oils in your food preparation. Above all, be sure to use all oil *very* sparingly. Keep in mind that while monounsaturated fats such as olive oil will be less likely to promote cellular oxidation, they will not have the possible benefit of reducing blood cholesterol levels and thereby reversing arterial deterioration. When buying oils, make an educated choice that is most likely to fit *your* body's needs.

Try to buy the cold-pressed, unrefined oils rather than the heat-processed, bleached ones, since processing destroys some of the nutrients contained in the oil, particularly vitamin E, the essential fatty acids, and lecithin.[16] In fact, the heating of oil for cooking also destroys these nutrients;[17] you'll get the most from these oils if you eat them fresh and cold—mix up an olive-oil dressing for your salad, for example. While you may not be able to find other unprocessed oils outside of health food stores, you can usually find "virgin" olive oil in most grocery stores. Be wary of buying "pure" oil; the word "pure" means that the oil is all one kind—for example, one hundred percent olive oil—and doesn't indicate the processing method.

Try not to use hydrogenated vegetable shortenings (Crisco and many margarines fall into this category). These are vegetable oils that have had hydrogen added to them to make them solid at room temperature. Although they contain no cholesterol, they may contribute to clogged sebaceous glands and thereby worsen acne breakouts. Also avoid fatty foods and condiments, such as ice cream and mayonnaise. (Try our recipe for lowfat mayonnaise on p. 55.)

7. *Include a tablespoon of wheat germ in your diet every day.*

The nutritional benefits of wheat germ are many. An ounce of wheat germ has as much *protein* as one egg. Wheat germ also provides *vitamin A*, the *B-complex vitamins* with the exception of B_{12}, and *trace minerals*. Most importantly, it's rich in *vitamin E*, the "anti-aging" vitamin. Vitamin E is needed in the formation of nucleic acids, so it's essential to the life of the body's cells. It also functions as an antioxidant, preventing fatty acids and vitamins from combining with oxygen and damaging or destroying cells. Any time you increase your dietary intake of polyunsaturated oils, you should also increase your intake of vitamin E to control peroxidation of their fatty acids. Vitamin E is also needed to prevent the destruction of vitamin A through oxidation.[18]

The authors have applied vitamin E externally to help heal scar tissue, sunburn, skin roughness, diaper rash, wrinkling, and a variety of other simple skin afflictions; they have even encountered doctors who recommend taking 400 I.U. of vitamin E daily to counteract scarring and long-term eczemas. Vitamin E is thought by some to fend off the depredations of age, especially wrinkling and the brown pigmentations known as "age spots" or "liver spots" that often appear as one gets older. Vitamin E is sometimes referred to as the "sex vitamin" because of its apparently beneficial effect on sex hormone activity; male rats deprived of vitamin E become impotent, and female rats similarly deprived can't conceive, but when they start receiving E again, these problems clear up. Vitamin E also seems to be a real help in countering the effects of menopause and birth control pills. Actually, studies indicate that vitamin E affects all glandular activity.[19] Be sure you get enough from wheat germ or other sources.

All in all, wheat germ is a nutritional bargain, and it's easy to integrate a tablespoon of it into your daily diet. It can be mixed with other grains or flours, used as breading instead of bread crumbs, added to meat loaf or meatballs, sprinkled on hot or cold cereals, and stirred into drinks like the brewer's yeast shake on p. 27.

8. *Substitute whole-grain flours and whole-grain products for refined-flour products wherever possible.*

Whole grains are an important source of *B vitamins, fiber* or *"roughage,"* and the mineral *magnesium.* When eaten in combination with dairy products or legumes, they are a good source of *protein* as well (the milk products or legumes contain amino acids that balance those found in the grain, so together they provide complete protein). Refined, "enriched" white-flour products are not a good substitute for natural whole grains because only some of the nutrients removed in processing are restored, in synthetic form, through "enrichment," and the natural bulk provided by the whole grain is removed. Many researchers now believe that the high incidence of cancer of the colon in countries like the United States is attributable to the lack of dietary fiber in the refined flours we eat.

One mineral often lacking in diets high in refined-flour products, polished rice, white sugar, etc., is *magnesium.* Like calcium, magnesium is present in the bones of the body and functions as a protector of the nerves. Without magnesium, soft body tissues tend to calcify; then atherosclerosis, arteriosclerosis, which is arterial hardening through calcification, high blood pressure, and heart attacks become possible threats.[20] You need magnesium to utilize proteins, fats, and carbohydrates, and for proper functioning of the enzyme systems.[21] A diet high in whole grains and cereals will insure you'll get plenty of this essential mineral.

You may have heard that a diet high in carbohydrates will make your skin break out. Nowadays, though, the opposite is believed to be true. If you eat plenty of *complex carbohydrates* like whole grains, you're likely to obtain fewer calories and less protein from foods high in saturated fat, which has been implicated in the sebum buildup that creates acne.[22] You may enjoy clearer skin and find that it's easier to lose weight, too, since whole grains are bulky and filling, but not highly caloric. What you should limit in your diet are *simple carbohydrates*, especially table sugar. Table sugar contains little or no nutrition, as you'll learn in the next chapter; it's truly "empty calories."

Over the last ten or fifteen years, Americans have become much more conscious of the health benefits of eating whole grains, so you shouldn't have trouble finding whole-grain breads, brown rice, whole-grain pasta, and whole flours in your local market. Just use them instead of the refined foods you may have been using; you'll quickly learn to love the rich, nutty taste of natural grains.

If you have the time and inclination, the most satisfying way to convert your family to whole grains is to make homemade bread; when the aroma of baking bread begins to permeate the house, you won't be able to keep them away!

Although it hasn't been scientifically proven, there may be a special benefit to your skin in eating buckwheat. Buckwheat is rich in *rutin*, which is sold in vitamin form as a panacea for broken veins. Rutin is a bioflavonoid which decreases the fragility and permeability of the capillaries. If you want to clear up spidery capillary lines on your face or body, perhaps eating buckwheat pancakes, buckwheat pasta, or kasha will help.

Remember to keep your unprocessed flours, cereals, bran, grains, wheat germ, etc., under refrigeration. They can become rancid, otherwise.

9. *Include 2 tablespoons of bran in your diet every day.*

You're probably already aware of the value of bran as *"roughage"* in your diet, and you'll be glad to know it has nutritional merit as well. Two tablespoons a day will insure healthy digestion and bowel regularity, and it's believed to reduce the risk of intestinal cancers. Bran is also high in *RNA* and contains some niacin—not bad nutrition for a leftover!

Breakfast can be a treat with the following recipe to look forward to, and you'll know you're doing something good for your body as well as your taste buds.

BREAKFAST CEREAL

2 tablespoons raw bran
2 ounces nuts or seeds (almonds, sunflower seeds, etc.)
2 ounces raisins
2 ounces wheat germ
2 ounces yogurt

Mix all ingredients together and eat with a spoon. Yummy!

10. *Eat 2 eggs a week.*

Eggs shouldn't be avoided just because they contain cholesterol. They're an excellent source of complete *protein, A, B, and D vitamins, copper, phosphorous, potassium, iron,* and *unsaturated fatty acids.* You've already learned how important protein, unsaturated fats, vitamins A, B, and D, and iron are to your diet and your skin. You might also be interested to know that copper functions as a catalyst in the synthesis of hemoglobin and is needed for the manufacture of RNA; potassium, in conjunction with sodium, regulates the fluid balance in the body, transmits impulses through the nervous system, and is responsible for normal muscle contraction; and phosphorous is necessary for calcium absorption and the metabolism of fat and glucose.

Eggs also contain *lecithin*, that miraculous food we discussed earlier. The important thing to know about the lecithin in eggs is that it emulsifies cholesterol. Provided you eat no other saturated fats on a regular basis, the lecithin in the egg will emulsify the cholesterol in the egg, allowing you to include two eggs in your weekly diet without increasing the risk of heart disease. Be sure that you cook the egg in unsaturated or polyunsaturated fat, and skip the traditional bacon or sausage you might be used to having with it. Also, if you use eggs in homemade muffins, cornbread, pancakes, or breading count each of these uses as one of your egg allowances. Of course, if you've been given instructions by your doctor to eliminate eggs from your diet, be sure to follow his advice.

There does seem to be a nutritional difference between fertilized eggs and sterile ones; fertilized eggs are preferable because of their higher vitamin and mineral content, but hard to come by outside of rural areas.

11. *Eat a 3- to 4-ounce serving of legumes once or twice a week.*

Dried legumes, such as pinto beans, split peas, kidney beans, and garbanzos (chick peas), are high in *RNA*. In fact, a 3½-ounce serving of pinto beans or lentils has more RNA than an equivalent amount of liver.[23] When eaten in combination with dairy products, grains, or seeds, they provide complete *protein*, which is why vegetarians rely on them as a protein source, instead of meat. You, too, can benefit from eating legumes instead of meat once or twice a week because they contain no saturated fat and provide trace minerals not found in meat, such as *potassium*. They're also a lot easier on the pocketbook.

A good Mexican or Indian cookbook should provide you with all the inspiration you need for preparing balanced and scrumptious meals with dried peas and beans. Another way to provide solid nutrition inexpensively with legumes is to serve homemade split pea, lentil, or bean soup with a crusty whole-grain bread. What better way to fill up on a wintry day!

Dried legumes, most of which must be soaked overnight before they are cooked, are preferable to canned, precooked ones. The texture is better (canned beans tend to be mushy), you can control the amount of salt they contain, and their nutritional content hasn't been lowered through overcooking.

Be sure to avoid any legume products, such as canned refried beans or canned pork and beans, which have been prepared with saturated fats. In fact, we've recently discovered that mashing two cups of cooked pinto beans, then cooking them again in a skillet with a couple of chopped jalapeno peppers, spices to taste, and two or three tablespoons of water is a good way to completely eliminate the oil or fat from the traditional refried bean dish. Try these "reboiled" beans as an alternative to refried beans; we think you'll agree they're as good as or better than the recipe you're used to.

12. *Substitute textured soy products for heavy meat products in your cooking.*

We'd like to give a salute here to soybeans. Soy flour, which can be used in lieu of or in combination with grain flours, is rich in *B vitamins*, and is a good source of *protein*. In addition, there are some very good soy products on the market which serve as meat substitutes and can be used when you want to eliminate saturated fats from your diet. Soy "sausage," soy "ham," etc., are acceptable-tasting substitutes for real pork products. Textured soy protein can be substituted for ground beef in spaghetti sauce, chili, meat loaf, burgers, and virtually any dish that calls for ground meat. And we've found textured soy "beef" and "pork" pieces an excellent substitute for real meat in Oriental stir-fry cooking. Try to locate the products—there are many on the market—having no artificial additives, flavorings, or colorings.

One wonderful soy product that's gaining in popularity is *tofu*, Oriental soybean curd. Tofu takes on the flavor of anything you put on it, so its versatility is unlimited. Oriental cooks use it in soups and stir-fry dishes; we've also found it a satisfying source of protein in sandwiches and casseroles, en brochette with vegetables, in homemade mayonnaise, or in desserts. Some of our favorite tofu recipes can be found on page 54.

13. *Eat two servings of vegetables a day, specifically a 3- to 4-ounce serving of spinach, asparagus, garlic, onions, mushrooms, radishes, or beets every day, or a 3- to 4-ounce serving of broccoli, cauliflower, kale, and green peppers every day; eat an additional vegetable daily.*

All fresh vegetables are highly nutritious, especially if they're organically grown, and they are the very best source of the *enzymes* helpful to digestion. Spinach, asparagus, mushrooms, radishes, scallions, cauliflower, onions, and celery are reputed to be good sources of *RNA*.[24] We suggest a 4- to 6-ounce serving of at least one of these vegetables once a day. A vegetable salad with fresh spinach or celery as one of the greens, and mushrooms, radishes, and onions as garnishes, is a succulent option.

AN ODE TO GARLIC
In days of old
Garlic was sold
With onions to wear as a charm.
Health would abide
'Cause no germs reside
On someone who smells like a farm!

It's been amply demonstrated that the old wives' tradition of using garlic and onions as health amulets has some basis in fact: both of these vegetables have antibacterial properties. And recent medical findings indicate garlic acts as a blood thinner and prophylactic against heart attacks. (Not to mention that you surely won't be troubled by vampires if you eat enough garlic!)

At a meeting some years ago, one of the authors was proselytizing about the benefits of eating sardines and garlic when one of her closest friends took her aside and said, "There's nothing worse than a reformed foodaholic. Now, because we're so close, I'm going to tell you what no one else will. And that is, we're all tired of hearing about the miracle of sardines. So please write a book about it instead of talking about it." The authors will always be grateful to sardines and garlic—they helped plant the seed for this book!

Broccoli, cauliflower, kale, and other vegetables with stems that form a cross are known as *cruciferous* vegetables. They're loaded with *vitamin C*, the great detoxifier, and have recently been identified as protectors against varous types of cancer. Another extremely rich vegetable source of vitamin C is green pepper. Some brands of vitamin C supplements actually include extracts of green pepper.

Vitamin C functions as a strong defense against viruses and toxic materials —a good reason for taking extra vitamin C when you have a cold. It's long been known as the scurvy-preventer; in addition to bleeding gums, bloody diarrhea, and pulmonary and kidney trouble, scurvy is marked by wrinkled, saggy, sallow skin, and severe bruising.[25] Vitamin C is also an antioxidant, helping to prevent oxygen molecules from combining with the body's cellular material and thus damaging it. This function is extremely important since one major theory of aging is that cell deterioration is at least in part a result of oxidation, the same process that makes metals rust or paper turn yellow from exposure to air. Oxygen, of course, is essential to the normal energy reactions that go on within the cells, but sometimes unstable oxygen molecules get into the act and begin to react with the material of the cell itself, disrupting the cell's reproductive processes. An adequate intake of vitamin C tends to reduce the chances of these unstable molecules combining with the cell's materials.

Vitamin C is a great healer and may enhance the effect of other medications. Researchers at the National Cancer Institute have done studies demonstrating that five to ten grams daily of vitamin C improve the body's ability to produce lymphocytes, which fight cancer as well as other forms of infection.[26] And dentists often recommend increased amounts of vitamin C for their patients with gum disease, to improve the rate of healing.

Finally, vitamin C is essential to normal collagen synthesis, [27] which is important for strong bones and wrinkle prevention. If you have bleeding gums or bruise easily, you should increase your intake of vitamin C; you'll be doing your skin a favor at the same time.

Beets are an important part of the diet because, according to Dr. Frank, they contain an amino acid which helps the body to create nucleic acids on its own, plus an enzyme necessary to brain function.[28] If you're fond of beets, cold borscht once a week can be a treat; you'll find a recipe on page 51. Using beets as a salad garnish is another good way to include this vegetable in your weekly eating plan.

Green and yellow leafy vegetables, and carrots, rutabagas, and sweet potatoes are high in *vitamin A*, good for combating skin dryness, roughness, and acne.

Avoid overcooking vegetables, since a lot of nutrition is lost in the cooking water; steam vegetables when they can't be eaten raw to minimize the depletion of vitamins. Vegetables stir-fried briefly in a little vegetable oil are tasty and retain most of their nutrients. As a general rule, though, for optimum nutrition, all fruits and vegetables should be eaten fresh, with as little cooking as possible. Frozen food is a poor substitute for fresh; canned food is really a last resort.

14. *Eat an ounce of sprouts every day.*

Sprouts of alfalfa, mung or soy beans, peas, oats, wheat, sesame, etc., are good sources of *vitamins B* and *C*. Add them to salads, breads, or sandwiches. They can usually be found in the produce section of your grocery store, or you can sprout your own in your kitchen for even fresher, more nutritional sprouts.

15. *Eat two 4- to 6-ounce servings of fresh, dried, or frozen fruits or the equivalent of this amount of fruit in fruit juices every day.*

Fruits provide *enzymes* helpful to digestion, as well as *vitamins* and *minerals*. Drink unsweetened juice once a day and eat a fresh fruit at some other meal. Two of the best sources of *vitamin A* are cantaloupe and apricots, which are therefore very good for combating dry, rough skin. Citrus fruits are high in *vitamin C* and the bioflavonoids. The latter are found in the same foods as vitamin C and work in support of C in its many functions. So, citrus fruits have a special value as detoxifying foods. Furthermore, citrus fruits have recently been found to increase production of anti-cancer enzymes in the body.[29]

Fruit contains the natural sugar, fructose, which is usually readily tolerated by the body; for this reason, dried fruits are an acceptable occasional alternative to candy as a sweet snack. Fruits such as dried raisins, peaches, and apricots, are also high in *iron, calcium*, and other nutrients; a 3½-ounce serving of dried apricots provides over twice the adult Recommended Daily Allowance (RDA) of vitamin A!

Freshly squeezed fruit juices are always preferable to those made from frozen-juice concentrates, but if fresh aren't available, frozen are better than nothing. One caution about fruit juices is that they may be more concentrated in sugar than whole fruits. If you squeeze juice from fresh fruit, you'll become aware of how much fruit is necessary to make up a glass of juice; to avoid using your entire daily allotment of fruit in one serving, you may wish to dilute your juice with water. Frozen fruits are also an acceptable choice in cooking (for example, in Oriental dishes) as long as they aren't the primary source of nutrients. Use them instead of syrups on pancakes, or put them in the blender with a little honey and make your own fruit syrups.

16. *Eat an ounce or 2 of nuts and seeds as occasional replacement for other sources of protein.*

Nuts and seeds are high in the trace mineral *zinc*, essential to insulin production and metabolism and in *phosphorus*, contain *vitamins B* and *E* and other minerals, and are good sources of *protein*. Sesame seeds in particular are also rich in *calcium* and *lecithin*. And like wheat germ, raw nuts and seeds contain the germ, the source of life. So throw a few seeds and nuts on your salads or into your cereals, homemade breads, or stir-fried vegetables.

Because nuts and seeds are high in protein, you'll probably want to use them as an occasional replacement for other sources of protein in your diet. Use the method on page 15 to determine how much protein is right for you. When you decide to include nuts in your daily diet, just eliminate an equal amount of some other protein. Then you can eat the nuts without feeling guilty.

Although seeds and nuts contain a lot of oil and should therefore be used sparingly, they're also a healthy occasional snack for your growing children, as long as they're not salted. Nuts and dried fruits are a good replacement for the cookie jar.

17. *Substitute blackstrap molasses, honey, fructose, or aspartame for sucrose (table sugar).*

We're going to talk at length about table sugar in our chapter on the things you should avoid for the health of your skin. For the present, we'd like to say that refined sugar is something you need to lose your taste for as soon as you possibly can.

Most refined sugar is manufactured from sugarcane. There's nothing wrong with freshly cut sugarcane; like any other fruit, it contains many valuable vitamins and minerals, plus enzymes to help in its assimilation. But all of these nutrients are removed when the sugar is refined, leaving nothing but simple carbohydrates.

The by-product of the refining process is blackstrap molasses, which contains all the vitamins and minerals that were refined out of that table sugar you're going to learn to avoid. You can use blackstrap molasses with a fairly clear conscience if you need a sweetener in cooking because it's very high in *B vitamins*. One of the authors believes that including it regularly in the diet has helped turn her hair from gray to dark again. If you ever eat it directly from the spoon, be sure to clean your teeth thoroughly, as it can promote dental caries even more rapidly than table sugar when taken in this fashion. Recently, molasses with cane syrup added has been put on the market; this product doesn't have as high a nutritional content as unadulterated blackstrap molasses. Read the label on the product you buy to be sure it hasn't been cut with cane syrup.

Another acceptable sweetener is honey; however, because recent research indicates that glucose (found in honey) has a tendency to raise blood-sugar levels even more rapidly than does sucrose (table sugar),[30] it would be wise to go very lightly on this sweet. Also, babies under one year of age can get botulism from honey, so it's not a good choice for small youngsters, either. Nevertheless, honey is highly nutritious, containing *aspartic acid*, used to treat fatigue and insomnia. Unstrained, unrefined honey also contains pollen, which is high in *protein, water-soluble vitamins*, many *minerals*, and the *gonadotropic hormone*, a plant hormone similar to the human pituitary hormone gonadotropin, which stimulates the gonads. As a consequence, honey has, in our folklore, the reputation of being an aphrodisiac. You can substitute honey for sugar in most recipes; use about one-third less than the sugar called for in the recipe, then adjust to taste.

However, any sweet taken to excess is not going to be good for your body or your skin, so if you have a sweet tooth, you may need to keep it under control with aspartame or powdered fructose for a while. Eventually, as your body becomes more balanced, you'll lose your taste for sweets and be content without them.

18. *Drink six to eight 8-ounce glasses of pure water every day in addition to any other fluids you drink.*

On a diet high in RNA, fluid intake must be kept high to prevent uric-acid levels from increasing. Water will also help keep your elimination systems freely functioning and remove impurities from the body. One young friend of ours began a weight loss regimen that required her to drink two 8-ounce glasses of water before every meal. In addition to losing weight, her acne cleared up for the first time since she reached puberty.

It's as important to drink water and give the skin moisture from within as it is to stay in a moist environment; dryness from either within or without causes wrinkles, so older women especially need to follow this health rule. Remember that human beings are descended from fish, and the chief component of our bodies is water. So the best way to moisturize the skin is from within.

The best water is mineral water from natural springs, though this isn't commonly available in most parts of the country, except through special purchase. Try to avoid drinking tap water which has any such detrimental additives as water softening agents or aluminum compounds. There are several types of water-filter systems on the market which attach easily to the faucet and which eliminate many impurities from the water supply. If you feel really uncomfortable about your tap water, you can usually obtain spring water in gallon jugs at grocery stores, or in larger sizes, with rentable dispensers, from health food stores.

We've already mentioned milk and juice as good sources of nutrition. For reasons which we'll explain in the next chapter, coffee, teas which contain caffeine, and carbonated soft drinks should be avoided; hot herbal teas such as rosehips and ginseng, which have no caffeine, can be good substitutes, especially in the morning with breakfast, or as helpful relaxants at night.

Some warnings about herbal teas are in order here. Be sure the teas you buy are packaged by legitimate companies, as there have been recent reports of cases in which people became ill from drinking improperly dried herbal teas. Also, some herbal teas can produce unpleasant pharmacological reactions; for example, senna and aloe are cathartics: the ever popular chamomile can be allergenic in people sensitive to such plants as ragweed; dandelion is a diuretic; and peppermint has been linked to cancer of the stomach and esophagus.[31]

Note that on any diet high in RNA, alcohol is a no-no because it tends to increase the risk of acidic urine. We'll discuss the other dangers of alcohol at length in the next chapter.

19. *Take vitamin, mineral, and RNA supplements.*

If you've been ill, vitamin and mineral capsules of therapeutic strength will help set you on your way toward a better-balanced body. And many doctors believe that since the nutritional value of much of our food is suspect because it either has been grown in depleted soil or has lost many of its nutrients during its transportation across the country, everyone should supplement his or her diet with extra vitamins and minerals. An Idaho potato just isn't as nutritious by the time it gets to Texas as it was when it left Idaho; a Texas grapefruit has lost a lot of its vitamins by the time it winds up on a breakfast table in Vermont. So, while the better part of our nutrition should come from the food we eat, we urge you to investigate for yourselves the value of vitamin and mineral supplements, particularly antioxidants like vitamins A, B_1, B_5, B_6, C, and E, the bioflavonoids, the minerals zinc and selenium, and certain amino acids. Since everyone is different, we can't tell you how much of or even whether a certain supplement is right for *you*. But we hope you'll want to get personally involved in your own youth extension, and with the help of a good internist and nutrition expert, find out for yourself what *your* body needs to keep it balanced and in optimal condition. You will certainly want to increase your intake of many of these vitamins when you're under stress; just remember that increased use of one supplement generally requires increased use of others, to retain proper balance. And, once again, do consult a professional before adding supplements to your diet; many vitamins and minerals are toxic if taken in excessive quantities.

You may at times want extra calcium for your nerves; good sources are calcium carbonate, the least form of which is the digestive aid Tums, and calcium gluconate, in which the calcium is organic and hence highly usable by the human body.

If you opt to use them, vitamin supplements should be taken with your meals because vitamins are catalysts, which help you better utilize the food you eat. If you take them *before* breakfast you'll lose fifty percent of their nutritional value before midday. You may even want to consider taking supplements that apportion your daily requirements into four parts, to be taken with each meal and again at bedtime, to keep a steady supply of nutrients in your system throughout the day. Further, be aware that vitamin supplements do have calories; know the caloric content of the vitamins you take, and adjust your intake of other foods accordingly, on an eating program that's right for *you*.

Another possible addition to your diet, from the shelves of your health-food store, are various digestive enzymes, such as papain, bromelain, lipase, and cellulase. Many products presently on the market combine several enzymes, each of which works on a different substance—proteins, starches, fats, or fiber. Studies show that taking enzymes with meals tends to lower triglyceride (bloodfat) levels, so you may want to add some digestive enzymes to your daily diet, especially at any meal where you may eat a lot of fat. In addition, enzymes will help you digest proteins and carbohydrates more efficiently. And if you have digestive trouble from taking yeast, it's probably because you lack the enzymes necessary for digestion. Chewing enzymes after a meal will help solve these problems.

RNA-DNA supplements in tablet or liquid form are available at most health-food stores; made from yeast, they may not be necessary if you take yeast itself. It's recommended that you take them under a doctor's supervision and pay close attention to your water intake to prevent uric-acid levels from becoming too high.

And finally, please remember, before changing your diet radically, check with your doctor.

FIGURE-8 DIET PLAN: SAMPLE OF DAILY MENUS

The following one-week menu is provided as a demonstration of how easily foods on the Figure-8 diet can be incorporated into a simple daily eating plan.

SUNDAY

Breakfast
1 cup orange juice blended with 2–4 tablespoons brewer's yeast and 1 to 2 tablespoons lecithin
2 bran muffins
1 poached egg
1 cup skim milk

Lunch
3 to 4 ounces spinach and mushroom salad with garlic dressing, garnished with wheat germ, bean, alfalfa, or wheat sprouts, and sesame seeds
3 to 4 ounces sardines or oysters
1 cup buttermilk or skim milk

Dinner
3 to 4 ounces broiled chicken dark meat or curried chicken (see recipe, p. 48)
½ cup brown rice or curried rice (see recipe, p. 47)
3 to 4 ounces steamed cauliflower

3 to 4 ounces steamed asparagus
3 to 4 ounces apricots, cantaloupe, or grapes

* Throughout the day, drink six to eight 8-ounce (1 cup) glasses of water.

MONDAY

Breakfast
16-ounce ounce brewer's yeast milkshake (recipe on p. 27)

Lunch
      sardine sandwich with mustard on bran bread, garnished with
      alfalfa, bean, or wheat sprouts
  1 cup cold beet borscht (recipe on p. 51)
3 to 4 ounces mixed citrus fruit

Dinner
3 to 4 ounce serving of chicken livers with Italian sauce (recipe on p.
    47)
  1 cup whole-wheat pasta
3 to 4 ounces spinach and mushroom salad with yogurt-dill dressing,
    garnished with sunflower seeds
3 to 4 ounces steamed fresh green beans
3 to 4 ounces fresh peaches, nectarines, or grapes

* Throughout the day, drink six to eight 8-ounce (1 cup) glasses of water.

TUESDAY

Breakfast
  1 cup grapefruit juice blended with 2–4 tablespoons brewer's
    yeast and 1–2 tablespoons lecithin
3 to 4 ounces cooked whole grain cereal with wheat germ and bran
    added
  1 cup skim milk

Lunch
3 to 4 ounces canned sardines or a 3–4 ounce serving sardine loaf
    (recipe on p. 24)
3 to 4 ounces marinated cucumbers and onions (recipe on p. 50)
3 to 4 ounces fresh fruit stirred into 2 ounces plain yogurt

Dinner

3 to 4 ounces lentil soup made with celery and onions (recipe on p. 50)

1 cup lettuce salad with chopped green peppers and garnished with bean, wheat, or alfalfa sprouts, and sunflower seeds

1 slice whole-grain bread

1 cup skim milk

* Throughout the day, drink six to eight 8-ounce glasses of water.

WEDNESDAY

Breakfast

16-ounce brewer's yeast milkshake

Lunch

4 to 6 ounces vegetable salad with garlic dressing, garnished with beets, a chopped egg, wheat germ, sesame or sunflower seeds, and alfalfa, bean, or wheat sprouts

2 bran muffins or 2 toasted slices of bran bread

1 cup fresh orange, grapefruit, or tomato juice, or 1 cup tomato soup

Dinner

3 to 4 ounces baked red snapper, cod, salmon, or mackerel

3 to 4 ounces steamed kale

3 to 4 steamed carrots with parsley

½ cup brown rice

3 to 4 ounces fresh fruit cup

* Throughout the day, drink six to eight 8-ounce glasses of water.

THURSDAY

Breakfast

1 cup orange juice blended with 2–4 tablespoons brewers yeast and 1–2 tablespoons lecithin

3 to 4 ounces yogurt/bran/wheat germ breakfast cereal (recipe on p. 33)

1 cup skim milk

Lunch

½ cup cottage cheese with 3–4 ounces fresh cantaloupe or apricots and other fruits as desired

3 to 4 ounces canned or fresh salmon, mackerel, or shellfish of your choice

1 slice whole-grain bread or 1 whole-grain muffin

Dinner

3 to 4 ounces sliced roast turkey or chicken dark meat

3 to 4 ounces onion-corn stuffing made with whole-grain bread cubes (recipe on p. 51)

3 to 4 ounces lettuce salad with garlic dressing, garnished with wheat, alfalfa, or bean sprouts and sunflower, sesame, or flax seeds

3 to 4 ounces steamed broccoli with yogurt-dill dressing (recipe on p. 48)

* Throughout the day, drink six to eight 8-ounce glasses of water.

FRIDAY

Breakfast

16-ounce brewer's yeast milkshake

Lunch

nut-butter sandwich on bran bread (see recipe on p. 49), garnished with alfalfa or wheat sprouts

½ cup fresh carrot juice

3 to 4 ounces fresh orange and grapefruit slices

Dinner

1 cup apricot nectar

3 to 4 ounces salmon or mackerel croquettes with wheat germ as part of the breading

3 to 4 ounces spinach and mushroom salad with garlic dressing, garnished with sunflower, sesame, or flax seeds

3 to 4 ounces steamed potatoes with parsley

* Throughout the day, drink six to eight 8-ounce glasses of water.

SATURDAY

Breakfast

½ cup grapefruit juice blended with 2–4 tablespoons brewer's yeast and 1 tablespoon lecithin

2 to 3 buckwheat pancakes (see recipe on p. 52) with wheat germ

½ cup fresh berries blended with honey to be used as pancake topping

1 cup skim milk

Lunch

3 to 4 ounce canned sardines, or equivalent in sardine hors d'oeuvres (see recipe on p. 24) on bran-toast squares

1 to 2 tablespoons nut butter on raw sliced yellow squash or zucchini

3 to 4 ounces mixed fruit with 2 ounces yogurt stirred in

Dinner

6 to 8 ounces stir-fried "beef," broccoli, and bean sprouts with soy-beef pieces substituting for regular beef (see recipe on p. 52) (this recipe may also contain onions and any other vegetables that appeal to you)

1 cup steamed brown rice

1 cup skim milk

* Throughout the day, drink six to eight 8-ounce glasses of water.

FIGURE-8 DIET FOODS:
A SAMPLING OF RECIPES

YEAST SPREAD

In Israel during Austerity 1948–58 when meat was scarce and liver unavailable, a version of this recipe was served in lieu of the traditional Jewish chopped liver.

1 onion, finely chopped
1 clove garlic, crushed
1 tablespoon oil
½ cup wheat germ
1 cup milk

4 tablespoons unsweetened brewer's yeast
1 hard-boiled egg, grated
  salt and freshly grated black pepper

Fry the onion and garlic in the oil until it just begins to brown. Mix in the wheat germ. Add the milk and the yeast, and bring to a boil, stirring constantly. Add the egg and salt and pepper to taste; heat briefly, and serve on crackers as you would chopped liver.

CHICKEN LIVERS ITALIENNE

Prepare your favorite Italian tomato-based spaghetti sauce without adding any meat. Quick fry chicken livers (¼ pound per serving) in a little olive oil for 30 seconds to three minutes on each side, depending on how rare you like them. Do not overcook. Cover with the rich tomato spaghetti sauce and serve.

CHILI

3 cups pinto beans
10 cups water
3 teaspoons chili powder
2 to 3 teaspoons honey
1 chopped onion
1 clove garlic
2 bay leaves

Simmer all ingredients in a crock-pot for about ten hours or overnight. An hour or so before serving, add

1 cup soy-burger bits *or* ½ pound
  ground calf heart mixed
  with ½ pound ground beef
1 can whole tomatoes
1 small can tomato paste

Serve with hot flour or corn tortillas, or hot corn bread or corn muffins.

YOGURT-DILL DRESSING

½ cup plain yogurt
1 small scallion, chopped fine
1 teaspoon fresh chopped or dried dill

Mix yogurt with scallion and dill and serve as a dressing on salads or cooked vegetables.

GARLIC DRESSING

1 clove garlic
¾ teaspoon lemon juice or vinegar
2 tablespoons olive oil
2 tablespoons yogurt
⅛ teaspoon dry mustard
freshly ground pepper to taste

Crush garlic. Mix with lemon juice and oil. Add yogurt, stirring until well blended. Add mustard and pepper. Serve on salads or cooked vegetables.

CURRIED CHICKEN

4 tablespoons vegetable oil
2 teaspoons curry powder
2 small cloves garlic, crushed
4 medium chicken thigh/leg pieces
1 large onion
2 medium tomatoes, cut into pieces
1 cup pineapple chunks
1 cup chicken stock
1 cup yogurt
freshly ground pepper to taste

Heat oil in large skillet. Add curry powder and garlic and stir. Place chicken in skillet and cook over medium heat until brown on one side. Turn chicken and add onion. Brown chicken on other side. Add tomatoes, pineapple, bouillon, yogurt and pepper. Stir. Simmer covered until chicken is tender, about 30 minutes.

NUTRITION AND VITAMIN THERAPY

SAFFRON-BROWN RICE

2½ cups water
1 tablespoon tamari soy sauce
1 cup brown rice
½ teaspoon curry powder

Boil water; add soy sauce and saffron. Add rice and turn heat to low; do not stir rice. Cover pot and cook for 50 minutes or until water is absorbed.

HONEY-BRAN MUFFINS
(makes 1 dozen)

1 cup whole wheat flour
1 cup coarse bran
1 tablespoon baking powder
dash salt
¼ cup vegetable oil
1 egg, lightly beaten
¼ cup honey
¾ cup milk
1 mashed banana, or 1 large chopped apple,
  or ½ cup chopped dates or raisins

In a medium-sized mixing bowl, combine flour, baking powder, bran, and salt. Pour oil into a small bowl, add egg, milk, and honey, and mix well. Stir liquid ingredients into dry ingredients until well blended. Add fruit, if desired. Bake at 400°F for approximately 20 minutes.

WHEAT GERM-BRAN BREAD
(makes 4 loaves)

3½ cups whole-wheat flour
¾ cup nonfat dry milk
5 teaspoons salt
2 packages active dry yeast
2¾ cups very warm water
1 cup plain yogurt

¼ cup honey
¼ cup molasses
2 tablespoons vegetable oil
4 cups unbleached flour (approximately)
1 cup wheat germ
1 cup bran
1 egg, beaten

In a large mixing bowl, combine whole-wheat flour, dry milk, salt, and dry yeast. Combine water, yogurt, honey, and molasses in a saucepan and heat to 115–120°F. Add liquids to dry ingredients and beat thoroughly. Add 2 cups unbleached flour and vegetable oil, and beat again. Stir in wheat germ and bran. Add enough additional flour to make a soft, pliable dough. Knead about 5 minutes. Leave in a warm place and let rise until doubled. Punch down. Divide into 4 sections. Divide each section into 3 parts; shape each into a 12-inch rope and braid. Cover and let stand until doubled. Brush with egg and bake at 350°F for approximately 30 minutes.

CUCUMBERS AND ONIONS

4 medium cucumbers
2 medium onions
½ cup wine vinegar
1 tablespoon honey
1 teaspoon paprika

Slice cucumbers and onions very thin. Combine vinegar and honey, and pour over vegetables. Sprinkle with paprika. Chill for an hour before serving.

LENTIL SOUP

2 cups lentils
8 cups water
1 cup chopped celery
1 large onion, sliced and halved
3 tablespoons chopped parsley
1 bay leaf
1 teaspoon powdered cloves

1 clove garlic, diced
    salt and freshly ground pepper to taste
2 cups diced potatoes

Wash and drain the lentils, sorting out any stones or unusable beans. Place them in a pot of cold water, and gradually bring them to almost a boil. Add celery, onion, parsley, bay leaf, cloves, garlic, and salt and pepper. Cover and simmer for about 2 hours. Add potatoes and continue simmering for another half hour.

WHOLE-WHEAT ONION-CORN STUFFING

12 ounces dried whole-wheat bread cubes
 1 cup chopped celery
 1 large onion, diced
 8 eggs
 ½ cup wheat germ
 1 cup chicken stock
 1 can corn, with liquid
    salt, freshly ground pepper, and sage
    or poultry seasoning to taste

In a large mixing bowl, combine all ingredients. If mixture seems dry, add more eggs and stock until it is very moist. Use as stuffing for turkey or chicken, or bake separately as you would corn bread, and serve as a side dish with fowl.

BEET BORSCHT

1 grated fresh beet
2 fresh beets cut in quarters
1 quart water
1 tablespoon vinegar
1 tablespoon honey
1 tablespoon salt
½ teaspoon peppercorns
1 small onion
    lemon juice to taste
    yogurt

Boil all ingredients until vegetables are tender; remove cut beets. Serve hot or cold; if served cold, top each serving with a tablespoon of yogurt.

BUCKWHEAT PANCAKES

¾ cup buckwheat flour
2 teaspoons granular yeast
2 tablespoons water
1¼ cups warm milk
2 egg yolks
  salt to taste
1½ tablespoons vegetable oil
2 tablespoons yogurt
2 egg whites

Place flour in a medium-sized mixing bowl. Dissolve the yeast in the water; add to the flour. Add milk, egg yolks, and salt, and stir to blend. Cover and let stand in a warm place about 2 hours. Add vegetable oil and yogurt. Beat egg whites until stiff and fold in. Bake on a hot griddle. Use about ⅓ cup batter for each pancake.

"BEEF" AND BROCCOLI

1 package (5 oz.) vegetarian soy
  "beef" steaklets or chunks
1 teaspoon dry sherry
1 teaspoon soy sauce
1 teaspoon water
2 teaspoons cornstarch
2 teaspoons cooking oil

Cook vegetarian "beef" according to the directions on the package, let cool, and pour off any remaining water. Then marinate in a mixture of dry sherry, soy sauce, corn starch, and water. Add the oil, mix, and let stand. Then prepare the following:

2 small green peppers
1 pound broccoli
1 green onion (optional)
1 large yellow onion
  other vegetables of choice,
  such as celery, mushrooms, etc.
1 cup bean sprouts

Cut up green peppers into one-inch squares; cut up broccoli into flowerettes; skin remaining broccoli stalks, and cut them into ¼-inch rounds. Cut onions up into wedges and then separate into layers. Chop up green onion and other vegetables into small pieces. Put to one side. Then combine the following to make a cooking sauce:

½ cup broth or water
1 tablespoon soy sauce or oyster sauce
1 tablespoon cornstarch

Let these ingredients stand for a few minutes in a small container, and meanwhile collect the following:

2 tablespoons cooking oil
1 teaspoon freshly ground ginger
1 teaspoon crushed garlic
¼ teaspoon cayenne pepper
(optional, for a Szechuan flavor)

In a large fry pan or wok, add 1 tablespoon oil and heat to high temperature (about 375°F). When oil is hot, add ginger, garlic, and cayenne pepper. Add soy "beef" and cook (stir-fry) for 1½ minutes. Remove from pan. Add 1 tablespoon oil and then onions and green pepper; stir-fry for 30 seconds; add broccoli and any other vegetables, and ¼ cup water. Cover and let steam for five minutes; reheat "meat" briefly, then move ingredients to side of pan. Stir cooking sauce, and pour into pan. Stir continuously, until sauce boils and thickens; turn down heat and mix all ingredients to coat. Serve with steamed brown rice.

SARDINE PÂTÉ

½ teaspoon curry powder
pinch coriander
pinch pepper
2 tablespoons safflower oil (if mixture is dry, use more oil)
2 cloves garlic, minced
2 onions, chopped
1 pound (4 cans) sardines in water
4 shallots, chopped

Sauté onions, shallots, and garlic until golden brown. Chop sardines in blender until smooth. Add everything except dill to pan, mix, and heat thoroughly. Drain off oil. Purée in blender until smooth. Chill until of spreading consistency. Top with dill and serve.

BEAUTIFUL SKIN

HONEY TOFU "CHEESECAKE"

2 eggs
1 pound 6 ounces tofu
2 tablespoons lemon juice
½ cup honey
1 teaspoon vanilla
1 teaspoon grated lemon peel
2 tablespoons vegetable oil margarine
¾ cup graham cracker crumbs
½ cup fresh or frozen fruit
2 tablespoons honey

Put 1 egg and half the tofu and lemon juice in a blender; blend one minute until smooth and creamy. Pour into a mixing bowl; repeat with other egg and other half of tofu and lemon juice. Add honey, vanilla, and lemon peel. Melt margarine and stir in crumbs; press crumb mixture into bottom and sides of 9-inch pie-plate. Fill with tofu mixture. Bake at 325°F for approximately 50 minutes, or until knife inserted in the middle comes out clean. Remove from oven and cool at room temperature. Cover and chill in refrigerator for at least 3 hours. Before serving, top with ½ cup fresh or frozen fruit that has been blended with 2 tablespoons honey.

TOFU TAMALE PIE

1 medium onion, chopped
1 green pepper, chopped
2 cloves garlic, minced
2 tablespoons oil
1 pound tofu, mashed
2 cups chopped tomatoes
2 cups corn, fresh or frozen
⅔ cup water
1 tablespoon chili powder
½ teaspoon salt
½ teaspoon cumin
1 cup corn meal or masa harina
8 ounces jack or cheddar cheese

Sauté onion, pepper and garlic in oil. Stir in tofu, tomatoes, corn, water, chili powder, salt, cumin, and corn meal. Bake for 45 minutes at 350°F. Remove from oven and top with cheese. Bake 15 minutes longer.

HOMEMADE LOW-FAT MAYONNAISE

   4 ounces tofu
   1 tablespoon oil
  ⅛ teaspoon dry mustard
   2 tablespoons lemon juice, or 1 tablespoon
      each lemon juice and vinegar
  ⅛ teaspoon paprika

Blend all ingredients in blender. Thin with water as necessary. Keeps for about a week in the refrigerator.

STEP 1: NUTRITION AND VITAMIN THERAPY CHECKLIST

1. As you review the list below, check off the foods and supplements you already eat with Figure-8 plan regularity:
- Liver or other organ meats once a month
- Sardines four or more times a week
- Other seafood or poultry dark meat four or more times a week
- Brewer's yeast, 2 to 4 tablespoons daily
- Lecithin granules, 1 to 2 tablespoons daily
- Skim milk and some nonfat cultured milk product, 16 to 18 ounces daily
- Thin vegetable oils instead of hydrogenated or animal fats (remember to use *very* sparingly)
- Wheat germ, 1 to 2 tablespoons daily
- Whole grain products instead of refined flour products
- Bran, 1 to 2 tablespoons daily
- Eggs, two a week
- Legumes, 3 to 4 ounces at least once or twice a week in place of other protein
- Soy products instead of red meats in your cooking
- Spinach, asparagus, onions, mushrooms, radishes, celery, or beets, one or two 3- to 4-ounce servings every day

- Peppers, broccoli, cauliflower, or kale, a 3- to 4-ounce serving every day
- Other vegetables, a 3- to 4-ounce serving every day
- Sprouts, an ounce daily
- Citrus fruits, 3 to 4 ounces daily
- Apricots or cantaloupe, a 3- to 4-ounce serving twice a week
- Other fruits, a 3- to 4-ounce serving daily
- Nuts and seeds as occasional replacement for other protein (use sparingly because of their high fat content)
- Blackstrap molasses, honey, fructose, or aspartame as substitutes for table sugar
- Pure water, six to eight 8-ounce glasses daily
- Multivitamins, as appropriate for you

2. If you don't already own one, purchase an inexpensive kitchen scale for measuring and weighing portions; you will need to get an idea of what constitutes the required serving size of the various foods on the list.

3. If you aren't yet a liver lover, treat yourself to a new cookbook; French and Oriental cooks prepare liver and other organ meats in interesting ways.

4. Ditto for grains and legumes; Mexican and Indian cookbooks would be good choices here.

5. Ditto again for seafood and fish; a good general cookbook on seafood and fish preparation may help you find new ways to fix these treasures from the sea. And every good ethnic cookbook has its own way of preparing fish and seafood, so shop around.

6. Each week for a month, make a two-part list, using one sheet of paper divided into two columns. In the first column, write down every time you eat one of the foods listed in the Figure-8 Diet Plan, with appropriate portions. This will help you determine how close you have come to your goal for the week. At the end of the week, use the second column to write down all the foods in the Figure-8 Diet Plan that you didn't include or eat enough of. Pay extra attention the following week to including those foods in your diet.

7. Check some of the following out of your local library, or pick up paperback copies at a bookstore:

Jane Brody, *Jane Brody's Nutrition Book* (New York: Bantam, 1981).
Linda Clark, *Stay Young Longer* (New York: Jove/HBJ, 1977) and *Face Improvement Through Exercise and Nutrition* (New Canaan, CT: Keats, 1973).
Adelle Davis, *Let's Eat Right to Keep Fit* (New York: Signet, 1970).

Dr. Benjamen S. Frank, with Philip Miele, *Dr. Frank's No-Aging Diet* (New York: Dial Press, 1976).

Frances Moore Lappé, *Diet for a Small Planet*, (New York: Ballantine, 1971).

Jon N. Leonard, Jack L. Hofer, and Nathan Pritikin, *Live Longer Now* (New York: Putnam, 1976).

Michael Lesser, *Nutrition and Vitamin Therapy* (New York: Bantam, 1981).

Nathan Pritikin, with Patrick M. McGrady, Jr., *The Pritikin Program for Diet and Exercise* (New York: Bantam, 1980).

David M. Reuben, *The Save Your Life Diet* (New York: Ballantine, 1976)

8. Be patient! You can expect the *real* changes in skin tone and health improvement to begin about three weeks after you've begun following the *full* diet plan. So if you choose to work into the diet slowly, just remember to give yourself a little extra time before you start expecting real improvement.

9. Be positive! At every meal, remember to affirm that your new way of eating is an adventure in creativity that will make for a younger, healthier you. *Bon appétit!*

---

[1] Michael Lesser, *Nutrition and Vitamin Therapy* (New York: Bantam, 1980), pp. 131–133.

[2] Adelle Davis, *Let's Eat Right To Keep Fit* (New York: Signet, 1970), p. 55; Michael Lesser, *Nutrition and Vitamin Therapy* (New York: Bantam, 1980), p. 90.

[3] Benjamin S. Frank, with Philip Miele, *Dr. Frank's No-Aging Diet* (New York: Dial Press, 1976), pp. 29–30.

[4] Benjamin S. Frank, *Nucleic Acid Therapy in Aging and Degenerative Diseases* (New York: Psychological Library, 1969); and Benjamin S. Frank, with Philip Miele, *Dr. Frank's No-Aging Diet* (New York: Dial Press, 1976), pp. 49–51.

[5] Benjamin S. Frank, with Philip Miele, *Dr. Frank's No-Aging Diet* (New York: Dial Press, 1976), p. 104.

[6] Ibid., p. 104.

[7] Adelle Davis, *Let's Eat Right To Keep Fit* (New York: Signet, 1970), pp. 71, 75, 81.

[8] Linda Clark, *Stay Young Longer* (New York: Jove/HBJ, 1977), p. 177.

[9] Ibid., pp. 181–183.

[10] Adelle Davis, *Let's Eat Right To Keep Fit* (New York: Signet, 1970), p. 107.

[11] E. Cheraskin and W. M. Ringsdorf, Jr., with Arline Brecher, *Psychodietetics* (New York: Stein and Day, 1974), pp. 90–92.

[12] Michael Lesser, *Nutrition and Vitamin Therapy* (New York: Bantam, 1980), pp. 108–111.

[13] Adelle Davis, *Let's Eat Right To Keep Fit* (New York: Signet, 1970), p. 218.

[14] Ibid., pp. 42, 45–46.

[15] Durk Pearson and Sandy Shaw, *Life Extension* (New York: Warner Books, 1983), pp. 366–369.

[16] Carlton Fredericks, *Eating Right for You* (New York: Grosset and Dunlap, 1972), pp. 212–214; and Michael Lesser, *Nutrition and Vitamin Therapy* (New York; Bantam, 1980), p. 105.

[17] Roger J. Williams calls attention to several studies which indicate that heating polyunsaturated oils for cooking may be associated with an increase in the incidence of atherosclerosis. *Nutrition Against Disease* (New York: Pittman Publishing Corp., 1971), pp. 269–270.

[18] Adelle Davis, *Let's Eat Right to Keep Fit* (New York: Signet, 1970); and Carlton Fredericks, *Eating Right for You* (New York: Grosset and Dunlap, 1972), pp. 130–137.

[19] Michael Lesser, *Nutrition and Vitamin Therapy* (New York: Bantam, 1980), pp. 98–101.

[20] Ibid., p. 113.

[21] Adelle Davis, *Let's Eat Right to Keep Fit* (New York: Signet, 1970), p. 173.

[22] Gustave H. Hoehn, *Acne Can Be Cured* (New York: Arco, 1978).

[23] Benjamin S. Frank, with Philip Miele, *Dr. Frank's No-Aging Diet* (New York: Dial Press, 1976), p. 104.

[24] Ibid.

[25] Michael Lesser, *Nutrition and Vitamin Therapy* (New York: Bantam, 1980), p. 73.

[26] Ibid., p. 79.

[27] Ibid., pp. 71–72.

[28] Benjamin S. Frank, with Philip Miele, *Dr. Frank's No-Aging Diet* (New York: Dial Press, 1976), p. 103.

[29] Jane Brody, *Jane Brody's Nutrition Book* (New York: Bantam, 1981), p. 442.

[30] Gina Kolata, "Dietary Dogma Disproved," *Science*, 220 (29 April 1983), pp. 487–88.

[31] Jane Brody, *Jane Brody's Nutrition Book* (New York: Bantam, 1981), p. 246.

Step Two:
Elimination of Common Poisons

We Hope This Won't Inconvenience You, But . . .

Now that we've told you all the good things you should put in your body to make your skin young, healthy, and beautiful, we're going to tell you about some things not to put into your body, just to make sure your skin stays that way. The items on our list fell into two basic categories: those which are bad because they can damage the body's hormone system, and those which are bad for other reasons. The bugaboos are as follows:

Bad for Your Hormone System
Tobacco
Alcohol
Drugs
Caffeine
Sodium in the form of salt and other food additives
Refined sugar products

Bad for Other Reasons
Processed foods
Muscle meats and other high-fat foods
Highly spiced foods
Refined flour products
For acne sufferers, foods rich in iodine and bromine
Crash diets

A Brief Word about Hormones

Because so many of these common poisons damage the endocrine or internal glandular system of the body, you should have a basic understanding of what that system does and why it's important to your skin. The endocrine system secretes hormones into the bloodstream that act as chemical messengers in triggering functions important to the entire body. This complex system influences nearly every aspect of your body's development and performance, including growth, height, and weight, the development of all secondary sex characteristics, sleep patterns, fear and flight responses, the immune system, mental abilities, behavioral tendencies, libido, creativity, humor, and personality traits. The figure below shows the position of the major endocrine glands in the body.

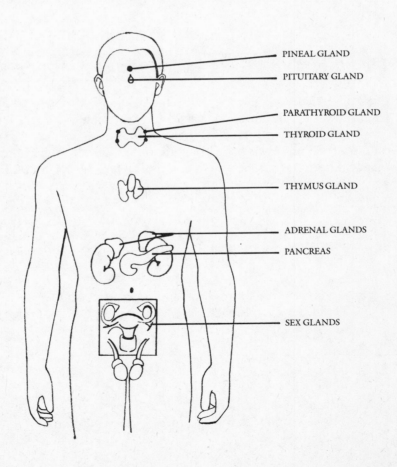

PINEAL GLAND

PITUITARY GLAND

PARATHYROID GLAND

THYROID GLAND

THYMUS GLAND

ADRENAL GLANDS

PANCREAS

SEX GLANDS

Since the hormones secreted by the endocrine glands play a part in regulating nearly every bodily function, and since a hormone imbalance can cause a variety of skin afflictions from acne to collagen breakdown, it is important to be aware of the many ways in which we may do harm to our hormone systems. According to Dr. John Wolf, Chief of Staff of Dermatology at Baylor College of Medicine, there is much research going on currently as to what causes changes in hormone levels, and what the ramifications of such changes may include. Acne, for example, is in part caused by interaction of the male androgyn sex hormones with the sebaceous glands. These hormones are produced in both males and females. They tend to be produced at excessively high levels during puberty; this is why so many teenagers have acne. Pregnant women also get acne occasionally, due to similar imbalances in their hormonal systems.

While all the factors contributing to glandular imbalances and hence skin afflictions have yet to be pinpointed, it is known that one major way the endocrine system may be damaged is through chronic stress (see Step 7), the cumulative effect of which plays a significant part in many illnesses. Another equally common way in which we disrupt the body's hormone balance is through the habitual ingestion or use of toxic substances. These common poisons can overload one or more of the body's glands and cause a domino effect in the glandular system. It's to these dangerous substances that we now turn our attention.

COMMON POISONS AT-A-GLANCE
The chart below cites those common poisons you'll want to avoid for the health of your skin and the major types of damage they can do.

Common Poison	Major Type of Damage to Skin and Body
Tobacco	Constricts blood vessels and thereby dries skin's outer layers; chokes skin's oxygen supply by combining hemoglobin with carbon monoxide; contributes to use wrinkles around eyes and on and around lips; stresses the adrenals and the pancreas and thus contributes to premature aging; depletes body's supply of vitamin C; produces acid smoke which pollutes skin's environment; contributes to many degenerative and often fatal diseases.
Alcohol	Upsets body's insulin balance; creates vitamin deficiencies; dilates skin's blood vessels, thus contributing to the condition called rosacea; damages liver and thereby contributes to premature aging; extreme and prolonged overuse is often fatal.

Common Poison	Major Type of Damage to Skin and Body
Aspirin	Can cause internal bleeding; stimulates adrenal production of aldosterone.
Acetaminophen	Can cause liver and kidney damage.
Ibuprofen	Can cause reactions similar to those of aspirin.
Laxatives	Can cause numerous vitamin deficiencies by rushing nutrients out of the body; overuse results in dependency.
ACTH	Can cause potassium deficiencies, resulting in edema; affects the body's blood-sugar level; affects the pituitary and adrenal glands.
Cortisone	Can cause potassium deficiencies, resulting in edema; affects the body's blood-sugar level; can cause acne; affects the body's collagen; affects the pituitary and adrenal glands.
Diuretics	Can cause potassium deficiencies, resulting in edema.
Antibiotics	Can destroy healthy bacteria in the bowel, causing diarrhea; can bring about vitamin deficiencies; some can cause sun sensitivity.
Sulfa drugs	Can disrupt the body's enzyme systems; can result in eczema.
Tranquilizers	Can cause allergic rashes and skin shedding.
Birth control pills	Can create skin disorders due to deficiencies of folic acid, vitamin B_6, and vitamin E; can result in brownish pigmentation; disrupt the body's natural hormone balance and sexual cycle; discontinuing their use can cause acne.
Dilantin (sometimes used to treat epilepsy)	Can cause acne breakouts in some people; can cause folic acid deficiency, resulting in "mask of pregnancy."
Caffeine and Theobromine	Stimulate the adrenals and disrupt the body's insulin balance; can contribute to anemia; if very hot, can contribute to rosacea.
Salt and sodium products	Can create potassium deficiencies and thus stress the adrenals, resulting in possible edema, hypoglycemia, indigestion, premenstrual syndrome, hypertension (high blood pressure), stroke, and kidney failure in predisposed individuals.

Common Poison	Major Type of Damage to Skin and Body
Refined sugar	Contributes to hypoglycemia, diabetes, obesity, acne, and possibly many degenerative diseases; disrupts the normal adrenal-insulin balance.
Additives in processed foods	Can cause hyperactivity, allergic reactions, blood vessel dilation, and possibly other so-far-unknown reactions.
Muscle meats and other high-fat foods	Contain cholesterol and saturated fats which can clog veins and arteries; may contribute to the sebum buildup that results in acne.
Spicy foods	Can cause blood-vessel dilation and ruptured capillaries just under the surface of the skin.
Refined grains	Can create deficiencies of B-complex and E vitamins.
Foods rich in iodine and bromine	Can worsen acne in sensitive patients.

Tobacco

Of the various ways of using tobacco, cigars and pipes are statistically less harmful than cigarettes. Because they are more difficult to inhale, they contribute primarily to upper respiratory ailments and mouth cancers rather than the more serious lung cancer. But since most women who smoke prefer cigarettes, we'll address this to the cigarette smokers in our audience.

We're sure you know by now that cigarette smoking contributes to the incidence of heart disease, emphysema, and stroke, as well as to cancer of the lips, mouth, and larynx, esophagus, lungs, and bladder. New evidence of its dangers is being uncovered all the time; as recently as June of 1983, studies demonstrated that smoking was a causative factor in the increased incidence of gum disease. In addition to contributing over time to atherosclerosis, recent studies indicate that smoking causes muscle contractions in the walls of the coronary arteries, thus contributing even more markedly to a weakened heart system. The American Lung Association directly attributes more than 300,000 deaths a year in the United States to a specific type of lung cancer that comes only from cigarette smoking. Babies exposed to nicotine in utero tend to be smaller at birth and are more likely to die shortly after birth than are babies of non-smoking mothers.[1] And according to Houston plastic surgeon Dr. Thomas Biggs, cigarette smoking is as damaging to the skin as sun exposure, and is in fact the most significant factor in premature aging; he says he is able to tell from 20 feet away, by a person's color, if that person is a smoker. Dr. Biggs relates that he encountered a patient whom he hadn't seen in many months. He immediately congratulated the woman for having given up smoking. Taken aback by this seemingly psychic observation, the patient asked how Dr. Biggs knew; the doctor replied he could tell by the woman's healthier color.

Tar and nicotine are poisons. If you put poison into your body, you place additional stress on all the body's systems. In addition to performing its regular jobs, your body has to struggle to eliminate the poison and compensate for the body functions that the poison interferes with.

One of the ways in which smoking poisons the body is by constricting the blood vessels, allowing less blood to get through. This dries out the skin's outer layers and contributes directly to the development of wrinkles. The carbon monoxide in tobacco also combines with the hemoglobin in the blood, preventing the hemoglobin from picking up oxygen the tissues need for metabolism. So smoking chokes off the skin's blood supply in two ways.

As a response to the poisons in the inhaled smoke, the adrenal glands release epinephrine (adrenalin), causing blood pressure to rise, the heart rate to increase, and blood-sugar production to be stepped up. This chain of events accounts for the "rush" one feels after the first few inhalations. But insulin secretion follows, automatically lowering the blood-sugar level again, so the hormone system gets a kick without any nutritional support to balance it. This process is similar to what happens when you take in caffeine or sugar, as you'll see below.

A further hormonal response to smoking explains why it is often so difficult to quit. The nicotine in cigarettes stimulates the brain to secrete a hormone called beta-endorphin. Endorphins are believed to have an effect similar to opiates or tranquilizers; they make you feel calmer, happier, and more peaceful. Smokers come to rely on this pleasant "buzz" and tend to get cranky and hostile when they try to quit smoking.[2]

In addition, two cigarettes reduce the body's vitamin C content by fifty milligrams, the average amount of C contained in an orange, so if you're even a half-pack-a-day smoker, you'd need to eat five oranges every day to replenish your supply of vitamin C.[3] Remember that vitamin C depletion produces scurvy, and a symptom of scurvy is wrinkling.

Smoking masks the taste of food by altering the taste buds. And nicotine causes the skin on the hands to turn yellow.

Burning tobacco releases carbon, polluting the air and contributing to the dirt in your skin's environment. Many brands of American cigarettes are made of tobacco which has had a kind of sauce added to it in the curing process. This "sauce" may contain sugar, flavorings, saltpeter, and other chemicals that are supposed to improve its aromatic qualities and evenness of burning.[4] Sugared tobacco produces a highly acid smoke, which is even more damaging to the skin and lungs than regular tobacco smoke.

And as if all that weren't enough, long-time smokers invariably develop use-wrinkles around the eyes from squinting to keep the smoke out and on and around the lips from puckering. Unfortunately, once you hit forty, these creases become practically irreversible; heavy smokers are likely to look ten to twenty years older than their nonsmoking counterparts.

Alcohol

Alcohol is another substance with which many Americans habitually poison themselves. Like smoking, drinking alcoholic beverages depletes the body's store of essential nutrients, especially B-complex vitamins, and affects the body's insulin level. Heavy drinking can create huge vitamin deficiencies and eventually ravages the internal organs, particularly the liver. This internal damage registers on the skin, and especially on the face, in bloating, puffiness, ruddiness or splotchiness, and eventually in wrinkling. And alcohol is very drying; if drinking alcohol makes you feel thirsty, you can be sure your skin is equally thirsty.

Although there is no doubt that heavy drinking is extremely dangerous to your health, some controversy now surrounds even moderate or light "social" drinking. Alcohol dilates the blood vessels; this is the reason alcoholics often have splotchy, red complexions. Some doctors believe that one to two ounces of alcohol a day will relax and open up the blood vessels, improving circulation and reducing the risk of coronary disease. Many other doctors believe, however, that over the long term, any benefits will be outweighed by damage to the liver and possibly other internal organs. Furthermore, this dilatation of the blood vessels carries a risk for your skin. It results in a flushing effect called *rosacea*, known in layman's terms as "drinker's flush" (think of the people you know who turn red when they've been drinking—W. C. Fields came by his red nose this way!) and ultimately causes the tiny capillaries in the face to break, creating unattractive, spidery lines under the skin.

The harmful effects of alcohol are the same whether you're imbibing hard liquor, wine, or beer. Although they differ in strength, one serving of each generally has the same amount of alcohol: an ounce of the hard stuff contains as much pure alcohol as a four-ounce glass of wine or a twelve-ounce can of beer. So don't fool yourself into thinking that because you drink wine or beer you aren't getting as much alcohol—serving for serving, the results will be the same.

It's often said that beer is a nutritious drink, but this is a myth—at least in this country. It's true that natural, locally brewed beer does have some nutrients. When one of the authors lived in a small village in Germany a couple of decades ago, the local brewery had a beer-delivery service; in Germany where everybody drank beer, the beerman had the same status as the American milkman of bygone days. Beer was considered wholesome, made from natural ingredients, full of vitamins, unpasteurized and unadulterated with any artificial additives. Like all natural foods, it had to be consumed quickly or it spoiled. Nursing mothers and young children drank it; doctors recommended it, even for babies; it was a staple food. Unfortunately, such beer simply isn't available in this country, even through imports. American beer, unlike locally brewed German beer, is mostly empty calories and additives that make it ferment and foam; it lacks the nutrients of natural German beer. Most wine today is also fermented with sugar and contains other possibly harmful additives. Do you really want to put unnatural chemicals into your body? And don't forget that even natural wines and beers, like the local beer from the village brewery in Germany, contain enough alcohol to damage your body as much as they benefit it.

While it's true that limited imbibing of alcohol (a drink or two a day) is sometimes recommended to improve the circulation, as we mentioned above, many authorities think even this minimal amount of alcohol over time can damage the liver. If, as occasionally happens, your doctor prescribes moderate drinking to improve your circulation, we recommend that you ask him if you can try a less risky method of accomplishing the same end: regular exercise (see Step 3). If you are in doubt about the best course of action, consult another doctor for a second opinion. We feel that the known detrimental effects of drinking (and possibly other effects, still unknown) far outweigh the potential benefits.

Drugs

Unnatural chemical compounds of any sort don't belong in your body. Narcotics like cocaine and heroine will do extensive damage to nearly every body system and ultimately put you in an early grave, making it unnecessary for you to worry any further about your skin. Amphetamines and barbiturates are nearly as dangerous. Hallucinogens, such as marijuana and hashish (those ever-popular brownie ingredients) and LSD, may not kill you, but they may permanently alter your state of mind and body, including your memory and your fertility. And if you smoke pot or hash, they'll have the same effect on your lungs and skin as tobacco. Several such drugs and their associated skin problems are noted in the chart below.[5]

Type of Drug	Effect on the Skin
amyl nitrates* ("sniffers" or "poppers")	Impede oxygen consumption and assimilation; as a result the skin turns blue from oxygen starvation. Over long term, interference with oxygen utilization results in cellular deterioration and premature aging.
marijuana	Can worsen already existent acne and cause allergic skin reactions such as hives.
barbiturates	Can cause allergic rashes and skin flaking or peeling, plus blisters around the mouth and on other parts of the body.
amphetamines ("uppers")	Can result in allergic rashes; tend to dehydrate the body, causing dry lips and mouth, chapping, and possibly sores; can contribute to wrinkling.
heroin addiction	Causes premature aging, including dark circles under the eyes and wrinkling from collagen breakdown; heroin addicts have a secondary risk of developing scars, abcesses, blisters, or infections at injection sites.

* Not to be confused with amyl nitrites, salts of nitrous acid, which may be prescribed as medication to relieve arterial pressure in spasmodic diseases.

We assume that most of you are too health-conscious to use hard drugs in the first place. The drugs we really want to call your attention to are those you may be addicted to without knowing it, namely the common over-the-counter ones like aspirin or other painkillers, various kinds of laxatives, sleeping pills, and the like. Also, we want you to note the potential dangers of some common prescription drugs like cortisone, antibiotics, tranquilizers, diuretics, and birth control pills so that if they're prescribed for you, you can at least be aware of their possible side effects on your skin.

The most common over-the-counter preparations used in this country are aspirin and similar painkilling compounds, laxatives, and sleeping pills. These drugs are supposed to normalize body functions; if the body is kept in balance through proper diet, exercise, and rest, none of these preparations will ever be necessary.

Aspirin, though one of the most useful medicines on record, is nonetheless a toxic substance: it increases the adrenal production of hydrocortisone, which is useful as an anti-inflammatory agent, but it can, if taken in large quantities over a prolonged period of time, cause internal bleeding. If you have a headache, mild arthritis pain, or any other minor discomfort, a couple of aspirin tablets may help, but follow it a few hours later with vitamin C, the great detoxifier, to help mitigate the aspirin's negative effects. Avoid using aspirin frequently for a long period of time; if you suffer from frequent headaches, arthritis, or back pain, see your doctor.

Acetaminophen (Tylenol), touted as a painkilling replacement for aspirin "without aspirin's damaging side effects," is not an anti-inflammatory agent, which makes it useless for any pain that is the result of inflammation. While it doesn't cause the internal bleeding that aspirin can, it may nevertheless cause liver and kidney damage if taken over a prolonged period.

Ibuprofen, now available over the counter under the brand names Nuprin and Advil, is an aspirin-like pain reliever often used in the treatment of arthritis and menstrual cramps. It shouldn't be used by anybody who cannot take aspirin.

Recent evidence concerning the eating disorders of bulimia (alternate bingeing and purging) and anorexia nervosa (self-starvation) has called attention to the abuse of laxatives as an adjunct to dieting; victims of these disorders often pump themselves full of laxatives, after eating, to push the food through their bodies before the nutrients and calories can be absorbed. Excessive use of laxatives can cause malnutrition and bowel spasticity; the body becomes so dependent on the laxative that the normal excretory mechanism will not function without this chemical assistance. Furthermore, each cell needs a balance of sodium and potassium; if this balance is drastically disrupted—as it can be through heavy laxative usage, vomiting, or self-starvation—shock and heart failure can result. At the very least, these eating disorders are setting the stage for the possibility of deficiency diseases and premature aging.

Occasional use of laxatives may be warranted, but some kinds are better than others. Over-the-counter laxatives rush food out of the body before its nutrients can be broken down and used. Mineral-oil compounds have the added disadvantage of leeching from the system all the fat-soluble vitamins (A, D, E, and K), so that huge deficiencies of these elements can occur. *Never* use mineral oil for *anything*. It's far preferable to remedy the problem through proper diet, and especially through the use of bran, which will add bulk to the stool without inhibiting the absorption of nutrients.

For those with a tendency toward constipation, we suggest a five-part remedy; these steps have all been recommended to us by physicians.

1. Take at least 2 tablespoons of brewer's yeast (to which calcium and magnesium have been added in the proportions noted in Step 1) every day, either in the milk shake we've already recommended or stirred into a glass of strongly

flavored juice. Sometimes this small amount of improvement in nutrition and B-vitamin intake will be sufficient to balance the elimination system.

2. Add a quart of pure water to your present daily fluid intake. (If you presently drink six to eight 8-ounce glasses of water as suggested in Step 1, you shouldn't be constipated.)

3. Exercise vigorously for at least 20 minutes each day (see Step 3). Exercise stimulates the bowels.

4. Add 4 or more ounces of live-culture yogurt or acidophilus milk to your diet every day to get some healthy bacteria working in your system.

5. Add two tablespoons of bran to your daily diet, either sprinkled on cereal or added to cooked items. The bran will give you some bulk without causing diarrhea.

As for sleeping pills, we believe that once you improve your nutrition, begin to exercise on a regular basis, and learn to relieve stress through a positive mental outlook (see Steps 7 and 8), you'll be able to throw those remedies away. For the occasional night when sleep doesn't come, use nature's relaxants: calcium supplements. Just chew a few calcium tablets (you'll need to decide for yourself how much is right for you), have a cup of warm milk, and within a few minutes you'll be ready to snooze. And the best part is waking up in the morning, refreshed and with no chemical aftereffects.

Among the commonly used prescription drugs, ACTH (the standard abbreviation for the adrenocorticotrophic hormone) and cortisone both cause large amounts of potassium to be excreted in the urine, thus creating potassium deficiencies and an excess of sodium in the body. The tissues then overcompensate by holding fluids, and edema, or water retention, results. The same is true of diuretics, which are often taken as weight-loss remedies: potassium is excreted in the urine; this potassium loss results in sodium excess, with further fluid retention and edema as the eventual result.[6] Within a couple of days, the body is back where it was before. Diuretics not only do not help get rid of real weight, they don't even get rid of water weight for very long. If at any time you are required to take diuretics for medical reasons such as high blood pressure or hypertension, or if ACTH or cortisone have been prescribed by your doctor, you should balance their usage with potassium-rich foods such as oranges and bananas.

ACTH and cortisone are both produced naturally by the pituitary and adrenal glands. They help regulate the body's blood-sugar level. If the body is temporarily imbalanced, one of these drugs may be prescribed. Cortisone, for example, is often given for the collagen diseases such as rheumatoid arthritis and rheumatic fever. Unfortunately, taking either ACTH or cortisone can cause acne breakouts in some people, since both drugs stimulate the pituitary and adrenal glands to increase their own production of these hormones.[7] It's easy to see how anything but their most carefully monitored use can result in disruption of the body's hormone balance, with concomitant effects on the skin.

Antibiotics such as streptomycin, Aureomycin, and penicillin destroy the healthy bacteria of the intestines and can cause diarrhea, bringing about the same vitamin deficiencies as do laxatives. Some antibiotics, such as tetracycline, can cause skin marking if you go in the sun while taking them. Sulfa drugs disrupt the functioning of the body's enzymes and can result in eczema. Some of the negative effects of these drugs can be mitigated by taking them with certain foods; for example, after taking antibiotics it is helpful to eat yogurt, in order to replace the healthy bacteria in the bowel (large intestine). Sometimes, antibiotics must be taken to combat illnesses, but we hope that our readers will become sophisticated medicine takers and learn to offset with nutrition the dangers in the medicines they must take.

Tranquilizers, like barbiturates, can cause allergic rashes and skin shedding.[8]

Birth-control pills increase the body's need for folic acid, vitamin B_6, and vitamin E, a lack of any of which can cause a variety of skin disorders (see Step 1). The most common skin problem occuring from use of birth control pills is the sudden appearance of a splotchy, gray-brown, random pigmentation, similar to the phenomenon known as the "mask of pregnancy" in pregnant women. Certain sedatives and dilantin (sometimes used to treat epilepsy) can result in the same skin disorder; dilantin can also cause acne outbreaks in some people.[9] Progesterone, which now predominates in many of the newer oral contraceptives, may also aggravate acne. However, Dr. Roy Knowles, Associate Professor of Dermatology at the University of Texas at Houston, says that for some women who experienced minimal acne before taking the pill and none at all while taking it, stopping the pill may actually induce acne by throwing the hormone system back into a state like that of adolescence. The period of time taken for this syndrome to pass varies with each individual.

Whether or not to take birth control pills must be a matter of each woman's *educated* choice. The pill has given women more control over their reproductive systems than they ever had before, but it does alter the body's natural chemical/ hormonal balance. We would like our readers to be aware of side effects on the skin. Some of these effects, such as brownish pigmentation from folic acid deficiency, can be mitigated by taking vitamin supplements. Some others, like excessive bleeding, cannot.

Because there are literally thousands of drugs which might at one time or another be prescribed for you, we want to encourage you to become aware of the possible side effects of every drug or chemical compound you put into your body. You're the only one who can build your future health, longevity, and beauty. Whenever a doctor prescribes any medication, ask him what are its short-term and long-term effects.

Caffeine and Theobromine

Most coffee, tea, and cola drinks contain caffeine; chocolate contains a similar drug called theobromine. Like tobacco, caffeine and theobromine give you a lift because they stimulate the adrenals and hence increase the heart beat; unfortunately, the same boost that helps you wake up and get moving will disappear quickly because it is chemically rather than nutritionally induced: the adrenal secretions raise the blood-sugar level briefly, so you'll feel stimulated, but subsequent insulin secretions, without any nutrients to go to work on, will quickly lower the blood-sugar level, sometimes below where you started, which makes you crave that second cup of coffee as little as thirty minutes after you finished the first. Also, the increased insulin production can increase both hunger and skin disorders. And remember that anything which stimulates the adrenals unnaturally is ultimately going to age you prematurely.

Caffeine and theobromine are proven contributors to fibrocystic disease (sometimes called cystic breast disease or cystic mastitis).[10] Also, caffeine inhibits the body's ability to absorb iron. One of the authors had the unpleasant experience of developing anemia because she was taking an "extra strength" aspirin compound laced with caffeine, which inhibited her absorption of iron. So don't lean on caffeine drinks to keep you going; get your lift from wholesome fruits, vegetables, whole grains, and proteins, and switch to caffeine-free herbal teas and carob, instead of coffee and chocolate. (But beware of decaffeinated coffees and teas; the chemical used to extract caffeine is known to induce liver cancer!)

Another warning about these common beverages comes from Dr. John Wolf of Baylor College of Medicine. Rosacea, mentioned above with respect to alcohol usage, is at least partially a result of dilation of the blood vessels. It is characterized by blushing and, eventually, when the blood vessels remain constantly open, by spidery looking broken capillaries. Dr. Wolf says that drinking any extremely hot beverage can worsen this disorder almost as readily as can alcohol consumption, so let whatever you drink cool down a bit first.

There are sugar-free and caffeine-free carbonated drinks on the market, but we can't recommend soft drinks at all because of their high phosphoric acid content, strong enough to erode metal nails and human teeth.[11] On a scale of nutritional values from one to ten, they'd rate a minus number!

Salt

As we noted in Step 1, potassium and sodium need to be balanced in the body in order for it to remain healthy, and an excess of one will cause the other to be excreted. Earlier, we warned you that ACTH, cortisone, and diuretics could create potassium and sodium imbalances. Similar imbalances can result from the excessive sodium content of the overrefined, overprocessed, typical American diet. And, again, it's the adrenals that bear the brunt of sodium abuse.

Where is sodium to be found? In practically every processed food on the market. Salt was originally used as a preservative. Nowadays, with refrigeration in nearly every home, we no longer need it for that purpose, but we have become hooked on the taste of it in practically all prepared foods. Sodium nitrate is often used as a preservative in prepared meats like bacon and frankfurters; salt or monosodium glutamate (MSG) are used to enhance flavors; baking soda *and* salt can be found in prepared mixes; canned foods contain added salt unless they specifically claim to be salt-free, and then they're often relegated to the dietetic shelves of the supermarket (and, of course, they'll cost more because they're *special*); and carbonated drinks are enormously high in sodium—that's why they're called "soda pop"!

There are times when the body's sodium level needs to be high. During stress, sodium is retained by the body to raise the blood pressure, which forces nutrients from the blood into the tissues to help them meet the demands of stress. This increase in blood pressure is normal, natural—and *temporary*. As soon as the stress is removed, the extra sodium is excreted, and the blood pressure returns to normal.

But if the diet is extremely high in sodium, potassium is excreted and an imbalance results. Without potassium, glucose can't be changed into energy and the muscles can't contract; if the cells contain an unnatural amount of sodium, which brings water with it, the result is edema. Also, when potassium is low, hypoglycemia, or low blood sugar, can occur. The body with an excess of sodium reacts as if it were under stress, and a number of disorders can result, ranging from indigestion and the discomforts of premenstrual syndrome to hypertension (prolonged high blood pressure), stroke, and kidney failure.[12]

Remember that anything which unbalances the hormone system over a period of time will cause premature aging. So unless you have abnormally low blood pressure and are under a doctor's orders to keep your sodium intake high, get rid of your table salt and became aware of the hidden sodium in the foods you eat, especially prepared "convenience" foods.

Sugar

The human body was created to live in harmony with its natural environment. And of all the unnatural elements which can create disharmony in our bodies, the worst offender is refined sugar, or sucrose.

Does the body need sugar? Yes, and the body turns the food you eat into exactly the kind of sugar it needs: glucose. Does the body need refined sugar? Emphatically *no*! Not a spoonful; not a granule! According to investigative researcher William Dufty, the ingestion of refined sugar is directly responsible for a multitude of ills, including hypoglycemia (low blood sugar), diabetes, obesity, and acne, and indirectly responsible for just about every other disease. Why? Because refined sugar plays havoc with the endocrine balance and creates such wear and tear on the adrenals that they become totally incapable of handling stress; endocrine exhaustion results in early aging and various degenerative diseases, and may even be a contributor to forms of mental illness.[13] In fact, Dr. E. M. Abrahamson and A. W. Pezet suggest that a sugar tolerance test should be given to all persons suffering from psychological and psychosomatic illnesses; as they note, "It is high time that we realized that *blood sugar* is as important as an indication of health or disease as blood pressure or blood temperature."[14]

Refined sugar is not a whole food—its nutrients and the enzymes necessary for its proper utilization have been refined out of it. When the body processes glucose from the food you eat, it does so slowly, maintaining a proper balance of glucose and oxygen in the blood. If you eat refined sugar, it goes directly to the intestines where it is quickly absorbed into the bloodstream, upsetting the glucose-oxygen balance. The adrenals react as they would to stress, marshaling all the forces that must come into play when the body requires energy for quick action; the pancreas tries to counter the sugar upsurge by producing large quantities of insulin to help bring the glucose level up to counter the stress. If the adrenal-pancreas balance breaks down, the result can be diabetes or its opposite, hyperinsulin (hypoglycemia).[15]

Although different bodies react in differing degrees to the ingestion of refined sugar, the strength of your hormone system is largely determined by diet. Of course, some people are born with healthier adrenals than others and can stand abuse longer; by the same token, some people with a strong genetic makeup can survive smoking, drinking, and munching candy into their nineties. But even though they are surviving, their quality of life would be improved without these contaminants. In the long run, if you feed your system poison in the form of refined sugar, it will take its toll in your appearance, and sooner or later you can expect to show signs of premature aging, including decaying teeth, weak gums, susceptibility to illness, degenerative diseases of various kinds, and structural damage to the collagen layer of the skin. And, as we've noted, you may eventually develop diabetes, which Houston endocrinologist Dr. Alan Leiser says can be identified by such skin horrors as necrobiosis or tissue death, pigmentation changes, and skin atrophy. Just remember that for two hours after eating sugar, your immune system is less efficient than normal, making you susceptible for that period of time to the onslaught of viruses and other forms of illness. Since every illness is a stress which can age you, why court disaster? Give up refined sugar and look forward instead to a longer and healthier life.

The largest abuser of sugar in this country is processed food. If you get serious about giving up sugar—and we urge you to do so, for the health of your skin—you'll need to read every list of ingredients on every item in your pantry. There's sugar in ketchup, salad dressings, many canned items, prepared mixes, some frozen foods, coffee creamer, and so on. If a food has a label, read it carefully, if it has additives, preservatives, colorings, salt, sugar, or anything you don't recognize as being natural and wholesome, don't put it in your shopping cart. Nutritionist Carlton Fredericks recently suggested in a television interview that you should shop around the periphery of the supermarket, where you'll generally find produce, meats, fish, and dairy products, and avoid the shelves in the middle, which contain mostly processed foods. You'll end up eating more fresh fruits, meats, vegetables, and grains, and you'll be healthier for it.

Other Common Foods to Avoid

All of the substances above can cause premature aging by stressing the endocrine system and unbalancing the hormone levels in your body. Not every potentially harmful substance that you ingest will affect your body in this way. We'd like to point out some others that, while not directly interfering with your endocrine system, will ultimately prevent you from attaining optimal health.

Additives in Processed Food

At a dinner party some years ago, one of our authors offered her guests hot beverages after dinner. One woman opted for Sanka, laced with nondairy creamer and artificial sweetener. Then, after tasting it, she smiled and said, "Umm, my compliments to the chemist!"

All too often, these days, we may find ourselves eating or drinking artificial chemicals instead of natural foods, as if we were robots rather than humans. The idea that the body is a machine may be responsible for our constant abuses of it. But we aren't indestructible; we're really quite fragile. Machines are replaceable, but we own only one body for this lifetime.

The average American adult ingests annually not only 126 pounds of sugar and other sweeteners, hidden in processed foods, and fifteen pounds of salt, but at least ten pounds of hidden chemical stabilizers, neutralizers, emulsifiers, etc., as well,[16] largely in "convenience" foods. These foods—whether canned, dried, frozen, or in any other form—contain large amounts of preservatives and "flavor enhancers," including ingredients that prevent mold and bacteria from growing in the food, emulsifiers and texturizers to keep the texture from breaking down, artificial coloring and flavoring, and so on. In the short term, these additives may not have noticeable effects on your body, although studies have shown a possible causal relationship between many so-called safe food additives and hyperactivity in children. And some, like monosodium glutamate, can cause flushing, the result of blood vessel dilation. But even if you don't break out in hives on the spot, these adulterants can have a cumulative effect.

These nonnutritive additives are not food, and are just what their name says— not nutritious. We feel they shouldn't be consumed by the human body. No one knows exactly what their long-term effects are; most of them haven't been around long enough. So why risk your health unnecessarily? The foods that contain these additives usually contain large quantities of sugar and salt as well, and ounce for ounce they're far more expensive than fresh or homemade foods, so for body and budget, they're best avoided altogether.

Muscle Meat and Other High-Fat Foods

Another class of foods to avoid are those high in animal fat: the muscle meats of beef, lamb, and pork, high-fat dairy products, the saturated oils of palm or coconut, or any food made with lard, such as pâté or pie crust (unless, of course, you create your own with low-fat alternatives; see Step 1 for suggestions). These foods are high in cholesterol or saturated fats or both, and eating them consistently may clog your veins and arteries. Some researchers theorize that they create wastes in the body that are very difficult to clean out and increase the chances of contracting various degenerative diseases; it is known that as we age, the triglyceride (blood fat) level increases after any meal containing fat and stays high about five times longer than in people in their twenties or younger,[17] suggesting that we have less ability to utilize the fat we eat as we get older. And as we mentioned in Step 1, saturated fats may contribute to the sebum buildup that causes acne.[18] And we and many others have found that giving up sugar and alcohol is easier if you give up heavy meats and fats at the same time. For some reason, meats like beef and pork tend to inspire a craving for sweets, and alcohol can create a craving for heavy meats like steaks and chops.

Spicy Foods

Highly spiced foods can be dangerous for some people. Like alcohol, they can dilate the blood vessels and rupture capillaries under the skin, leaving the face a network of lacy, spidery lines. If you find that your face flushes after eating very spicy foods like hot curries or Szechuan dishes, or if you are prone to these capillary lines, cut back on spices. Some people are less sensitive than others, so the degree of spiciness that is acceptable will vary from person to person.

Refined Grains

Finally, try to avoid refined-grain products. "Man cannot live by bread alone" is a particularly valid observation if the bread is made from refined flour. While whole grains are rich in B vitamins, vitamin E, trace minerals, and bulk, full of life and energy, and can transmit these virtues to the person who consumes them, refined grains, on the other hand, are devoid of life and precious nutrients—even rats avoid them! Admittedly, an attempt has been made to "enrich" these lifeless foods through the addition of vitamins. But why eat foods that have been de-vitalized and then "replenished" with only a tiny fraction of their initial nutrients? Since science still hasn't identified all the nutrients in our foods, no amount of "enrichment" of processed foods can make them as nourishing as their natural equivalents.

For the sake of your health—and your skin—become aware of everything you put in your mouth. If it's made from refined, bleached flour, you can be sure that all you're getting is empty calories, with perhaps a few synthetic vitamins added. The same is true of polished rice—all the nutrients have been taken out along with the intermediate and inner shells. Eat wheat germ and rice polishings instead of refined grains, and you'll reap the benefits in health for years to come.

Iodine-Rich Foods: A Special Word to Acne Patients

Doctors generally warn acne sufferers to avoid foods rich in iodine or bromides. The biggest offenders seem to be shellfish, seaweed, and kelp, and of course iodized salt. Iodine affects the thyroid gland, and you know by now that glandular imbalances affect the skin. If you suffer from acne, it would be wise to observe your reactions to any foods rich in iodine or bromine, and to avoid them altogether if you notice adverse reactions.

Crash Diets

While we're warning you about the various things you should and shouldn't put in your mouth, we'd like to mention one other item—crash-dieting. Fad diets may help you lose pounds quickly, but they also tend to rob the body of essential nutrients and to create imbalances. Unless the diet you follow contains a sufficiency of proteins, fats, and complex carbohydrates, chances are good you'll gain back any weight you may lose. And according to Dr. Alan Garber, Chief of Diabetes–Metabolism, the Methodist Hospital, and Professor of Medicine at Baylor College of Medicine, if you lose weight too rapidly, you'll lose not only fat tissue but muscle tissue as well. As a result, protein will not be properly synthesized to rebuild healthy skin tissue, and there won't be time for the body to mold itself into a new configuration. And dieting ups and downs stretch the skin irreversibly. As a result, you'll end up with sags and wrinkles, and you'll look older instead of younger. Moreover, fad dieting won't help you learn new eating habits to keep the weight off permanently. So take it slow and steady and stay healthy in the process.

Breaking the Habit Barrier

Living correctly is simply a question of habit—breaking harmful old ones and forming healthful new ones. If you can develop a zest for eating and living right, you'll find that breaking and reforming habits is much easier. For some of us, breaking a habit is best done "cold turkey." For others, a more gradual approach works better. It depends on your personality and the nature of the habit. If the habit is a true addiction like heavy drinking or smoking, cold turkey may be the only way. With ordinary bad habits like eaitng too much sugar, it's often easier to modify your behavior in stages.

Below you'll find a checklist with some suggestions you may want to try to help you eliminate the foods and other substances with which you may be poisoning yourself. You'll be replacing them at the same time with new ones, as explained in Step 1. If you prefer to go cold turkey with any of these substances, please feel free to do so. If you can come up with some other procedure that you feel will work better for you, by all means use it. For example, doing it with a friend, as a competition, can be fun and rewarding. Houston T.V. personality/talk show hostess Warner Roberts and one of our authors made a pact to give up white flour and sugar. And to give herself even more incentive, Warner went on the air and told her television audience about the pact. Not only did she and our author find the competition a successful means of kicking the habit, but a tremendous number of people phoned in or wrote that they, too, were joining the competition!

To eliminate the stress of going cold turkey on everything at once, our other author set up a schedule whereby she gave up an item at a time: caffeine one month, salt the next, sugar the next, and heavy meats the next. The main thing is, don't give up! Until your new living habits have taken hold, a little backsliding now and then is to be expected. Don't berate yourself for these occasional slips; your goal is behavior modification, not self-flagellation. Just chalk up the slips to experience and get yourself back on track.

If you now smoke or drink heavily, your first priority has to be getting these problems under control. You've probably tried to quit smoking or cut back on your drinking before. This time, though, you're going to succeed, because the incentive is stronger! (Both of the authors are former smokers, and we know that with enough incentive, you, too, can stop.) Think about why your previous attempts didn't work, or worked only temporarily. Imagine all the temptations you are going to face over the next few months and how you might deal with them.

And use all the crutches you feel are necessary. Would a support group help? A quit-smoking seminar? Prayer? Hypnosis? Scare tactics can be constructive: taking a good look at a smoker's lung tissue or the liver of an alcoholic suffering from cirrhosis may be just the thing needed to push you into quitting. Or buy a self-improvement tape geared toward breaking the habit you now engage in and play it regularly—there are many such tapes on the market. Or learn to substitute—remember the Greek actor Telly Savalas as "Kojak," who sucked a lollipop in lieu of smoking? (We suggest you chew sugar-free gum instead.) Or get in touch with your body through meditation and imagery (see Steps 7 and 8); visualizing the body's tissues and their responses to the new care you are taking of them can be wonderfully cleansing. This can help you get excited about caring for your greatest treasure, your body. As the Bible says, it is a temple wherein the spirit resides. Why not have all the benefits God intended for you? You're entitled!

STEP TWO: ELIMINATION OF COMMON POISONS CHECKLIST

1. Check off the things you've already eliminated from your life:
   • Cigarettes
   • Alcohol
   • Drugs you use on a regular basis (list them)
   • Caffeine and theobromine (coffee, tea, chocolate, cola)
   • Salt/sodium
   • Refined sugar
   • Processed foods
   • Beef, pork, lamb, and other high fat foods
   • Highly spiced foods (if they affect you)
   • Refined flour products
   • Foods containing iodine or bromines (if they affect you)
   • Crash dieting

From the following suggestions, choose the ones that are right for you:

2. Devote at least a week to getting yourself ready emotionally to make whatever changes in life-style may be necessary. During that week, make a list of everything you eat or drink, every cigarette you smoke, every aspirin, digestive aid, etc., that you put in your mouth. At the end of the week, go back and check off the things you want to eliminate. After that, set a goal to accomplish each week—and stick to it.

3. If you're tackling an addiction to cigarettes or alcohol and you find yourself fighting a craving, substitute some other activity, such as exercise or meditation or even brushing your teeth, for the action of taking the cigarette or the drink. Psychologists believe that many eating disorders and chemical abuses are self-punishing mechanisms. If you think your particular problem may involve self-punishment, try transferring your attention to some other form of "punishing" yourself that is really not damaging. For example, if you hate spending money, go buy a dress; if you hate exercise, go run!

4. Try substituting fancy nonalcoholic drinks for alcoholic ones. A Virgin Mary can be just as festive as a Bloody Mary, and you won't suffer any unpleasant aftereffects; you can be a better participant at a party if you're conscious.

5. Make a list of all the nonprescription drugs you take. In any instance where you can easily do so, substitute a natural remedy for the chemical one—

for example, extra vitamin C for cold medicines; milk and calcium tablets instead of sleeping pills or pain killers; digestive enzymes for antacids; bran for laxatives.

6. If you're taking any prescription drug, find out how it acts and what its side effects are. Drugs sometimes come with a detailed description in the package; read it carefully. For others, call your doctor's office for information. (Sometimes it's hard to coax an intelligent explanation out of a doctor or nurse. Be polite but be persistent; you have a right to know what those drugs are doing to you.)

7. Your decision to take any prescriptive medication, from birth control pills to antibiotics, must be the joint decision of you and your physician; just be sure it's an *educated* decision on your part. If you must take any medication with negative side effects, find out whether there are any vitamin supplements or food items that can mitigate those effects without disrupting the benefits of the medication. And find out how you can balance *your* body so that medication becomes less necessary in the future.

8. Keep track for a week of how much caffeine and theobromine you're ingesting in coffee, tea, colas, and chocolate drinks and snacks. Then methodically cut your consumption in half the next week, and in half again the week after. Keep halving your consumption until you're caffeine-free. Take brewer's yeast or a protein powder in juice or milk when you need an energy boost. Slowly eliminating from your diet the items that stimulate the adrenals and the pancreas should keep you from suffering blood-vessel constriction; your body will eventually become balanced, and you will no longer need chemical stimulants.

9. Take an honest look at your sodium intake. Go through your cabinets and assess what you've been eating—canned soups, bouillon cubes, pretzels, cake mixes, and just about all prepared foods are high in salt or sodium. And remember that you also want to avoid all the chemical preservatives with which prepared foods are loaded. So read labels, and if salt, sodium, or preservatives are part of the ingredients of the items on your shelves, don't keep them around. Then go to the medicine chest and get rid of those antacids that are high in sodium. Vow never to buy those food or drug items again.

10. Do some more detective work in your cabinets to find out how many products contain sugar—it's a hidden ingredient in many seemingly unsweet prepared foods, like ketchup and gravies. If sugar, sucrose, corn syrup, etc., are listed as ingredients, use the product sparingly or throw it out. Don't tempt yourself by buying sweet bakery products or baking sweet things. Buy or bake some wholesome whole-grain bread instead.

11. Replace the roasts, chops, and steaks in your diet with seafood, organ meats, poultry dark meat, and legumes combined with grains or nonfat dairy products. You'll improve your nutritional intake and save money at the same time.

12. If you enjoy very spicy dishes, observe their effect on you. Do you get a little flushed after a hot, spicy meal? If so, you're risking spidery capillary lines on your face. Moderate your intake of spices.

13. Take polished rice, white flour, white bread, and refined flour bakery goods off your shopping list; replace them with brown rice, whole-wheat flour, whole-grain breads, whole-grain pastas, whole-grain bakery goods (not sweet ones), and possibly some less familiar foods: soy flour, wheat germ, bran, and bulgur wheat (also called cracked wheat). Buy small quantities and don't let things sit on shelves too long; that way you won't have to worry about the products not containing preservatives.

14. If you're prone to acne, observe your reaction to bromine- and iodine-rich foods. If there seems to be a connection between your intake of these substances and your blemishes, stop using iodized salt and limit your intake of seafood, particularly shellfish and kelp, substituting instead other foods from Step 1, such as liver and organ meats, the dark meat of poultry, or RNA-rich legumes.

15. If you should slip in your resolve to reform your eating, drinking, and smoking behavior, don't allow the slip to turn into a landslide. Be forgiving of your slipping and stumbling, and just start again with a firmer resolve. Loving yourself enough to build a healthier, more beautiful body is the whole point of the Figure-8 program, so love yourself enough to forgive yourself when the inevitable slipups occur.

16. Some further reading to help motivate you:

E. M. Abrahamson, and A. W. Pezet, *Body, Mind, and Sugar* (New York: Pyramid Books, 1976).

Deborah Chase, *The Medically Based No-Nonsense Beauty Book* (New York: Alfred Knopf, 1974) (discusses the negative effects on the skin of alcohol, tobacco, and drugs).

William Dufty, *Sugar Blues* (New York: Warner Books, 1975) (discusses the negative effects of sugar, alcohol, tobacco, and preservatives).

Gustave H. Hoehn, *Acne Can Be Cured* (New York: Arco, 1978) (discusses the negative effect of saturated fats on skin conditions).

Martha Whittlesey, *Killer Salt* (New York: Avon, 1977).

[1] Jane Brody, *Jane Brody's Nutrition Book* (New York: Bantam; 1981), p. 352.

[2] Sandy Rovner, "Psychosomatic: The New Meaning," *Washington Post Health*, April 3, 1985, p. 11.

[3] Michael Lesser, *Nutrition and Vitamin Therapy* (New York: Bantam, 1980), p. 76; Adelle Davis, *Let's Stay Healthy* (New York: Signet, 1981), pp. 322–323.

[4] William Dufty, *Sugar Blues* (New York: Warner Books, 1975).

[5] This chart is based on the statements of Deborah Chase, *The Medically Based No-Nonsense Beauty Book* (New York: Alfred Knopf, 1974), pp. 159–160.

[6] Adelle Davis, *Let's Eat Right to Keep Fit* (New York: Signet, 1970), pp. 189–191.

[7] For a full discussion of complications which may arise from the use of ACTH and cortisone, see E. M. Abrahamson and A. W. Pezet, *Body, Mind, and Sugar* (New York: Pyramid Books, 1976), pp. 170–174.

[8] Deborah Chase, *The Medically Based No-Nonsense Beauty Book* (New York: Alfred Knopf, 1974), p. 160.

[9] Ibid., p. 83.

[10] Jane Brody, *Jane Brody's Guide to Personal Health* (New York: Avon, 1983), p. 647.

[11] William Dufty, *Sugar Blues* (New York: Warner Books, 1975), p. 178.

[12] Adelle Davis, *Let's Eat Right to Keep Fit* (New York: Signet, 1970), pp. 189–194; Michael Lesser, *Nutrition and Vitamin Therapy* (New York: Bantam, 1980), pp. 117–118.

[13] William Dufty, *Sugar Blues* (New York: Warner Books, 1975), pp. 69–73.

[14] E. M. Abrahamson and A. W. Pezet, *Body, Mind, and Sugar* (New York: Pyramid Books, 1976), p. 194.

[15] William Dufty, *Sugar Blues*, (New York: Warner Books, 1975) pp. 46–47; and E. M. Abrahamson and A. W. Pezet, *Body, Mind, and Sugar*, (New York: Pyramid Books, 1976) pp. 43, 165.

[16] Jane Brody, *Jane Brody's Guide to Personal Health* (New York: Avon, 1983), p. 61.

[17] Don Mannerburg and June Roth, *Aerobic Nutrition* (New York: Hawthorn/Dutton, 1981).

[18] Gustave H. Hoehn, *Acne Can Be Cured* (New York: Arco, 1978), p. 31.

Step Three:
Exercise

When you have time for a little recreation, do you grab your tennis racket and head for an hour on the court? Or is your idea of fun an hour or so in front of the television? If, like many Americans today, you're already physically active, that's great—you're giving yourself longer life, better health, more energy, firmer muscle tone, and glowing skin. If, however, you haven't yet pushed yourself out of your easy chair and embraced the active life, we'd like to help you up.

Oh, we've heard all the objections to regular exercise: "It's boring." "It hurts." "I don't have time." "I'll look funny." "I've never been good at any sport." "I'm too old/tired/weak to start." But if you'll read on, we think we can convince you that the end justifies the means, and what's more, there are dozens of ways to get the exercise you need, if only you'll become aware of them. All it takes is a few minutes a day and a little common sense.

Exercise doesn't just mean the difference between looking like plain Jane and looking like Jane Fonda. It strengthens your heart, enlarges your lung capacity, stimulates your bowels, and improves your circulation, helping every body system to function at its peak. As exercise helps you get oxygen to every cell and flushes out wastes and impurities, your skin will develop a healthy, youthful glow—the mirror of your improved well-being.

The Importance of Exercise

An interesting study on longevity by endocrinologist Dr. Hans Selye indicates the importance of exercise. Dr. Selye placed a hollow tube in living animals and cultivated live animal cells within it. When the cells in the tubes were left alone they died within one month because their natural wastes accumulated in the tube and killed them, but when waste products from the cells were washed away daily, the cells lived on, and neither aged nor died. Dr. Selye's experiment demonstrated that if waste is carried away from the cells, the cells will live indefinitely.[1]

This information indicates that aging may be slowed down by improving waste removal. Other scientists have come up with similar findings. Since exercise flushes wastes out of the cells, it rejuvenates the entire body.[2]

The old cliché that our bodies are like machines is in some ways quite accurate. When a machine is left unused and unoiled, it falls to rust and ruin through a process called oxidation; the same process, it seems, takes place in the body without exercise. If the machine is used and oiled daily, it can run for decades, even centuries. Scientists are finding the same to be true of the human body if it is exercised and cared for properly. Dr. George Mann of Vanderbilt University investigated males, fifteen to fifty years old, of the Masai people in Africa, who walk approximately twelve miles a day herding cattle. He divided the men into ten-year age groups. His findings were that the size of the coronary arteries increased with each decade of life, and that the arteries were too large to clog.[3]

The implications of findings like these are dramatic. Man was not built in the age of automation. The machines he has created to do his work for him have given him too much leisure. As a result, he has become a victim of his very creations. His machines become ever more efficient, while his own body rusts from disuse.

Dr. Vladimir Karenchevsky, long considered the father of longevity research, suggests that man was created to last a healthy, happy, active, one hundred and five years. The people of Abkhasia and Azerboijan, two communities in southern Russia, work in the fields until they die at approximately one hundred and twenty years of age. In Tibet the Hunza tribe averages an active life span of one hundred and thirty years, as do the Vilcabambam Indians of South America. The Australian Aborigines can follow a kangaroo for days, and the Indians of Mexico can run as far as one hundred and fifty miles.[4] More and more, we read and hear about ski instructors like Leland Osborn, who is ninety-two years of age, runners like Ruth Rothfarb who is eighty-two, news commentator Dorothy Fuldheim who is broadcasting on television at ninety, and people celebrating their one-hundredth wedding anniversary. What is the tie that binds these people from all around the world together? It would appear that the common thread running through all of their lives is exercise. By using your legs as nature intended, you push the blood up through the muscles and to the heart. Over time, your heart, like your other muscles, becomes stronger and more efficient. The heart develops collateral circulation which can, in fact, divert the flow of blood from arteries that have become blocked by plaque. It is this collateral circulation that can save your life in the event of a heart attack, and you will have the added bonus of a speedier recovery.[5]

There have been innumerable studies to support this thesis, and one rather famous one was conducted on 120,000 railroad employees. A portion of them were desk-bound clerks, another segment were moderately active switchmen, and a third group were very active section men. The inactive clerks were found to have a third more heart attacks than the moderately active switchmen and about twice as many heart attacks as the very active section men.[6] Findings such as these demonstrate dramatically that exercise is a significant contributor to a longer and healthier life.

Other Benefits of Exercise

In conjunction with longevity, dynamic or aerobic exercise also adds to your overall feeling of well being. By helping you manage stress, it contributes to mental health. For many years, runners have been aware of the feeling commonly referred to as "runner's high." But only recently has medicine begun to understand this phenomenon. Dynamic exercise increases the level of epinephrine on your body, making you feel energetic and alert. Exercise also stimulates the brain to secrete the peptide beta-endorphin; after approximately ten minutes of aerobics, the level of this hormone doubles in the brain. Beta-endorphin is a natural tranquilizer that takes the edge off unpleasant stimuli. Aerobic exercise, by increasing the level of endorphins in your body, makes your thoughts clearer and more organized, increases sensitivity, and literally raises your consciousness.[7] The increased flow of blood to your brain improves its memory and overall functioning.[8] Ten minutes of running, jogging or brisk walking daily could very well take the place of one hour on a psychiatrist's couch.[9]

Consequently, aerobic exercise has been highly recommended for women with premenstrual syndrome and patients with depression, anxiety, stress disorders, and a very unusual mental disorder called anhedonia. This condition is the result of a chemical imbalance in the brain; people who suffer from this problem are unable to experience any happiness. The only cure is vigorous exercise. By raising the body's level of endorphins, exercise makes anhedonia patients feel more content and joyful. The same physiological response can help normal people relieve feelings of anxiety or depression through exercise.

In effect, a type of biofeedback develops through aerobic exercise. You become more in touch with your body and aware of your breathing. You can call upon this awareness, while under duress, to calm both your mind and your body. People who exercise consistently are much better able to manage the stress in their lives.

Still other advantages of dynamic exercise include the following, all of which have been demonstrated through controlled studies:

1. Weight control—exercise burns fat, speeds up metabolism, burns calories, and tightens muscles.[10]

2. Increased stamina and energy level.[11]

3. Improved strength of the heart muscle and increased heart efficiency—exercise makes the heart beat more efficiently, saving as many as 10,000 beats in a night's sleep.[12]

4. Lengthened blood-clotting time (an effect which reduces the risk of spontaneous blood clotting) and an enhanced ability to dissolve blood clots; both effects are useful in preventing heart attacks and in reducing the risk of future attacks in heart attack victims.[13]

5. Improved stamina of people who have already had heart attacks and/or who suffer angina pectoris.[14]

6. Reduced blood pressure, a major contributor to stroke and cardiovascular disease.[15]

7. Reduced triglycerides in the blood and lower high-density lipoprotein cholesterol[16]—exercise is a great prescription for alleviating atherosclerosis.

8. Lower uric-acid levels[17]—exercise helps prevent gout.

9. Regulation of insulin production—exercise helps control diabetes,[18] and the prediabetic conditions of hyperglycemia and hypoglycemia.

10. Greater elasticity of the arteries—exercise is a superior treatment for varicose veins and spider veins.[19]

11. Prevention of osteoporosis and help for osteoarthritis sufferers—exercise keeps body movement fluid and strengthens the bones that weaken with age, because it improves the body's utilization of calcium.[20]

12. Deeper and sounder sleep.[21]

13. Improved bowel regularity.[22]

14. Stimulation of pleasure—exercise enhances the quality of life.[23]

15. Creation of a sensuous, tingly feeling similar to that experienced after sexual climax, plus improved sexual response and stamina.[24]

16. A stronger and more flexible body.[25]

17. Faster recovery after illness or injury.[26]

18. Reduced menstrual cramping, and easier pregnancy and childbirth.[27]

19. Protection of the body from cancer.[28]

20. Protection from degenerative diseases[29]—exercise is an effective elixir for the prevention of aging. If you are in excellent physical shape, you stand taller, feel better, and generally exhibit the characteristics of youth, such as muscle tone, vitality, and energy.

21. Improved skin condition.[30] If your circulatory system is operating at its maximum, then all of your cells and organs will function in top condition, and, of course, your largest organ is your skin. No other part of your body so reflects what is going on inside it. Judging by the skin's color, texture, and appearance, a trained observer can diagnose a liver disorder, a thyroid dysfunction, a hormone imbalance, a lack of proper rest, a deficient diet, a blood disorder, an allergy, an overexposure to the elements, an infection, a fungus, a virus, and various other conditions. The skin is the mirror to the body, reflecting its general health.

Exercise cleanses the skin by flushing out impurities through perspiration. It stimulates the circulation, bringing life-giving oxygen to the cells. It tightens and lifts the muscle bundles in motion under the skin. A well-exercised skin is thus firm, rosy, and glistening. Nathan Pritikin calls physical exercise "far more beautifying than any surgical face lift."[31]

What If You Don't Exercise?

It's a law of nature that anything not used will deteriorate. The following study demonstrates the validity of this truth. Young athletes were put to bed for 20 days, during which time all of their vital signs began to slow down in direct proportion to their lack of activity. Their oxygen intake capacity, red blood cell count, and their heart pumping capacity diminished, all because of a reduced level of exercise.[32] Other studies indicate that lack of exercise creates a negative calcium balance; young athletes put to bed for 36 weeks lost 4% of their total calcium.[33]

If you stop exercising, your muscles atrophy, your joints stiffen and lose their flexibility, your capillaries constrict, and the flow of blood through your tissues is curtailed.

The following story, related to us by a doctor at the Pritikin Center, is a lesson in point. After a massive heart attack, a man was told he would be bedridden for the rest of his life. Unwilling to accept such a prescription, he decided to kill himself. So he went outdoors and began running as fast as he could. Suddenly he became dizzy, and as darkness overcame him, he fell to the ground. The next morning he awoke outdoors—cold, but alive. Still determined to fulfill his quest, he set out again the following evening, and as before, he collapsed. Upon awakening the second morning, he noticed that he had run a little farther than the night before. But he still couldn't face life as an invalid, and night after night he went on trying to end it all. Then one morning, he realized he was actually feeling better. A trip to the doctor confirmed his perception; our little man, instead of killing himself, had saved his own life.

Medicine is filled with similar stories. Several years ago, one of our authors ran her way back to health. It all started with minor hemorrhoid surgery that turned into a major month's stay in the hospital. For unknown reasons, every body system began to fail, and nothing would turn the tide, short of going home. Another month's stay in bed caused further weakness, and a two-year decline in health followed. Increasingly frustrated and depressed by her sedentary life, she deteriorated further, until at last she got a new prescription: "Run for your life."

A few decades ago, men in our culture were told not to engage in any form of strenuous exercise after the age of forty; even tennis in one's middle years was considered taboo. We were told that every heart had an assigned number of beats; the more you used up, the closer you came to the Grim Reaper. Only now have we come to realize how important dynamic exercise really is; rather than using up your heart beats, exercise actually preserves them.[34] Health is entering a new age, the age of aerobics, where the focus is on the heart, and the goal is to strengthen it and make it more efficient. In the final analysis, the heart is the master muscle and its energy is like love: the more you give away, the more you have to keep.

Move with Your Mood

So, you believe it's impossible to find the time to exercise? Well, not to worry. Aerodynamics experts have proved it's impossible for the bumble bee to fly, but he does.

In the beginning—before Jane Fonda's workout—man exercised by moving any of his approximately 635 muscles, walking through the jungle, reaching for bananas, and running after his mate. As the Babylonian king said, nothing is new under the sun, and exercise still consists of simply moving—which can be practiced, by the way, while either awake or asleep. Contrary to popular belief, you can keep your job, keep your friends, and even keep up with your social life. Ah, you say, so where's the rub? When is that other sneaker going to drop? Never, we say—for exercising is nothing more than focusing on when you move, and pushing yourself a little harder.

Chin up, ordinary mortals—there are many paths to fitness. They include going up the stairs, walking to your car, shopping in your favorite mall, and even the old basic housework number. Think about it: our parents and grandparents didn't have bad skin or ugly bodies, even without a morning jog or an aerobics class. What they did have was manual labor. They walked, and plowed, and churned, and scrubbed, and generally moved about more than we, the luxury generation, do. Those feet were made for walking, and that's really all they have to do. How you look and how you feel are strictly up to you.

Consider, if you will, that all movement can increase your muscle flexibility and strength, and that consistently vigorous movement will improve your cardiovascular and respiratory capacities. So a morning of housework or gardening can be really beneficial in contributing to your overall physical fitness. Do you do windows? Score a plus for improved flexibility. Wash and wax your car, and the bending, stretching, and scrubbing will contribute to both flexibility and strength. Paint the house and you'll also increase your cardiovascular and respiratory capacities. Even typing, or operating a computer or a word processor can improve flexibility of arms, hands, and fingers, though if you sit during working hours, you'll want to add some daily activities to exercise your derrière—and your heart—as well.

How about having a little fun while you get fit? Playing a musical instrument improves flexibility—do it in a marching band with your local civic organization and you'll exercise your heart and lung muscles. Backpack a picnic lunch to your favorite recreation spot—walking on level ground can improve your heart and lung endurance and contributes to both strength and flexibility—after which you can reward yourself with a leisurely midday meal. Dancing is a super exercise—even a slow two-step will improve flexibility, while a square dance or a rhumba can really get your heart and lungs moving. And note that professional dancers are generally scrawny creatures with good skin and enormous appetites. We even have one friend who combines dancing with routine chores; she turns on her stereo and tap dances in place while she fixes dinner (just like Ann Miller on a soup can!). So you really can be fit just doing routine things—provided you move, move, move, and you do it every day.

For those of you who *do* like sports, fit some sporting activities into your schedule on a regular basis. Play golf or tennis, swim, bowl, hike, or bike, ride horses or even throw horseshoes. You don't have to do the same activity every day—allow yourself some freedom and make your activity suit your mood. If you're frustrated or annoyed, take out your emotions on the raquetball court; if you're feeling lethargic, just go for a walk (after a bit of a walk, you won't be quite so lethargic). Through trial and error you can find activities you're likely to stay with and enjoy, and having fun with exercise makes sticking with it no sweat. How you spend your time is strictly up to you. Just use common sense and choose exercises that are right for your age and your physical condition. The key to success is in keeping track of what you do, and being sure you do enough to get your lungs and heart in action and your limbs moving regularly for improved flexibility and strength.

35 Minutes a Day Keeps the Doctor Away

So, you ask, if fitness allows for all kinds of activities and movements, just how much exercise of what type constitutes a minimum requirement? The consensus seems to be that any exercise is better than none, and that, especially for those who have sedentary jobs and don't have a chance to do housework or much else, about thirty-five minutes a day, preferably taken at one time, is a good amount to aim for.

On the basis of this recommendation, we have devised the Figure-8 Exercise Plan, which you'll find below. Hawaii's famous exercise guru Sandra Colter explains that there are three basic types of exercise in a good program: stretching, strengthening, and endurance. That's why we've been emphasizing that whatever you do, you need to be sure you contribute to your flexibility, strength, and heart/lung capacity. Sandy says that twenty minutes of your exercise program should be spent on stretching and strengthening and fifteen minutes on endurance for a total of 35 minutes of exercise a day, preferably five times a week.

On the basis of this recommendation, we have devised the Figure-8 Exercise Plan, which you'll find below. If you already do some form of stretching or strengthening exercises on a regular basis, you may want to look at our remarks on aerobic/endurance exercises. If you do aerobics, you may simply want to check out our stretching and strengthening exercises. And if you're still shopping for an exercise program to fit your total body needs, we hope you'll try the whole plan for a few weeks—then pick and choose whatever seems right for you, making sure that every day you have enough activity of the three recommended types.

Two provisos are in order before you start. It's important to begin an exercise program slowly, gradually building up to your maximum potential over a thirty-day period, and exercising every other day at first to prevent sore muscles and hurt pride. And always remember to check with your doctor for medical clearance before embarking on an exercise program.

Where to Exercise and What to Wear

It's been said that half of life is just showing up, and it's certainly true that if you like where you're going you're more likely to be there! Location is everything!! So know your own style. If you don't like exercising with others, don't worry about being a closet fitness freak—just find a place where you can go it alone regularly. Workaholic personalities can maximize their time by watching the news or returning phone calls while using a treadmill or stationary bike. Social butterflies will enjoy the buddy system; if there are enough of you to meet on a regular basis, you might begin a neighborhood "exercise-in." Outdoor lovers can meet at the beach or in their own backyards and enjoy exercising in harmony with nature. And for personalized instruction, you might prefer your local gym or nearby dance studio. Whichever you choose, do it to music; think how motivated Bo Derek looked as she exercised to "Bolero"!

Did somebody just say, "But I have nothing to wear!"? It's a cry that's been heard ever since Eve discovered the fig leaf. Well, here's one time when you really do have a valid reason for buying new and special clothing. It's important for your clothes to fit the sport and provide maximum comfort and safety.

When you do stretching and strengthening exercises, you'll want your clothing to be lightweight and to fit loosely. Leotards are appropriate, freeing the body to do exaggerated movements. Then, for walking, running, jogging, biking, and any other aerobic activities that stress your feet and legs, purchase a good pair of running shoes that will cushion and support your feet, and wear light, absorbent clothing. When biking, be sure to wear a helmet. And finally, when swimming, wear earplugs or a bathing cap and put alcohol in your ears as a precaution against swimmer's ear.

THE FIGURE-8 EXERCISE PLAN: STRETCHING

Regardless of whether you're twenty, thirty, or fifty, it's important to be flexible, and if you don't want to shrink in your golden years, start now to stretch your body. Reach for that can of soup in your pantry, bend for that tennis ball, and curl like a cat before you get out of bed in the morning. Stretching exercises include anything that adds to your flexibility, from dance to touching your toes. So be conscious of your body throughout the day, and you'll get your stretches in quickly and painlessly. In other words, don't kvetch . . . stretch!

More formalized stretching and strengthening exercises like those below should be done in a two-part series of eight movements each. Start at the upper torso and work down to the middle body, thighs, and legs. We've created some great exercises for you to choose from, divided by age and progressing in difficulty.

Beginner Stretching Exercises

People under thirty should stay at the beginner level for one week; under forty for two weeks. People in their forties and fifties should stay at this level for three weeks. Over sixty choose your own pace.

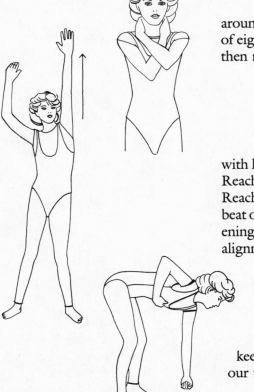

1. BEAR HUG—Reach your crossed arms around your neck and hug yourself to the count of eight, first with the right arm over the left and then repeat with the left arm over the right.

2. REACH FOR THE SKY—Stand straight with legs spread slightly and both arms in the air. Reach upward with one arm and then the other. Reach as high as you can comfortably go, to the beat of your own rhythm. This is great for lengthening the body and bringing everything into alignment.

3. PUNCH THE PIGGY—With knees bent keep the stress off of your back, punch towards our toes, alternating arms.

4. THE ACHILLES STRETCH—Beginning in a push-up position, supporting your body on your hands, walk your feet up until you are in a jack knife position. Keep your feet together and your heels apart and flat on the floor. Then move your feet in a walking motion, shifting your weight from the right side to the left side. Do this for two sets of eight.

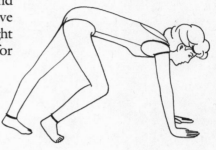

5. SLICE THE APPLE—Sitting with feet spread wide apart and back straight, reach both hands out in front of you. It is important in this exercise to reach forward from your chest, not your head, and to control the movements for your best stretch. Now place your right arm over your right ear and reach toward your left foot. Once again, control the movement so that you lead with your chest and not your chin. Repeat this stretch on your right side, with your left arm extended over your left ear. Remember to do each movement eight times on each side and out in front, and then repeat the whole exercise.

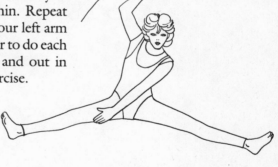

6. THE DOGGIE—Any resemblance between this exercise and a dog by a fire hydrant is purely on purpose. With your body resting on hands and knees, bring your right knee out to the side with a flapping motion and then back to center. Alternate right and left legs.

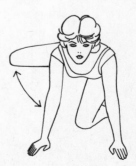

7. THE BACKSTROKE—While still on all fours, extend your right leg out behind you, and with toes flexed, lift your leg up and down for two sets of eight. Repeat this movement on the left side.

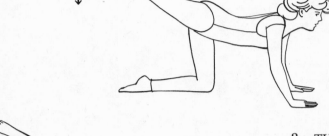

8. THE SIDESTROKE—Lie on your right side with feet outstretched, supporting your body by leaning on your right elbow. Now bend your right leg at the knee and press it behind you. Lift the extended left leg with toes pointed for two sets of eight. Then do another two sets of eight, alternating between the flexed and the pointed position with each lift. Repeat on the left side.

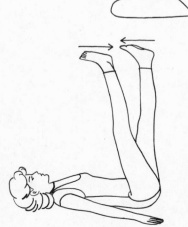

9. THE SCISSOR KICK—Lie on your back, with legs up in the air and feet flexed (toes *not* pointed). Now, to your own rhythm, imitate a scissor action, keeping legs parallel. Repeat eight times, and then do a second set of eight crossing one leg in front of the other. If your back is weak, support it with your arms placed under your buttocks.

10. THE CAT—Lie on your stomach with your lower body flat on the floor and your head and chest supported by your arms braced in the up position of a chin-up. Press your head back, chin to the ceiling, and stretch your lower torso and tummy. Do this exercise without arching the back.

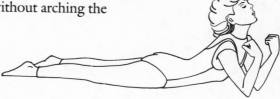

Advanced Stretching Exercises

After your allotted time at the beginner level, continue with the exercises above and add the ones below, substituting those marked "Advanced" for the more elementary version of the same exercise:

1. ADD AN INCH—Sit with back straight, leaning forward from your chest for balance. If you need extra support in sitting up straight, place both arms behind your back to act as a brace. Bend your left knee up to your chest, and extend your right leg out in front of you with the foot flexed. With slow, controlled movements, move the extended leg to the right and then back to center, in two sets of eight stretches. It is important to keep your foot flexed while doing this exercise. Next, bring your leg back to center, and still in the flexed position move your leg up as high as you can and down. Repeat the action with the left leg on the left side of your body.

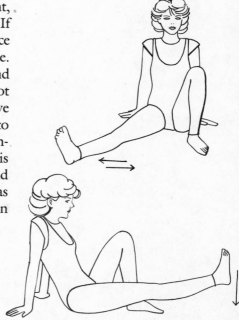

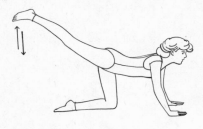

2. THE BACKSTROKE ADVANCED—Get down on all fours, extend your leg out behind you, and, with toes flexed, lift your left leg up and down for two sets of eight. Repeat this stretch on the left leg and then once again on both sides with toes pointed.

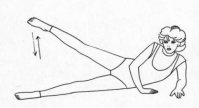

3. THE SIDESTROKE ADVANCED—On your side, with feet outstretched, support the right side of your body by leaning on your right elbow. Lift yourself on your elbow so that your body is at a 45° angle from the floor. Lift the left leg with toes flexed and move it up and down for two sets of eight. Then repeat the leg lifts, alternating between the flexed and pointed toe positions, for another two sets of eight. Repeat this stretch on the left side with the right leg.

Stretching is for all ages. Some familiar stretches not listed here which you might want to try are included in yoga, the Pilates system, calisthenics, and hydrocalisthenics (water exercises).

A final word about stretching. It really can lengthen your body without stretching it on a rack or hanging it upside down. The added flexibility gives you the spring of a young person into your eighties. Until you loosen up, you won't know what you're missing, but trust us—the new body awareness it brings will add a great dimension to your life.

THE FIGURE-8 EXERCISE PLAN: STRENGTHENING

Strengthening exercises (also called isometric exercises) not only build muscle power but also tighten and tone. It is important always to warm up with some stretching exercises before working on strengthening and to be conscious of isolating the muscle you are working on. Control and body alignment will prevent the jerky movements that can cause injury. Whatever your age, it is never too late to look your best, and the sooner you start, the longer your looks will last.

Beginner Strengthening Exercises

People under thirty should stay at each level for one week; under forty for two weeks. People in their forties and fifties should stay at this level for three weeks. Over sixty, choose your own pace.

1. TUMMY TUCK—A version of the old sit-up but with the knees bent and hands clasped behind the head for support, to spare the back. Do two sets of eight. Use the tummy muscle to raise and lower the body.

2. CLIMB THE ROPE—While still in the sit-up position, take your hands away from behind your head and reach first one hand and then the other *between your knees,* as you once again use your tummy muscles to raise and lower your body. Do two sets of eight.

3. SIDE TO SIDE—Still in the sit-up position, use your arms to rotate your body from side to side, for two sets of eight.

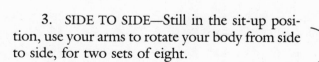

BEAUTIFUL SKIN

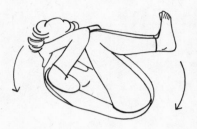

4. ROCK-A-BYE BABY—In the tummy tuck position with hands clasped behind your head for support and your chin tucked into your chest, raise your knees up to your nose and out again keeping ankles flexed. This will stimulate a rocking motion, and once again, you will be using the tummy muscles for support. Do two sets of eight.

5. MUSHY TUSHY—To tighten and lift the tushy muscles, lie flat on your back with your feet wide apart on the floor and knees bent. Now lift your pelvis up in a scooping motion. Move up and down for two sets of eight.

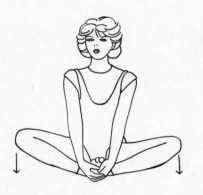

6. THE MUSHROOM—Sit in a modified Buddha pose, grasping your feet at the toes. Press both thighs down to their sides of the ground and up again to the count of eight—twice.

7. KICK THE AIR—Lying on your right side, with legs outstretched and head supported by your right arm, bend your right leg at the knee and move it toward the back of your body. Bend the straightened left leg at the knee and kick the leg in the air, as if you were climbing steps. Using that leg only, take four graduated steps up and four graduated steps down to the count of eight, and then do a second count of eight. Repeat with the opposite leg on the opposite side.

8. THE COSSACK—Standing with feet wide apart and your knees bent, bend over from the waist and grab your ankles. Now move your buttocks up and down in a slow rocking motion, being careful not to bounce. Do this for two sets of eight. Next, straighten the body while releasing your ankles, but keeping your knees bent, and lunge from side to side, first onto the right leg, and then onto the left leg. Again, do two sets of eight.

9. EN GARDE—Standing up tall with feet straight and together, lunge forward onto the right foot and then back into your original position. Then lunge onto the left foot and back. Repeat this motion for two sets of eight.

10. PLIÉ—Ballet students will appreciate the strengthening power of the plié. With torso erect and knees shoulder-width apart, bend at the knee in a half squat. Then return the body to its original position. Arms are extended gracefully out in front of you for balance.

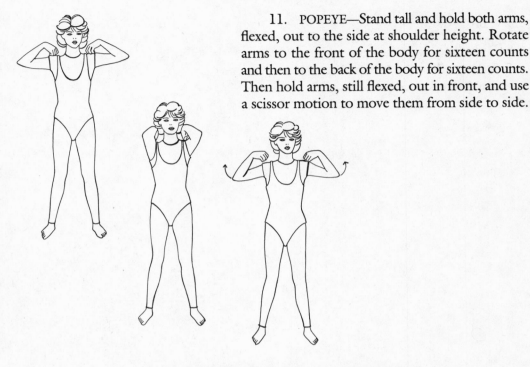

11. POPEYE—Stand tall and hold both arms, flexed, out to the side at shoulder height. Rotate arms to the front of the body for sixteen counts and then to the back of the body for sixteen counts. Then hold arms, still flexed, out in front, and use a scissor motion to move them from side to side.

Advanced Strengthening Exercises

After completing your allotted time at the beginner level, add these exercises to your daily routine:

1. ROCK-A-BYE-BABY ADVANCED—In the tummy-tuck position with hands clasped behind your head for support and your chin tucked into your chest, raise your knees, up to your nose, and out again, keeping ankles flexed. This will simulate a rocking motion, and you will be using the tummy muscles for support. Do this movement

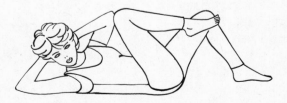

for two sets of eight. Now bring your right elbow to your left knee with one rock, and then your left elbow to your right knee with the next rock, alternating sides with each rock. Do this movement for two sets of eight.

2.   PUSH AND PULL—Using the tummy-tuck position, stretch your legs straight up in the air, lock them at the ankles and flex and bend the knees in a pumping motion, using the tummy muscles for traction.

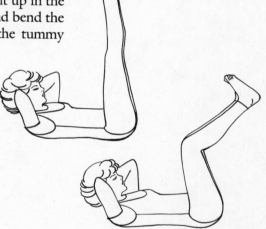

3.   RIDE THE BIKE—This exercise is for the most advanced tummy tuckers. Clasp your hands behind your head, pull your chin back, lift your legs six inches off the floor, and cycle with your legs as if riding a bicycle. After two sets of eight, supporting your lower back with your hands, lift your legs over your head and ride your bicycle in the air.

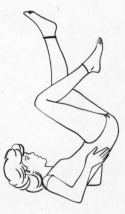

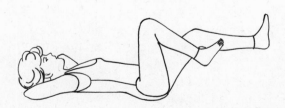

4. MUSHY TUSHY ADVANCED—To tighten and lift the tushy muscles, lie flat on your back with your feet wide apart on the floor and knees bent. Now tilt your pelvis up in a scooping motion. Move up and down for two sets of eight. Next, with knees still bent, close your legs at the ankles and move your pelvis up and down for two sets of eight. Then, with ankles together, knees still bent and pelvis tilted, close and open your legs at the knees for two sets of eight.

5. THE MUSHROOM ADVANCED—Sit in a modified Buddha pose, grasping your feet at the toes. Press both thighs down to their side of the ground and up again; do this for two sets of eight. Now sit on one leg while extending the opposite leg out in front of you, and then press the extended leg up and down for two sets of eight. Repeat this action on the opposite side.

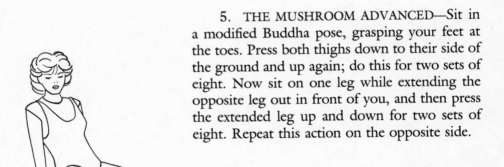

6. KICK THE AIR ADVANCED—Lying on your right side, with legs outstretched and head supported by your right arm, bend your right leg at the knee, and move it toward the back of your body. Bend the straightened left leg at the knee and kick the leg in the air, as if you were climbing

steps. Using that leg only, take four graduated steps up and four graduated steps down to the count of eight, and then do a second count of eight. Repeat with the opposite leg on the opposite side. Then swing both legs out in front of you at a 45-degree angle from your body and repeat the kick and climb action for two sets of eight on each side.

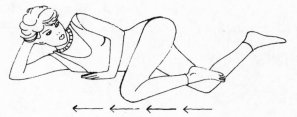

7. POPEYE ADVANCED—Stand tall and flex both arms out to the side at shoulder height. Rotate arms to the front of the body for sixteen counts and then to the back of the body for sixteen counts. Flex arms out in front, and use a scissor motion to move them from side to side (see page 100). Next, lift the arms with graduated scissor motions over the head and back to shoulder height for two sets of eight counts.

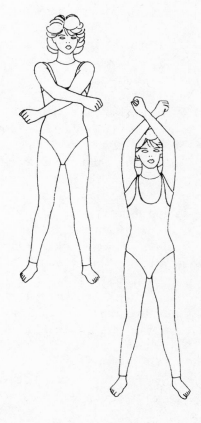

BEAUTIFUL SKIN

AND NOW FOR YOUR AEROBICS . . .

At the heart of a good exercise program is aerobic exercise. The word *aerobic* means "with oxygen," so all aerobic exercises make you breathe in more oxygen, pumping it through the body, feeding the cells, and flushing away the toxins. Aerobic exercise improves circulation and builds stamina by moving the arms and the legs and bringing the heart up to eighty percent of its heartbeat capacity, where it is sustained optimally for twelve minutes or more. This forces the heart to develop new blood vessels and thereby produces a more efficient heart muscle. The target heart-rate level is the focus of aerobics.

Dr. Kenneth Cooper of the Aerobics Center in Dallas, Texas, recommends the following simple way to determine your heart-beat capacity. First, subtract your chronological age from 220. This number tells you how many times your heart can beat per minute. Then take eighty percent of that number to obtain your target heart rate during an aerobic workout. When you divide this number by four, you get the heartbeat level for a 15 second interval, the time usually recommended for taking your pulse rate. A forty-year-old woman would thus have a target heart rate of 144 beats per minute ($220 - 40 = 180 \times .80 = 144$) or 36 beats per 15 seconds.

Dr. Cooper suggests taking the pulse by placing your fingers on your temple or your inner wrist, or over your heart, instead of on the artery of the throat, since pressing on that artery can slow the pulse rate by several beats per minute.[35]

Aerobic exercise is also the very best way to maintain normal body weight. The more you weigh, the more calories you use up during an aerobic workout. For example, a person who weighs 175 pounds would expend about a third more calories per minute than a person who weighs only 100 pounds, so the more you have to lose, the more you *can* lose by doing aerobics.

Once you get your heart working, the rest is easy, because the wonderful thing about aerobic exercises is that man was created to do them. What could be more normal than walking or running? No one is asking you to be an Olympic runner or race walker, but to march realistically to your own drummer. Find your sport and do it at your own pace, increasing a little each day until, before you know it, you'll have reached your own goal.

When doing aerobics, it's important to remember to always warm up for at least five minutes and to cool down for at least five minutes with the stretching exercises that focus on the Achilles tendons and leg muscles. Never start or stop cold, as it's too great a shock for the heart. Be kind to your body.

Listed on the following pages are some good aerobic exercises from which you can choose; or, if you're in a creative spirit, you can invent some of your own.

THE FIGURE-8 EXERCISE PLAN: AEROBICS*

Exercise	Equipment/ Special Need	Benefits	Drawbacks	Amount of Time	Frequency	Form
Walking	A good pair of shoes.	More efficient use of oxygen; stronger bones; loss of weight and body fat; relief from stress; better circulation.	If done outdoors, may be unpleasant in bad weather.	20 minutes, 12 minutes of which should be spent maintaining your heart rate at 80% of its capacity.	5 × a week	Follow your natural gait. Slowly increase speed and distance as you get into shape.
Jogging/ Running	Good jogging shoes and a clean bill of health which should include a stress test.	Same benefits as walking.	May cause shin splints, back injuries, pulled tendons, and pulled muscles, including facial muscles. If done outdoors, may be unpleasant in bad weather.	20 minutes	5 × a week	Run flat-footed with your body in alignment to avoid injury. Stretch for at least 5 min. before and after. Run only in clean air. Slowly increase speed and distance as you get into shape.
Biking	A bicycle or stationary bike. If outdoors wear a helmet.	Same benefits as walking.	If done outdoors, may be unpleasant or unsafe in bad weather.	20 minutes	5 × a week	Follow your natural form. Slowly increase speed and distance as you get into shape.

* Adapted from *Fit or Fat?* by Covert Bailey. Copyright © 1977, 1978 by Covert Bailey. Used by permission of Houghton Mifflin Company.

Exercise	Equipment/ Special Need	Benefits	Drawbacks	Amount of Time	Frequency	Form
Swimming	Access to a pool or lake.	More efficient use of oxygen; relief from stress; better circulation.	May not promote weight loss because the body will tend to conserve fat in the water to maintain its warmth.	12 minutes	5 × a week	Follow your natural form. Slowly increase speed and distance as you get into shape.
Jumping Rope	A ⅜″ nylon rope with a handle at each end	All the benefits of running, plus it's a lot of fun.	Strenuous; you must be aerobically fit before taking up this form of exercise. May cause leg injuries.	12 minutes	5 × a week	Skip rope 70–80 times per minute, hopping from foot to foot. Use a soft surface. Increase speed and jump for longer periods as you get into shape.
Roller Skating and Ice Skating	Skates that fit well.	All the benefits of running, with reduced trauma to legs and joints.	If you skate outdoors, the weather may limit your activity. Otherwise, the only drawback is that you'll be having so much fun that you may forget to get your heart rate up.	20 minutes	5 × a week	Follow your natural form. Remember to push your heart rate up to 80% of its capacity.
Cross Country Skiing	Cross country skis and poles.	All the benefits of running, plus it gives extra exercise to the arms.	A winter-only activity.	15 minutes	5 × a week	Glide on the snow. Remember to push your heart rate up to 80% of its capacity.

Exercise	Equipment/Special Need	Benefits	Drawbacks	Amount of Time	Frequency	Form
Rowing Machine	A rowing machine with a seat that glides.	Uses all of the main muscles of the arms, legs, abdomen and back; has all the benefits of running.	The machines are expensive.	15 minutes	5 × a week	Use your legs to push and your arms to pull.
Mini Trampoline	A mini trampoline	All the benefits of running with reduced trauma to legs and joints.	May cause pulled muscles.	12 minutes	5 × a week	Follow your own form. Increase speed as you get into shape.
Dancing	The proper shoes for either aerobic ballet or jazz dancing.	Combines fun and fantasy with the benefits of running.	May cause injury to legs, back, and joints, but less commonly than with running.	15 minutes	5 × a week	Take classes such as jazz, ballet, or aerobics for more structure and new inspiration. Dance to records or tapes at home.
Treadmill	A treadmill with a control for speed, distance and elevation.	Frees you from weather worries, as well as alleviating boredom by allowing you to talk on the phone, watch TV or listen to music while exercising.	A good treadmill may be costly.	20 minutes	5 × a week	You can walk fast or jog. Increase speed as you get into shape.

The First Act

F. Scott Fitzgerald said beautiful young people are an accident, but beautiful old people create themselves. So get busy and start building your work of art. It takes one month to see results from an exercise program, three months to make it a habit, and six months to get hooked. After that, the body alone will encourage you to go on, as it becomes dependent on exercise. There is a right exercise program for any age. Here is a six-week exercise program that is personally yours.

FIGURE-8 EXERCISE PLAN FOR SIX WEEKS

Workout for the Novice Exerciser in her 20s and 30s:

WEEK 1—20-minute workout

3 MINUTES deep breathing exercises and slow, easy stretches.

5 MINUTES cardiovascular conditioning (aerobics): jogging, easy kicks (using arms and legs), easy disco dance steps, jumping jacks, etc. Start out slowly, building to a faster beat, and slowly return to an easier pace, bringing heart rate down to normal.

10 MINUTES strengthening floor work—dividing time between abdomen and hips/legs (your thighs were worked during aerobics).

2 MINUTES cool down—relaxation, stretches, and breathing.

WEEK 2—26-minute workout

5 MINUTES deep breathing exercises and slow, easy stretches.

7 MINUTES cardiovascular conditioning (aerobics): jogging, easy kicks (using arms and legs), easy disco dance steps, jumping jacks, etc. Start out slowly, building to a faster beat, and slowly return to an easier pace, bringing heart rate down to normal.

12 MINUTES strengthening floor work—dividing time between abdomen and hips/legs.

5 MINUTES cool down—relaxation, stretches and breathing.

WEEK 3 and all weeks thereafter—35-minute workout

5 MINUTES deep breathing exercises and slow, easy stretches.

15 MINUTES cardiovascular conditioning (aerobics): jogging, easy kicks (using arms and legs), easy disco dance steps, jumping jacks, etc. Start out slowly, building to a faster beat, and slowly return to easier pace, bringing heart rate down to normal.

10 MINUTES strengthening floor work—dividing time between abdomen and hips/legs.

5 MINUTES for cooling-down stretches, and relaxing stretches such as yoga.

Workout for the Novice Exerciser in her 40s and 50s:

WEEKS 1 through 3—20-minute workout

3 MINUTES deep breathing exercises and slow, easy stretches.

5 MINUTES cardiovascular conditioning (aerobics): jogging, easy kicks (using arms and legs), easy disco dance steps, jumping jacks, etc. Start out slowly, building to a faster beat, and slowly return to an easier pace, bringing heart rate down to normal.

10 MINUTES strengthening floor work—dividing time between abdomen and hips/legs (your thighs were worked during aerobics).

2 MINUTES cool down—relaxation, stretches, and breathing.

WEEK 4 and 5—26-minute workout

5 MINUTES deep breathing exercises and slow, easy stretches.

7 MINUTES cardiovascular conditioning (aerobics): jogging, easy kicks (using arms and legs), easy disco dance steps, jumping jacks, etc. Start out slowly, building to a faster beat, and slowly return to an easier pace, bringing heart rate down to normal.

12 MINUTES strengthening floor work—dividing time between abdomen and hips/legs.

5 MINUTES cool down—relaxation, stretches and breathing.

WEEK 6 and all weeks thereafter—35-minute workout

5 MINUTES deep breathing exercises and slow, easy stretches.

15 MINUTES cardiovascular conditioning (aerobics): jogging, easy kicks (using arms and legs), easy disco dance steps, jumping jacks, etc. Start out slowly, building to a faster beat, and slowly return to an easier pace, bringing heart rate down to normal.

10 MINUTES strengthening floor work—dividing time between abdomen and hips/legs.

5 MINUTES for cooling-down stretches, and relaxing stretches such as yoga.

Exercise Tips for All Ages

1. *Don't wear makeup while exercising.* The skin is perspiring, giving off oil and releasing impurities from the system during exercise, so don't add makeup

to trap these waste products and force them back into the pores. Also, if you have skin problems, they can become more pronounced while you are perspiring; keep your face clean to avoid irritation. A sunblock is the only thing you should have on your face while exercising, and it should be used only if you are outdoors. Always wash your skin thoroughly after exercising.

2. *While warming up and cooling down*, it is important to stretch out to your limit, to move slowly, and not to bounce.

3. *During exercise, breathe out as you give your greatest effort.* Proper breathing will break down the lactic acid that builds up in the muscles while you exercise.

4. *Let your target heart rate be your guide.* After twelve minutes of aerobics, stop, find your pulse, look at the second hand on your watch, and count your pulse beats for fifteen seconds. Now multiply the heartbeats by four to find your heartbeats per minute. You should be working out at eighty percent of your heartbeat capacity.

5. *Stay at each level for as long as you wish*; this is not a competition. The suggested time for each level is just a guideline for your age group; you may want to choose a slower pace.

6. *Exercise consistently.* Exercise is not stored, and what you did last month can't help you today.

Focus on Your Face

Finally, we have some exercises designed expressly for your face, no matter what your age. Facial exercises *do* work. They are a form of isometric exercise that strengthens the muscle bundles under the skin, lifting and tightening your skin and features.

Just as you can help your skin with isometric exercise, you can also injure it with unnatural or unattractive movements. Pay attention to what your face is doing. If you're tense, relax your muscles; if you're squinting, get out of the sun, buy glasses or contact lenses, or stop smoking (those are the main causes of squinting, according to Dr. Thomas Biggs, a Houston plastic surgeon). When your mouth droops in a frown, smile for heaven's sake, if only because it takes fewer muscles to do so. A calm, happy face is always more attractive.

In the morning, in the evening, and during times of stress, practice facial exercises, and you'll immediately notice an improvement in your face, lessening the wrinkles you already have, while delaying those in your future. Everything we see on our faces has its beginning beneath the surface of the skin, and that's where wrinkles really come from.

When you've begun a series of exercises, you need to keep them up, because once you stop, wrinkles will return.

Select several of the exercises below and make them a part of your daily routine.

1. SCREAM! By releasing stress, you'll feel better, and you'll be exercising your face and neck. Try this ten times, twice a day. (Not recommended for city apartments—try singing instead.)

2. SING. Especially opera. (Have you ever seen a wrinkled opera singer? Think about it!) Like screaming, singing will release tension and exercise your face. Pick a pitch that is comfortable for you and sustain it for as long as you can, ten times, twice a day.

3. CHEW SUGARLESS GUM, or use the chewing gum motion. This is good for your face and neck. (If you don't feel comfortable chewing in front of anyone, do it in the privacy of your bedroom, when you're puttering around the house, or when you're doing some of your other exercises.)

4. ENJOY SEX, the greatest isometric exercise of them all, and by far the most pleasurable (see Step 4). Try this as often as, well, we'll leave that up to you.

5. FACIAL MASSAGE by a skilled masseuse who understands muscles can be very beneficial. Be certain, though, that your skin is never really moved, just pressed.

6. LAYING ON OF HANDS is the name we've given to a procedure that promotes good circulation. Using your fingertips, apply pressure to wrinkled areas on your face. Blood will rush to the area, bringing oxygen and flushing out impurities. Press with the fingertips of both hands, eight in all, the wrinkle you are working on. Hold the press to the count of five and repeat this motion fifteen times consecutively. Do this twice a day and when under stress.

7. FEED YOUR FACE. Lower your head below your body, on a slant board, or off your bed, twice a day for a few minutes. This will get your circulation going.

8. HEAD LIFTS. Lying on your back in bed, hang your head over the edge. Slowly raise your head and try to touch your chin to your chest. Then slowly lower your head back to its loose, hanging position. Repeat five times. This exercise is excellent for reducing the tendency toward saggy, droopy neck skin.

9. MAMA MIA! Make believe you have lost your teeth by wrapping your lips around them tightly. Now, to the count of ten, say, "Mama mia!" This is great for lines etched around the mouth.

10. PRETTY PINCH. Another exercise for reducing lines around the mouth consists of pinching your mouth together with your thumb and forefinger. Slowly move the pinch all around the mouth and back again.

11. HO-TEI. This exercise is named for the little round-tummied Oriental God of Happiness because that's who you'll look like when you do it. With eyes open, gently clench your teeth and grin as hard as you can, lifting your upper lips and cheek muscles. Try to use the muscles in front of your ears rather than the muscles around your mouth. Reach back as far as you can with your grin; imagine yourself grinning all the way to your ears. At the same time, contract your neck muscles. Hold for ten seconds. Release and relax. Work up to repeating this exercise ten times, a minimum of twice a day.

12. THE LION'S ROAR. Adapted from yoga, this exercise is helpful in reducing crow's-feet, developing the muscles of the cheeks, and toning the muscles of the neck and throat. Slowly widen your eyes and keep them wide through the exercise. *Very* slowly extend your tongue and hold it as far out and down as you can. Feel the muscles in your face, neck, and throat tense up. Become a lion in a silent roar. Hold for ten seconds. Slowly release and return to a relaxed state. Notice that as the muscles of your face and neck relax, they will be infused with blood. This is an excellent exercise for promoting improved circulation to the entire face and neck. Repeat five times.

13. RUN, RUN, RUN! Aerobics are a great form of exercise for your face. They act as a natural massage to stimulate circulation.

A Word of Encouragement

The body is very forgiving and will repay you well if you show it respect instead of neglect. You have the opportunity to get your body in balance through exercise, to turn Father Time around and send him jogging off in the opposite direction. It will mean a bit of work on your part, but anything worth having is worth working for. Aren't you worth 35 minutes of your time each day?

STEP 3: EXERCISE CHECKLIST

Check the things you do. Incorporate the others into your daily routine.

Always:
1. Exercise with a clean face.

2. Wash right after exercise.
3. Take proper precautions.
4. Wear appropriate clothing.

On a daily basis:
35-MINUTE WORKOUT
5 MINUTES deep breathing exercises and slow, easy stretches.
15 MINUTES cardiovascular conditioning (aerobics), sustaining your heart beat at eighty percent of capacity for twelve minutes.
10 MINUTES strengthening floor work.
5 MINUTES cooling-down stretches, and relaxing stretches such as yoga.

Facial Exercise and Massage
1. Chew gum.
2. Sing.
3. Do lip, face, and throat exercises.
4. Smile.
5. Apply pressure to pressure points.
6. Be conscious of what your face is doing and relax it.

---

[1] Maxwell Maltz, *Psycho-Cybernetics* (New York: Essandess, 1968), p. 238.

[2] Theories concerning retardation of waste production have been proposed by Carlton Fredericks, author and nutritionist, in *Eating Right For You* (New York: Grosset & Dunlap, 1972) and *Psycho-Nutrition* (New York: Grosset & Dunlap, 1976), wherein he popularized the use of such antioxidants as vitamins A, B complex, C, E, zinc, and selenium; New York physician Benjamin S. Frank, who has successfully used concentrated doses of nucleic acids to strengthen the cells as they repair and regenerate and whose work is described in this book for the medical community, *Nucleic Acid Therapy in Aging and Degenerative Disease* (New York: Psychological Library, 1969), and in his popular book with Philip Miele, *Dr. Frank's No-Aging Diet* (New York: Dial Press, 1976); Dr. Denham Harmon of the University of Nebraska Medical Center, who developed the free-radical theory of aging and whose work is discussed extensively by Durk Pearson and Sandy Shaw in their book *Life Extension* (New York: Warner Books, 1982), wherein a discussion can also be found of the use by the medical community of the intracellular enzyme SOD (superoxide dismutase), which destroys the superoxide free radical.

[3] Joy Gross, *30-Day Way to a Born Again Body* (New York: Rawson, Wade, 1979), p. 141.

[4] Nathan Pritikin with Patrick M. McGrady, Jr., *The Pritikin Program for Diet and Exercise* (New York: Bantam, 1979), pp. 69–70.

[5] Samuel M. Fox, "Relationship of Activity Habits to Coronary Heart Disease," in J. P. Naughton and H. K. Hellerstein, eds., *Exercise Testing and Exercise Training in Coronary Heart Disease*

(New York: Academic Press, 1974), pp. 12–13. Cited in Charles T. Kuntzleman and the Editors of *Consumer Guide, Rating the Exercises* (New York: William Morrow and Company, Inc., 1978), pp. 59–61.

6 H. L. Taylor, "Coronary Heart Disease in Physically Active and Sedentary Populations," *Journal of Sports Medicine and Physical Fitness*, 2:1962, p. 73, cited in Charles T. Kuntzleman and the Editors of *Consumer Guide, Rating the Exercises* (New York: William Morrow & Co., 1978), pp. 59–61; and Pat Stewart, ed., *U.S. Fitness Book* (New York: Simon and Schuster, 1979), p. 16. See also a somewhat different account of the same study in Nathan Pritikin with Patrick M. McGrady, Jr., *The Pritikin Program for Diet and Exercise* (New York: Grosset & Dunlap, 1983), p. 73.

7 Nathan Pritikin with Patrick M. McGrady, Jr., *The Pritikin Program for Diet and Exercise* (New York: Bantam, 1979), p. 81; Sandy Rovner, "Psychosomatic: The New Meaning," *Washington Post Health*, April 3, 1985, p. 11.

8 Kenneth H. Cooper, *The Aerobics Way* (New York: Bantam, 1977), p. 183.

9 Jane Brody, *Jane Brody's Guide to Personal Health* (New York: Avon, 1983), p. 87.

10 According to *New York Times* health columnist Jane Brody, exercise not only burns up calories directly, but the body continues to burn calories for as many as fifteen hours *after* exercise. *Jane Brody's Guide to Personal Health* (New York: Avon, 1983), p. 87.

11 It is a fact that the more you exercise, the more you are able to exercise. What's more, Dr. Kenneth H. Cooper, of the Aerobics Center in Dallas, Texas, indicates that dynamic exercise allows you to get more work done, including sendentary work like that involved in a desk job, with less fatigue. *Aerobics* (New York: M. Evans and Company, Inc., 1968), p. 29.

12 Ibid., p. 28.

13 Kenneth H. Cooper, *The Aerobics Program for Total Well-Being* (New York: M. Evans and Company, Inc., 1982), p. 118; and Jane Brody, *Jane Brody's Guide to Personal Health* (New York: Avon Books, 1983), pp. 86–87.

14 James F. Fixx says, "Of the heart patients who survive an initial attack, 4 to 6 percent die each year. However, if they start a medically supervised program of running and other exercises, the rate drops to well under 2 percent." *The Complete Book of Running* (New York: Random House, 1977), p. 227.

15 Dr. Kenneth H. Cooper and his colleagues conducted a study of the relationship of heart attack risk factors and fitness levels using 3,000 male volunteers with an average age of 44.6 years. The conclusion of their research was that as the fitness level of the volunteers improved, their risk factors were all reduced. See K. H. Cooper, M. L. Pollock, R. P. Martin, S. R. White, A. C. Linnerud, and A. Jackson, "Physical Fitness Levels Versus Selected Coronary Risk Factors," *Journal of American Medical Association*, 12 July, 1976, p. 166. Discussed in Charles T. Kuntzleman and the Editors of *Consumer Guide, Rating the Exercises* (New York: William Morrow and Co., Inc., 1978), p. 89.

16 Ibid., p. 166.

17 Ibid., p. 166.

18 *New York Times* health columnist Jane Brody notes that, "diabetics who exercise may have fewer blood vessel complications because the 'stickiness' of their blood cells is reduced." *Jane Brody's Guide to Personal Health* (New York: Avon, 1983), p. 87.

[19] Jane Brody cites swimming as the best dynamic exercise for countering varicose veins. Ibid., p. 109. Also, Mildred Cooper and Kenneth H. Cooper note that dynamic exercise is particularly useful in avoiding or reducing varicosities during pregnancy. *Aerobics for Women* (New York: Bantam, 1972), p. 32.

[20] Jane Brody, *Jane Brody's Guide to Personal Health* (New York: Avon, 1983), pp. 87 and 610–612. Further, Kenneth H. Cooper recommends calisthenics, aerobics, and weight-bearing exercises to strengthen bones and reduce the risk of fractures due to bone deterioration. *The Aerobics Program for Total Well-Being* (New York: M. Evans Co., Inc., 1982), pp. 115–116.

[21] Kenneth H. Cooper, *The Aerobics Program for Total Well-Being* (New York: M. Evans Co., Inc., 1982), p. 12.

[22] Ibid., p. 12.

[23] Ibid., p. 12.

[24] Dr. Cooper notes, "This is a subject for which quantifiable data are lacking, yet there does seem to be a positive relationship between aerobic conditioning and a satisfying sex life. Many times over the past 20 years, I have had patients volunteer the information that their sex lives have improved in response to regular physical exercise, and when both partners are involved, this relationship seems to be enhanced even more." Ibid., p. 201.

[25] Charles T. Kuntzleman and the Editors of *Consumer Guide* specifically recommend stretching exercises for improving flexibility. *Rating the Exercises* (New York: William Morrow and Company, Inc., 1978), pp. 59–61.

[26] Edward L. Fox, Donald K. Mathews, and Jeffrey N. Bairstow specifically note that exercise speeds recovery after orthopedic surgery and bone fractures. *I. T.: Interval Training for Lifetime Fitness* (New York: Dial Press, 1980), p. 7.

[27] Mildred Cooper and Kenneth H. Cooper, *Aerobics for Women* (New York: Bantam Books, 1972), pp. 30–33; and Kenneth H. Cooper, *The Aerobics Program for Total Well-Being* (New York: M. Evans Co., Inc., 1982), p. 12.

[28] Dr. Bruno Balke, of the University of Wisconsin, supervised an experiment on cancerous mice. He divided the mice into two groups. One group he exercised regularly on a treadmill, and the other group he did not. His findings demonstrated that the exercised mice had fewer tumors than the nonexercised mice, and some of the nonexercised mice died during the experiment.

[29] Pat Stewart, ed., *U.S. Fitness Book* (New York: Simon and Schuster, 1979), p. 16.

[30] Jane Brody, *Jane Brody's Guide to Personal Health* (New York: Avon, 1983), p. 88.

[31] Nathan Pritikin with Patrick M. McGrady, Jr., *The Pritikin Program for Diet and Exercise* (New York: Bantam, 1979), p. 74.

[32] Ibid., p. 75.

[33] Ibid., p. 75.

[34] See Kenneth H. Cooper, *The New Aerobics* (New York: Bantam, 1977), pp. 71–72, for his discussion of the myth of the "heartbeat bank."

[35] Kenneth H. Cooper, *The Aerobics Program for Total Well-Being* (New York: M. Evans and Co., Inc., 1982), p. 125.

[36] Adapted from: Covert Bailey, *Fit or Fat?* (Boston: Houghton Mifflin Co., 1978), pp. 38–45.

Step Four:
Sex

Human beings are naturally sensuous. We delight in the pink cotton-candy clouds and purple skies of a gorgeous sunset; we find peace in the soothing sounds of ocean waves breaking on the beach; we enjoy the scent of magnolias or lilacs or honeysuckle and are stimulated by the taste of exotic spices and tropical fruits. And we're tactile creatures; we love to hug and be hugged, to stroke a beloved's hand, to feel the pleasures of fur or velvet or silk, to be cooled by a fresh mountain breeze in summer or warmed by the nearness of a toasty open hearth in winter. In fact, the sense of touch is our most widespread sense because it's transmitted to us by the entire surface of our skin. And, under the right circumstances, that surface can become a source of sexual pleasure and even gratification. As an organ of sensuality, the skin is nearly as important as the genitalia. Its beauty and softness stimulate erotic responses in others; and, filled as it is with nerve endings, its capacity to give sensual pleasure is virtually limitless. According to some recent sex research studies, with proper mental transference and appropriate stimulation, any area of the body with tactile sense organs can become a source of orgasmic pleasure and release.

The relationship between skin and sex is really circular, and it's a delicious circle at that. Not only is healthy skin provocative and sexy, but sex is important to the care and feeding of your skin.

We doubt that your mother ever told you that, probably because she didn't know it. Only recently (within the last three decades) through the work of such researchers as Alfred Kinsey, William Masters and Virginia Johnson, Alice Kahn Ladas, Beverly Whipple, and John D. Perry, have women's sexual natures and capabilities become recognized. And only in the past five to ten years have the beauty benefits of sex been publicized.[1] So don't blame poor old Mom if you aren't—yet—as gorgeous as you deserve to be. What Mother didn't tell you, we will.

Tiresius Was Right!

Two particularly positive effects of the sexual revolution on almost everybody in this country (whether or not you carried a flag in the revolution!) have been (1) a better understanding of the sexual nature of women, and (2) an acknowledgment by the medical community that sex is good for your health.

With respect to the first of these points, a Greek myth tells the tale of what amounts to the first human sex change, wherein a chap named Tiresius accidently stumbled into a holy wood where humans weren't supposed to trespass. There he chanced to see two sacred snakes copulating, and—zap!—Tiresius was instantly changed into a woman! After spending a few years as a female, Tiresius one day found himself wandering again in the forbidden wood (perhaps he should have taken a course in map reading) and, predictably, he again saw the two snakes blissfully sporting. And—zap again!—Tiresius found himself again the man he had once been.

Sometime thereafter, Zeus, the ruler of all the Greek gods, and his wife Hera began to dispute the question of whether men or women enjoyed the sex act more. Zeus insisted that women did, and Hera petulantly maintained that men did. To settle the dispute, they naturally called upon Tiresius, because he had been both sexes. To Hera's vast dismay, Tiresius maintained that women have the ability to enjoy sex far more than do men. Hera was so enraged by this statement that she struck Tiresius blind; this, of course, kept him from ever again viewing any snakes.

Hera's rage not withstanding, it would appear that Tiresius was right, although for our Western culture, proof of women's sexual capabilities has been long in coming. It wasn't until the 1950s that Kinsey demonstrated women had sexual natures and needs equal in depth to men's, and in the 1960s, Masters and Johnson demonstrated that all women, if properly aroused, could be not only as orgasmic as, but even more orgasmic than men by virtue of their ability to climax one or several times with each sex act, provided they were properly stimulated, and by their ability to sustain a peak pleasure level. More recent research makes claims for multiple orgasms recurring over periods of up to two hours, and for single sustained orgasms of thirty minutes and more.[2] And the research of Ladas, Whipple, and Perry has demonstrated that women really can have vaginal orgasms—a point disputed by most earlier authorities (despite the fact that many women kept saying, "I do! I do!"). Such orgasms are at least in part the result of stimulation of the G spot (named for Dr. Ernst Grafenberg, the first contemporary physician to describe it), a place on the front vaginal wall which, when stimulated, can cause a deep, total body orgasm, generally reported as being different in kind from the more readily observable clitoral climax. And Ladas, Whipple, and Perry report that many women are even capable of the female equivalent of ejaculation. These women experience the rapid release of a clear or whitish fluid at the peak of orgasm, an experience that has a sensual effect all its own![3] So, physiologically speaking, we girls really are a lot luckier than was once believed, because we have so many possibilities for pleasurable release.

And the really nice part about having these various pleasure mechanisms is the further recent acknowledgment by the medical community that using them is *good* for you. Sexual activity is a specialized form of exercise and has the same physiological benefits of other forms of exercise—plus a few more. Most of the body's systems are stimulated and refreshed by sexual arousal and gratification. In addition, sex has psychological benefits ranging from relief of stress to the deep contentment that comes from sexual enjoyment shared with a loved partner. Both the physical and the mental benefits of sex have a wonderful effect on your skin, cleansing, nourishing, relaxing, and softening it. Perhaps that's why lovers and newlyweds have a special glow!

The Sexual Response Cycle

Masters and Johnson, in their book *Human Sexual Response*,[4] divide the sexual response of both sexes into four phases: *the excitement phase*, during which the sexual tension begins to mount in response to appropriate stimuli; *the plateau phase*, when sexual tension intensifies if effective stimulation continues; *the orgasmic phase*, usually the period of shortest duration in the cycle, when the blood vessels and muscles release the tension developed from the sexual stimulation; and *the resolution phase*, during which the individual returns, in a reverse pattern, to an unstimulated state. Generally speaking, the length of the excitement and resolution phases is roughly equivalent; these will normally be the longest phases of the sexual cycle, and the length of the excitement phase in any given sexual experience will determine the length of the resolution phase in that experience. The plateau phase is fairly brief in most people; the orgasm itself as Masters and Johnson observed it commonly lasts only a few seconds.

Masters and Johnson also divide the female orgasm into three states: (1) an intense sensual awareness radiating from the clitoris through the pelvis, and ranging in degree from mild to shock; (2) followed by a sensation of warmth, which begins in the pelvis, then spreads throughout the body; (3) followed in turn by throbbing or involuntary contraction of the vagina and lower pelvis. Contractions commonly range in number from three (mild) to ten (strong).

Masters and Johnson's observations of female sexual response were based on the effects of clitoral orgasm, and while their work gave many of us encouragement, reassurance, and maybe even some new goals to strive for, the picture wasn't yet complete. More recently Ladas, Whipple, and Perry have demonstrated that for some women vaginal or G-spot orgasms may in fact be even more pleasurable, longer in duration, and easier to restimulate than the clitoral kind.

The point is that practice, experience, a relaxed attitude, and just knowing what's possible can work wonders in helping both sexes—and women in particular—to repeat the orgasmic phase a number of times or to extend indefinitely the pleasure of this most intense experience. And either repetition or extension of the orgasmic phase is a desirable goal, since the more frequent or longer the orgasm, the greater the health, beauty, and skin benefits.

Sexercise: Fine Tuning of the Body Machine

Sex produces more beauty benefits than any other form of exercise; no other physical activity is as natural or affects as many parts of the body at the same time.

From our discussion on Step 3, you already know that during exercise, increased breathing improves oxygen intake to the lungs, thereby bringing this life-giving force into contact with the blood. And every exhalation removes toxins from the body. As exercise stimulates heart function, improved circulation brings the newly acquired oxygen to every cell of the body, and the skin takes on a healthy glow. Furthermore, improved circulation carries oil (sebum) and moisture (perspiration) to the surface of the skin, so the skin becomes hydrated and hence softer and more supple.

During sex, many of the same physiological changes occur.[5] In the excitement phase, the heart rate increases and blood pressure begins to rise. In the plateau phase, the heart might be expected to go from a rate of 80 to between 110–175 beats per minute. (It's been observed that the heart rate is somewhat more rapid during masturbation than during intercourse.) The systolic pressure may rise to as much as 140 to 180 mm Hg rather than the normal 120, and the diastolic pressure may increase to 90 or 100 mm Hg rather than the normal pressure of 80. During the plateau phase, the respiration also begins to increase. A further increase in both heart rate and blood pressure usually occurs during orgasm (systolic pressure as high as 150 to 200 mm Hg—diastolic pressure 100 to 120 mm Hg). Respiration may increase to as much as 40 breaths per minute; this is double the normal respiration rate. These increases in heart rate, blood pressure, and respiration are healthful for the body as a whole, offering exercise for the lungs and heart muscle, removing toxins from the body, and improving the general circulation. During the resolution phase, heart rate, blood pressure, and respiration return to normal.

During this final phase a film of perspiration will often appear on the body, a response that is directly proportional to the strength of the orgasm. Some women will, of course, perspire simply from the physical exertion of the sex act. In either case, the perspiratory response is healthy for the skin, helping to soften wrinkles and retard aging; it's one reason why a woman who has been thoroughly pleasured looks and feels dewy, smooth, and silky. So, while exercise can be thought of as toning, sexual activity might be considered as fine tuning for the sake of body— and particularly skin—beauty.

Another positive effect of sexual activity on the skin is the phenomenon described by Masters and Johnson as the *maculopapular sex flush*; "maculopapular" is a Latin word meaning "skin rash." This sex flush is actually a bright rash which begins to appear in some women during the excitement phase as the small blood vessels relax and blood and heat are brought to the surface of the skin. Masters and Johnson observed this sex flush in about seventy-five percent of their female subjects; only twenty-five percent of their male subjects exhibited a similar tendency.

In the excitement phase this flush usually appears on the stomach, face, neck, and throat, then spreads to the breasts. As the plateau phase progresses, the flush spreads over most of the other body surfaces—shoulders, arms, lower abdomen, back, thighs, and buttocks. Masters and Johnson observed that in general, the intensity of the flush tends to parallel the intensity of the sexual tensions of the woman involved, reaching its peak in depth of coloration late in the plateau phase. As a woman enters the orgasmic phase, the blush terminates, disappearing from the body surfaces during the resolution phase in reverse order from its appearance, i.e., from the buttocks, thighs, back, arms, and lower abdomen first, then more slowly from the breasts, neck, throat, face, and stomach. This sex flush is an excellent skin treatment, promoting blood circulation into the skin's outer layers.

Beauty expert Oleda Baker and her co-author Bill Gale have noted yet another beauty benefit of sexual activity in the isometric exercise that occurs automatically in all parts of the face and body during sex.[6]

In the excitement phase, the voluntary muscles and even some involuntary muscles become progressively more tense as a woman's movements become more restless and rapid. Responses are not restricted to the pelvic area, but can include flexing of arms, legs, buttocks, neck and shoulders.

As she progresses to the plateau phase, the sexually stimulated woman often reacts with facial grimaces, frowns, and scowls, flaring nostrils, widening of the eyes, and straining of the muscles around the mouth as it opens involuntarily in a gasping reaction to hyperventilation. The little muscles around the eyes and in the upper eyelids tighten, helping to smooth out lines on the outer corners of the eyes and keeping the lids from drooping. As the muscles around the mouth contract, the network of tiny muscles in the cheeks tightens up, filling out the creases that run from the side of the nose to the upper lip. The muscles on the side of the mouth become firmer, eliminating the tendency toward droopy bags. As the jaws clench and tense, the tendency to form jowls or a double chin lessens; etched lines that can form at the sides of the mouth are prevented. The neck stretches, particularly as orgasm approaches, firming the throat muscles.

Also during the plateau phase, the back arches, the thigh muscles tense, and the calves, feet, toes, hands, and fingers stretch and flex, exercising the whole body. Arm muscles flex, preventing upper-arm flesh from drooping. As the woman strives toward orgasm, muscles of the buttocks tense, firming the buttocks. At the same time, her abdominal and pelvic muscles tense; voluntary thrusting and tightening of the pelvis and stomach during intercourse and involuntary contractions both before and during orgasm are excellent exercises that help prevent flabbiness.

The breasts normally react to sexual stimulation with erect nipples during the excitement phase, followed by a twenty to twenty-five percent enlargement due to venous engorgement, a response that can remain for five to ten minutes after orgasm. (This response is more noticeable in women who have not breast-fed their infants.)[7] During the excitement and plateau phases, the chest muscles may flex rhythmically as the woman arches her back and presses against her partner; during orgasm, the rib cage may even expand. All such exercise improves muscle tone and firmness in the breasts.

During orgasm, all the isometric contractions and flexings are heightened; when the woman reaches her peak of excitement, she will involve her whole body in a thoroughly orchestrated orgasmic experience.

In the resolution phase, muscle tension rapidly dissipates unless stimulation begins again. If the body is allowed to rest, all sexual tension will disappear within about five minutes. But let us reiterate: it is to your advantage to prolong your orgasm or to continue stimulation after orgasm, whenever possible, because multiple or prolonged orgasms will maximize your beauty and health benefits and keep all your systems operating at an optimal level. In other words, if you want to live longer, try making love longer!

Hormone Balance

One myth concerning skin that's always been particularly prevalent is that too much sexual activity during puberty will cause pimples; actually, just the opposite is closer to the truth. There's a relationship between hormone balance and skin health, but it would appear that more sex rather than less is what keeps you glowing (and grinning).

A major difference between regular exercise of the aerobic type and sexual exercise is the effect of the latter on the endocrine system and the resultant effect the glands have on the body as a whole. When the glands are stimulated positively, as they are during the sex act, the hormonal changes that take place throughout the entire endocrine system promote the body's general health, to the extent that they may actually help prolong life and youth. In their book *Life Extension*, Durk Pearson and Sandy Shaw note: "Erotic self-image plays a major role in neuroendocrine function. (Youthful erotic stimulation has been shown to alter the neuroendocrine systems of old male and female rats and rhesus monkeys toward more youthful functioning.) Not only is staying young good for your sex life, a good sex life can help you stay young."[8]

An example of the benefits to health of sexual activity is the effect of regular orgasm on patients with arthritis. Rheumatoid arthritis, one of the collagen diseases, has been linked to adrenal exhaustion; aspirin is effective in relieving the pain of arthritis, largely because it gives the adrenals a little kick and gets the endocrine system moving to help relieve the pain. However, recent studies have observed that arthritis sufferers who experience frequent orgasmic release have notable relief of stiffness, pain, and other symptoms of the disease.[9] (Arthritic males may not achieve the same degree of relief from repeated orgasm as do females, possibly because of their different hormonal balance; they do, however, reap other physiological benefits.)

Since hormones are important to the working of all the body's cells, and since sexual activity gives a boost to the glandular system, it makes good sense to keep the glands humming through regular sexual exercise. You'll note that the functioning of the glandular system is circular: sexual activity would not be possible without neuroendocrine functioning; and neuroendocrine function is stimulated by sexual activity.

So get busy enjoying the benefits of healthy and frequent sex. To help you do so, we've devised some mental attitudes for you to learn to cultivate.

Mental Attitude #1: You Can't Wear Yourself Out.

Orgasmic bliss is one good thing you're unlikely to overdose on. In fact, studies show that the more you use your sexual faculties, the more acute, sensitive, and responsive you become. Conversely, the less you use your sexual abilities, the less capable you'll become of responding. So don't hide this light under a bushel: when it comes to sex, you've got to "use it, or lose it."

Dr. Alan Brauer in his sexual enhancement seminars recommends an orgasm a day for good health (to replace, perhaps, the apple in the old saw). On the Figure-8 program, we suggest that, circumstances permitting, a healthy adult should experience at least as many orgasmic periods as exercise periods: a minimum of three or four a week. (The maximum is up to you—go for it!)

Of course, some people, for one reason or another, cannot attain this goal, or may choose not to do so. But even most patients under a doctor's care can engage in sexual intercourse without fear of complications. In fact, all the doctors we consulted encouraged sexual activity and healthy, loving, supportive relationships as great aids to the retention of both beauty and youth. As one doctor joked, "About the only time sex might be bad for your skin is if you use whips and chains." But normal, healthy, happy sex gets everybody's vote of confidence.

And perhaps we should state here that you don't have to have intercourse to experience satisfying orgasms—any kind of stimulation that pleases you is OK. Some women have even reported attaining orgasm through fantasy alone. From the perspective of health and beauty, it really doesn't matter how the orgasm is created; the physiological benefits will still accrue. So enjoy! And the more often, the better, because you simply can't wear yourself out.

Mental Attitude #2: You Can't Take It with You.

It follows, then, that you should learn to use it here. Sex is a bit like money: it's unlikely you'll be able to use it anywhere except in this three-dimensional plane of experience. And your sexual nature is something you need to integrate with the rest of you if you are to become a total person. So don't wait to start coming to terms with this most important part of your adult self. If you aren't totally satisfied with this part of your life, it may be that you're letting someone else dictate your actions.

For example, is the "critical parent" part of you restricting you because of ideas learned in childhood or adolescence? Do you avoid variety in your lovemaking because "nice women do it only in the missionary position"? Examine such ideas to see if they are valid in the context of your grownup life.

The same goes for guilt, especially over things you may have fantasized or experienced in childhood; if you have guilt, does it really make sense in the context of an adult sex life? The late Presbyterian clergyman, Dr. Peter Marshall, wrote the following poetic words, "Next to hunger, the most powerful of human instincts is that of sex. You cannot escape from it, for you are made that way. It pulses in your blood, sings in your throat, and shines in your eyes. . . . There is nothing shameful about the sex urge."[10] If you have guilts, reread these words often.

Do you remain silent about your needs, for fear of what your partner may think of you? Communication of your needs is the only way to involve your partner in real emotional intimacy.

The point of all this is that any problems related to sex need to be solved so you can begin enjoying the benefits to health that accrue from pleasurable sexual activity.

If you're uncomfortable with your body or any portion of it, start reading some reputable sex manuals. Alexander Comfort's *The Joy of Sex* has pretty and explicit pictures to help you get used to seeing people giving pleasure to other people and to themselves. If you think you'd feel more comfortable knowing what's "normal" (always remembering that "normal" is a subjective term), *Human Sexual Response* by Masters and Johnson is reassuring, though the medical language is somewhat weighty. Ladas, Whipple, and Perry's *The G Spot* has been an eye-opener even for other sex researchers and will encourage you to learn for yourself what's the most comfortable and natural sexual approach for you.

Furthermore, some doctors have begun recommending four hugs a day for good health. A good, long hug (fifteen seconds or longer) has the physiological effects of (1) getting you to breathe deeply, thus oxygenating your blood, and (2) helping the body release endorphins, nature's pleasure chemicals, which decrease your sensitivity to pain, help you to resist illness, and improve your mental acumen.[11]

The happiest and healthiest adult relationships (and the longest lasting) are those that incorporate a high level of sexual activity and a high level of affectionate touching. Men whose wives give them warm good-bye kisses before sending them off to work in the morning live an average of five years longer than men who don't get kisses. Hugging, touching, cuddling, fondling, caressing, or simply holding—they all help to satisfy your skin's hunger to be touched. Feed that hunger, for your health's sake.

Finally, if for any reason you feel unworthy of receiving sexual pleasure and of reaping the benefits it can bring in terms of health, joy, beauty, and longevity, go to your mirror and say to the person you find there:

You deserve to be happy!
You deserve to be healthy!

You deserve a full measure of harmony, joy, beauty, balance,
and pleasure in your life!
You deserve to be a total person; all parts of you are
beautiful, and wholesome, and worthy of being loved.

If you're truly willing to learn about yourself and grow toward totality (and this means, by definition, coming to terms with your sexuality), you'll find very soon the effort you've expended will begin returning to you its benefits. Happy, loving sex is for the here and now.

Mental Attitude #3: You're Never Too Old.

One of the most popular—and unfortunate—misconceptions in our society is that with the onset of menopause and the termination of fertility, women cease to have sexual desire. This is another one of those unpleasant holdovers from the days when "nice" women were childbearers rather than sexual partners. The fact, though, is that a woman reaches her peak of interest in sexual activity in the twenties or early thirties and, barring any pathologies, remains there until her eighties and probably longer, provided she lives longer. Indeed, many women find that after menopause, they are even more interested in sex because they no longer need to worry about birth control. Dr. Joyce Brothers claims that often women in fact discover a whole new dimension to sex in their forties and fifties; they experience a new sense of freedom and a greater lack of sexual inhibition.[12] We know personally of men and women in their seventies and eighties who are still interested in sex and pursuing its pleasures actively. In fact, there's evidence to suggest that, into the nineties and even beyond, we never outgrow our need for sex!

A woman's ability to attain orgasm seems not to diminish any sooner than does her interest. In fact, Masters and Johnson reported no change in clitoral response levels into the seventies, the highest age of their research population. Responses may become somewhat slower, but recent reports on both men and women suggest that the slowing of response time from initiation of sexual activity to orgasm can be a real advantage; those who report an increase in sexual pleasure in later years (after 50) cite the lengthening of the excitement phase as a positive factor because it gives them more time to reach a peak of excitement, and, once attained, the peak can be maintained indefinitely. Men and women who continue enjoying sex in their later years very often consider themselves better lovers because they spend more time at loving.

Naturally, some physiologic changes will eventually take place in the body of the postmenopausal female due to hormonal differences, but for women who maintain a high level of sexual activity during their mature lives, discomfort due to these changes is usually minimal. So don't assume that you'll ever be too old to enjoy sex. If you're willing to turn off your age with the changes we suggest in the Figure 8 program, you'll be healthy, vital, young looking, and sexy for as long as sex is in style. So the next time opportunity knocks, just say to the one you love, "Come on, honey, let's go do something good for my skin!"

STEP 4: SEX CHECKLIST

At least three or four times a week? Give yourself a gold star. If not, try some of the things below. Just check the ones that appeal to you the most.

1. Acquire some of the following books from your library or local bookstore:
    William H. Masters and Virginia E.Johnson, *Human Sexual Response* (New York: Bantam, 1966).
    Shere Hite, *The Hite Report on Female Sexuality* (New York: Dell, 1981).
    Alexander Comfort, *The Joy of Sex*, (New York: Crown, 1972).
    Nancy Friday, *My Secret Garden*, (New York: Pocket Books, 1974) (on women's sexual fantasies).
    Nancy Friday, *Men in Love*, (New York: Pocket Books, 1978) (on men's sexual fantasies).
    Alice Kahn Ladas, Beverly Whipple, and John D. Perry, *The G Spot and Other Recent Discoveries About Human Sexuality* (New York: Dell, 1983).

2. Join your partner in a Jacuzzi, hot tub, or sauna, or get busy on mutual muscle massage.

3. While most authorities will tell you that no true aphrodisiacs exist, make a point of enjoying a few old standards like oysters or asparagus, now and then, noting to your beloved that there's a purpose to the cuisine. (An old New Orleans aphrodisiac dish called for eggs cooked with absinthe; you might just find that "absinthe makes the heart grow fonder.")

4. Play Ravel's *Bolero* or the "Liebestod" from *Tristan and Isolde* as background music; both of these well known pieces are supposed to parallel the love act from foreplay through orgasm.

---

[1] See, for example, beauty experts Oleda Baker and Bill Gale, *Twenty-Nine Forever* (New York: Berkley Publishing Group, 1977).

[2] See, for example, the currently popular work of Dr. Irene Kassorla in *Nice Girls Do* (New York: Stratford Press, 1980) and materials on the sexual enhancement seminars of researchers Alan Brauer and his wife, Donna Brauer, in Richard Rhodes, "The Age of the 30-Minute Orgasm," *Playboy*, 29:8 (August 1982), 130, 180–186. Both Kassorla and the Brauers recommend extensive stimulation prior to or instead of intromission and thorough satisfaction of the female partner first, since women in general have a much more difficult time talking themselves through foreplay to orgasm and especially to extended orgasm.

[3] Alice Kahn Ladas, Beverly Whipple, John D. Perry, *The G Spot and Other Recent Discoveries About Human Sexuality* (New York: Dell, 1983).

[4] William H. Masters and Virginia E. Johnson, *Human Sexual Response*, pp. 82–88, 182–188.

[5] Our discussion of physiologic changes during sexual arousal is based on that of William H. Masters and Virginia E. Johnson, *Human Sexual Response* (Toronto, New York, and London: Bantam, 1980); and James Leslie McCary, *Human Sexuality* (New York: Van Nostrand Reinhold Co., 1967).

[6] Our discussion of the isometric benefits of orgasm was inspired by that of Oleda Baker and Bill Gale, *Twenty-Nine Forever* (New York: Berkeley Publishing Group, 1977); rpt. in "The Beauty Orgasm," *Cosmopolitan* (special beauty edition, Summer, 1979) pp. 74–79. For a definitive description of myotonic response during the four phases of sexual activity, see Masters and Johnson, *Human Sexual Response*, pp. 291–297.

[7] James Leslie McCary, *Human Sexuality* (New York: Van Nostrand Reinhold Co., 1967), pp. 177, 182.

[8] Durk Pearson and Sandy Shaw, *Life Extension: A Practical Scientific Approach* (New York: Warner Books, 1983), pp. 654–655.

[9] Jane Brody, *Jane Brody's Guide to Personal Health* (New York: Avon, 1983), pp. 606–607.

[10] Quoted in Frank S. Caprio and Joseph R. Berger, *Helping Yourself with Self-Hypnosis* (Englewood Cliffs, N.J.: Prentice-Hall, Inc., 1963), p. 98.

[11] Jim Lytle, "A Loving Look at Bad (and Good) Hugs," *New Woman* (14, 5, May 1984), pp. 110–111.

[12] Joyce Brothers, *Better Than Ever* (New York: Simon and Schuster, 1975), pp. 143–144.

Step Five:

Cleansing, Moisturizing, and Makeup

For most women, applying makeup is the most enjoyable part of any skin care regime, because through makeup a woman can give herself a new face every day. But first, her skin has to be clean and moist so that her makeup can enhance her natural beauty instead of simply camouflaging her problems. In this chapter we outline a basic cleansing and moisturizing routine, and share makeup advice from makeup artist Roland Patino, whose work has appeared in *Town & Country* and whose ideas have been an inspiration to us.

Skin Deep

Knowing your skin type is the first step in solving any skin problems. It's easy to figure out what type you are. Simply wash your face, and look into the mirror. Try to identify the spots on your face that are dry, flaky, and red, and the spots that are oily and blemished. Now with clean hands, run your ring finger gently over your face. Feel the oily areas; feel the dry areas. If you are like most people you have a combination skin, and you can literally draw a T denoting the demarcation of dry and oily places which live together on the same face. The idea is to get them to live in harmony and peace. The oily area will extend across your forehead and down your nose to your chin; the rest of your face will feel much drier than this area, which we will refer to from here on as the T spot.

Cleanliness Is Next to Godliness

God created man in His image, and that image is covered with skin. A clean face is a must for good skin care, because your skin is the foundation for everything you put on your face. Just as a painter begins on a clean canvas, so you must begin on a clean skin.

We're all familiar with the barrage of gimmicky ways to clean the face. Use water; don't use water; use soap; don't use soap; use creams; don't use creams; and so on. Well, after seven years of research, we would like to report that a mild soap and tepid water are still the best cleansers around for almost everyone.

There is a right way to wash your face. First, splash your face with tepid water. Then lather your hands with a mild pure soap and work the soap into the skin, gently massaging the face in a counterclockwise motion. Work the soap upward and outward into the hairline. Splash your face twenty times with clean, tepid water to remove both dirt and excess soap; thorough rinsing is the key to a clean face. Be gentle under your eyes, as the skin there is paper-thin and easily damaged.

There are many safe soaps available. Look for soaps without deodorants or extra ingredients. Two good examples are castile soap and Neutrogena. Don't use glycerine soaps or creams; they contain humectants which take moisture right out of the skin.

We know that you've always heard that people with dry skin should never use soap. However, it isn't the soap that is responsible for either creating a dry skin condition or maintaining it. The soap remains on your face for a matter of seconds; if you rinse it properly, it won't be on your face long enough to dry it out. After washing, you will moisturize, which will eliminate dry-skin problems.

Don't Forget Your Eyes

After a long day, your eyes need some special attention. To remove your eye makeup before bed, dip a small cotton swab in a gentle, nongreasy eye-makeup remover. Don't use a tissue; it is made from wood pulp and could irritate the tender skin around your eyes. To clean your lashes, hold a tissue under them and use a cotton swab dipped in eye-makeup remover to gently dab off your mascara. After cleaning your lids and lashes, moisturize around your eyes to restore the sensitive tissue.

Exfoliation

Once a week you should exfoliate your skin while you are cleansing it. Exfoliation is simply gentle rubbing of the skin with a mild abrasive to slough off the old dead skin cells on the surface, making room for the healthy new cells that are regenerating under the surface. Exfoliation will remove scaly, flaky patches and leave your face feeling softer and smoother.

You can remove dead skin with a washcloth or with the slightly harsher Buf-Puf, depending on how sensitive your skin is. The Buf-Puf has a mildly abrasive texture and should be used with a light touch. Avoid exfoliating the skin around the eyes, as it is very sensitive and does not recover well. Be sure to rehydrate your skin afterwards by splashing water on it no less than twenty times, and don't forget to moisturize.

Funny Face

Once a month, use a masque to add a little zip to your complexion. Masques stimulate your circulation, remove dead skin cells, and firm up your skin. There are two main types of masques: clay and gel. Gels are usually prescribed for dry skin and clays for oily skin. Most of us, however, have both oily and dry areas on our faces—the oily "T" and the outlying dry areas—so we have to use both. Apply a clay masque to the oily areas on your face, and a gel masque to the drier spots. If your skin is basically dry, use a gel masque alone; if it's truly oily all over (which is unusual except in teenagers), use a clay masque. And just as with the Buf-Puf, you must protect the thin and sensitive skin under your eyes. Leave moisturizer around your eyes and be careful to keep the masque away from this tender area. On this day don't exfoliate—the masque is enough.

Now for a Word about Toners

Toners and astringents, if applied, should be used now, after cleansing and exfoliating, and before moisturizing. They contain alcohol and can be irritating to the skin. If the skin is dry or sensitive, they can cause pimples and rashes. So we recommend you use only mild toners and astringents on very oily surfaces (your T spot), if at all.

Facial Fallacy

Though we hate to spark negativism and controversy, we feel it is our obligation to speak up against the facial. Through our investigations we have found that not only do facials not achieve the benefits claimed for them, but they may also create wrinkles and stimulate the oil glands to cause breakouts. The less your face is handled the better, for moving the skin around can only disturb and destroy the sensitive network beneath. Actors and actresses who, because of their profession, must put on and take off makeup more often than normal, are also earlier candidates for face lifts. And once they come under a doctor's supervision, he will advise them not to have facials ever again. Another problem with facials is that blemishes are often disturbed or squeezed ineptly, and many is the horror tale of resultant infection and scarring. And if you believe facials can make your pores smaller, forget it. The idea that you can make your pores bigger or smaller is a fallacy. The only things you can actually do to your pores are clog them or cause them to scar. So, please, hands off!

Beauty Benefits

Three new products in our age of minor miracles are collagen, Product 15, and amino acids. We've found that all three will achieve good results when integrated into a sensible skin care program. Use these products on your wrinkle-prone areas and make them a part of your daily routine.

Collagen, often referred to by the trade name Zyderm collagen, contains purified bovine collagen in lidocaine and saline solution. When injected, it penetrates the skin and fills out the wrinkles. Although not all dermatologists agree, it is our opinion that collagen will also pump up the skin when applied topically.

Topical application is simple: just smooth soluble collagen onto your damp face and apply a moisturizer on top, to seal it in. It plumps up the tissue, and some doctors believe that it increases your own production of collagen. In our opinion, collagen is the best wrinkle cream you can buy. We have achieved especially good results with the La Prairie products, which contain a highly refined European collagen that penetrates the skin better than the other brands we have tried.

Injected Zyderm collagen fills out the wrinkles and keeps them smooth for approximately two years, more or less, depending on the individual (see chapter entitled "Alternate Measures"). If you opt for collagen injections, you must establish a regular maintenance program, just as you do for dyeing your hair or going to the dentist.

Product 15 is a true moisturizer discovered by several dermatologists in Florida. Applied topically, it penetrates the skin. There it draws moisture from beneath the skin and pushes it up 'and out, keeping wrinkles from forming. One brand is called Complex 15, available in many drug stores. It is a good choice for your daily moisturizer.

A process discovered in Japan involves applying amino acids to the skin's surface in the form of a cream. Amino acids are the building blocks of protein which, as you recall from Step 1, is the major structural component of all our cells. The amino acids are supposed to permeate the skin's surface, protect, and soften it, and to some extent repair wrinkles. Amino acids are found in many of the more expensive moisturizers and wrinkle creams today, including La Prairie.

Treat Your Skin from Within

Now you're ready to moisturize. But the first step in moisturizing your skin is something you should do all day long—drink plenty of water. We seldom stop to think that sixty-five percent of the body is water, that for nine months we lived and swam in amniotic fluid, or that man's ancestors originally came from the sea. Furthermore, the skin plays an important role in the elimination of fluid from the body, and its supply of moisture must therefore be constantly replenished. You should drink a minimum of six to eight glasses of water throughout the day to replace the constant loss of water from perspiration and elimination.

Lock Moisture In

From time immemorial, women have been aware of the need for moisturizers, and even in the Bible we read accounts of nomadic women covering their faces and bodies with olive oil to protect themselves from the hot desert sun. Just as a dry piece of leather or a prune or raisin is revitalized when soaked in moisture, so is the skin revitalized when it is kept moist. Today we know that a moisturizer will not put moisture back into the skin, but what it *will* do is lock in what moisture there is on the skin's surface. As a result, the skin beneath the moisturizer will stay soft and supple. Fewer wrinkles will develop, and those that do appear will not become dry and etched.

Until you are about thirty, you really don't need to moisturize your skin because your sebaceous glands are making enough oil to do the trick by themselves.

Of course you may be the exception to the rule. If you have drier-than-average skin early on, then by all means moisturize when you need to. Observe your skin carefully and respond to its needs. Moisturizing on top of your skin's own built-in moisturizer can cause pores to clog.

However, for most women thirty-five or over, moisturizing is a must. For best results, dampen your face and put a collagen cream on the wrinkle-prone areas (we recommend the La Prairie wrinkle cream containing collagen). Then apply a moisturizer. The collagen cream will plump up the wrinkles, and the moisturizer will seal the collagen and moisture into your skin. Be sure to purchase a moisturizer that will seal but not clog your pores—for most women, a light, greaseless product is best, one that doesn't feel sticky on your skin.

In summer, your skin may dry out from the sun, so be sure to moisturize the dry areas, and when you return from water sports, remember to reapply moisturizer to replace your skin's natural moisturizing protection. In the summertime, people with oily skin should use a lighter moisturizer because perspiration will keep the skin moist and may encourage breaking out. If vacation plans find you in an airplane, moisturize and drink lots of water because the air in the pressurized cabin is dry. In winter, thorough moisturizing may also be necessary, because the dry cold air outside combined with the dry, hot air in heated buildings will conspire to sap moisture from your skin.

A word of caution about hormone creams: Premenopausal women should not use them and postmenopausal women should be aware of the slight risk of skin cancer involved in using them. Though hormone creams do fill out your wrinkles, the effect is dependent upon their continual usage because the skin actually becomes addicted to the creams. Collagen creams are a better way to erase the wrinkles of women in early menopause, and collagen injections can be used in the later stages, if you like.

Remember always to moisturize in the morning, before putting on any makeup, to keep your skin soft and smooth; reapply moisturizer on trouble spots during the day, and always apply moisturizer at night. A sleeping body often rolls on its face, and as long as that face is moist, it will recover uncreased. And a final word of advice—if you sleep on a satin pillowcase, you'll wake up smooth!

FACE CARE

Now that we've gone over the basics, here's a simple program for keeping your skin clean, moist, and glowing.

NORMAL SKIN

Morning:
Wash your skin with a mild soap such as castile or Neutrogena. Rinse twenty times with tepid water. Keeping the face damp, apply a wrinkle cream such as La Prairie under the eyes and on wrinkle-prone areas. Put a moisturizer on top of wrinkle cream and dry areas with an up and out motion toward the hairline.

Night:
Remove your makeup with a gentle cream. Then wash and rinse as in the morning. Reapply wrinkle cream and moisturizer on dry spots (especially around the eyes).

Once a Week:
One night a week, exfoliate gently with a Buf-Puf and rinse twenty times with tepid water. Apply wrinkle cream and moisturizer as before.

Once a Month:
Use a facial masque (once again, we recommend the La Prairie products), applying a clay masque to oily areas and a gel to dry spots. Follow directions for the product you are using. Don't exfoliate the same day.

OILY SKIN

Morning:
Wash with a mild soap and rinse twenty times with tepid water. Apply a toner with a cotton swab to oily areas on your face (but not around the eyes). Rinse again and apply a moisturizer to dry spots, if necessary, working it up and out into the hairline (especially around the eyes).

Late Afternoon:
Remove all makeup from your face. Wash and rinse as in the morning. Reapply moisturizer and makeup to damp face.

Night:
Remove makeup with a light cream. Wash, rinse in tepid water, and moisturize as in the morning.

Once a Week:
One night a week, exfoliate gently with a Buf-Puf and rinse twenty times with tepid water. Keeping your face damp, apply moisturizer on dry spots (especially

around the eyes). If you have acne, see your doctor and use a prescriptive soap, lotion and acne treatment.

Once a Month:
Use a facial masque (we recommend the La Prairie brand), applying a clay masque to oily areas and a gel to dry spots. Follow directions for the product you are using. Don't exfoliate the same day.

DRY SKIN

Morning:
Wash your face with a mild soap such as castile or Neutrogena. Rinse twenty times with tepid water. Keeping your face damp, apply a wrinkle cream such as La Prairie to the dry areas of your dampened face. Next, moisturize over dry areas (especially around the eyes).

Night:
Remove makeup with a light cream. Wash, rinse in tepid water and moisturize as in the morning.

Once a Week:
One night a week, wash your face gently with a washcloth and rinse twenty times in tepid water. Apply a wrinkle cream and moisturizer (we recommend the La Prairie products) on dry areas over a damp face (especially around the eyes).

Once a Month:
Use a gel facial masque (we recommend the La Prairie products), following directions for the product you are using. Don't exfoliate the same day.

ALLERGIC SKIN

People with allergic skin should use hypo-allergenic products. However, they may be allergic even to those, because although hypo-allergenic products have few irritants, they are not entirely irritant free.

Tools of the Trade

Now for the fun part: makeup. Before you begin, gather together the necessary tools. You'll need three sponges, or one sponge cut into three sections, and five brushes: a powder brush, a blush brush, an eye brush, an eyeliner brush, and a lip brush. Our makeup artist, Roland Patino, recommends sable-tipped brushes for proper contouring and blending.

Keep It Clean

Begin with a clean face, clean hands, clean tools, and clean makeup. Makeup tools should be washed, dried, and stored in a clean, dry spot after each use, and makeup should be bought in small quantities, so that it can be discarded every six months or so. Cosmetics are a great home for uninvited bacterial guests to grow and flourish. Old, contaminated makeup can cause irritation, rashes, pimples, and infections to both the eyes and the skin.

A Word to the Wise

Do not make your own cosmetics, for the success or failure of any recipe is only as good as the skill of the chef. With too many variables and too few controls, the reward is not worth the risk.

However, there are certain things to look for when purchasing your makeup. Buy makeup from a reputable cosmetics firm that has been in business for a while; these companies are likely to have strict controls on production. Unless you have very dry skin, always use a makeup with a water base, which is easily removed and will not clog your pores. If you like to use powder, dust it on very lightly, as powder tends to fill in the lines and make wrinkles look more pronounced. Creams and gels are great because they are moist and give a dewy, youthful look to your makeup.

Makeup Workshop

Now the fun begins! As master makeup artist Roland Patino says, "Makeup is an art, and your face is a canvas." Although your bone structure places a few minor restrictions on your efforts, your face is essentially a blank slate to be drawn on as the spirit moves you. Approach your makeup in a spirit of creativity, and you'll discover a thousand different ways of bringing out your best. *You* are in control.

Follow the instructions accompanying the illustrations for tips on proper application.

Okay, Let's Play

After applying your moisturizer, allow your face to rest and set for approximately two minutes. Then apply a cover foundation or cover stick over your entire face to even out the skin's tones and trouble spots. The cover should be lighter than your makeup so that it won't interfere with the next step, highlighting.

Step 1: Conceal Imperfections and Even Out Skin Tone

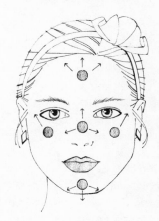

Dot a dab of coverbase on your forehead and blend it into your hairline. Dot a dab of coverbase on the right and left cheeks and, with up and out movements, blend it into the hairline over each ear. Put a dab of coverbase in the middle of your nose; blend half of it up into the forehead and the other half over the bridge of the nose and into the cheeks. Smooth a dot of coverbase on the chin down and out into the jawline and neck.

Step 2: Cover Dark Rings and Flaws

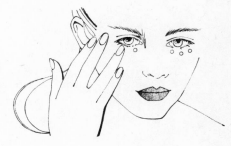

If you have dark circles, use a tiny amount of coverup under the eyes, applying it gently with your ring finger. Coverup will also diminish, if not totally cover, freckles, hives, blotchy skin and acne.

Step 3: Apply Foundation

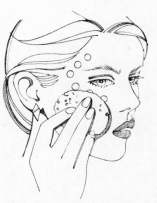

Always apply liquid foundation with a light touch. Put three dots of makeup base on each temple. Blend up and into the hairline on both right and left sides, using your fingertips and a sponge. Next apply three dots on top of each cheekbone, blending on each side across and up into your hairline. Go lightly under your eyes. Add two dots on your cheekbones, blending down your jawbone to your throat. It is important to have the same color tone from your jawline to your neck. Use as little makeup as possible under the eyes to keep tiny wrinkle lines from looking more pronounced. Now blend all over once more for a flawless finish.

Foundation Information!

Always use a water-base foundation, especially if you have oily skin, acne, or blocked pores. People with dry skin can use an oil-base foundation but if you do, be sure to clean your face well and remove all your makeup at the end of the day. Test it for color by putting it on your neck. If your skin tone leans toward pink, you should use a beige foundation, but if your skin tone is yellow, go forward with pink. If you have a suntan, don't use any foundation, but simply wear a colored gel. This will add a dewy, smooth look to your complexion.

Light and Dark

When you want to sculpt your face to achieve a particular effect, you can use highlighting on top of your makeup to achieve spectacular results. Highlighting is simply the use of makeup in lighter and darker shades. Use a water-base foundation two shades lighter than your normal color to strategically lighten the areas of your face that you wish to enhance, such as your cheekbones, and a darker shade to diminish and hide areas such as full cheeks or an enlarged nose. Light foundation will also diminish, if not totally cover, freckles, hives blotchy skin, and acne. Highlighting is the key to bringing out the beauty hidden in your face.

The first step is to camouflage the areas of your face that you are not happy with by erasing them with a darker shade of foundation. For example, you can hollow out puffy cheeks or make a wide nose look narrow. The second stage of highlighting is building the face. Do you want higher cheekbones, a larger forehead, a more pronounced chin or a different shape to your face? Well, you can have what you want by applying a light foundation on those areas to accentuate them. You can create the effect of a completely new face.

Day and Night

Day and night makeup are as different as day and night. Except for your foundation, which should be lighter at night, a general rule is "lighter during the day and darker at night." If you work in an office which uses artificial light, you must meet the problem halfway. And on the subject of office lighting, fluorescent light in particular is believed by some researchers to cause skin cancer,[1] and you should therefore protect yourself from its rays just as you would from the sun, so day or night in fluorescent light, use a sunblock.

For California Girls

If you have a suntan, don't wear makeup, but use a little blush gel. Never put dark on anything that is already dark; it will only look muddy. If your skin is tan, and therefore dried, a moist gel will add a little moisture and glow. All colors should be brighter, including lipstick, blush, and shadow, because your face must be treated as tan, and not normal. Change your colors to match the change in your complexion.

Eye Makeup

Eye makeup is next, and since eyes have long been considered a woman's greatest attraction, this is a very significant step. It's also the most fun! First you must honestly appraise the shape of your eyes: Are they big, little, almond-shaped, round? And so on. Then you will be able to dramatize the areas you want, as you create your eyes. The eye-clinic chart will help you contour your eyes correctly.

Here's a handy makeup tip: to correct eye makeup mistakes, dip a cotton swab in moisturizer and gently remove the excess makeup.

Step 4: Apply Eye Shadow

Apply your eye-shadow undercoat on clean eyelids. Use a neutral shade, from the top of the brow to the bottom of the lid. Next, put on shadow. Apply to the middle of the eyelid, stroking it outward a thin layer at a time to control the intensity of the color. *(continued on page 142.)*

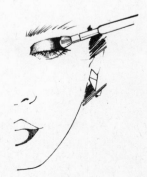

Eye Clinic

This chart will help you contour your eyes to correct any flaws that they may have, and to show them off to best advantage.

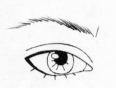
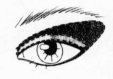

NORMAL EYES
· Put a lighter shade on the inner half of the lid.
· Blend in a deeper tone of the same color on the outer half of the lid. Put an even deeper tone in the eyelid crease, bringing the color to the outer edge of the brow down into the corner of the eye. Blend.
· Add mascara to the bottom halves of the upper and lower lids and smudge a bit of dark shadow or eye pencil under the mascara.

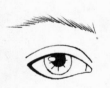
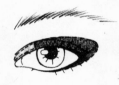

CLOSELY SPACED EYES
· Apply brighter eye shadow on the inner third and darker color on the outer two thirds of your eyelid.
· Blend color out beyond the outer corners of eyes.
· Use an eye pencil in a deeper shade around the outer half of the lashes on top and on bottom. Smudge for an even, finished look.
· Use mascara on the outer half of top and bottom lashes.

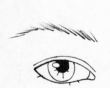
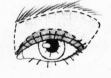

LITTLE EYES, LITTLE LIDS
· Apply light shadow from lid to brow bone.
· Apply a darker color, in the shape of an arch, from the lid crease down to lashes. Blend.
· Curl lashes.
· Use mascara on lash tips.

WIDELY SPACED EYES
· Apply shadow to the inner third of lids.
· Add an arc of a deeper-colored shadow from the inner corner of your eyes to the sides of your nose, ending beneath the large part of the eyebrow.

- Put a lighter shade of the same color or a complementary shadow on the outer two-thirds of the eye from the eyelash up to the brow bone. Blend.
- Use mascara on full top and bottom lid, stressing the center by applying most heavily there.
- Line the full eyelid, both top and bottom, with a dark shade of pencil and smudge.

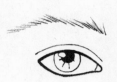
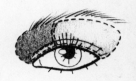

BIG EYES WITH BIG LIDS
- Shadow lids with a smokey shadow.
- Apply three tones of the same color shadow in three vertical lines. Put the medium shade on the inner lid, the darkest shade on the outer lid up to the browbone, and the lightest shade in the middle third of the lid. Blend together.
- Line eyes with a deep shade of eye pencil—for example, smokey gray—from the middle third of the lid out, drawing your line as close as possible to the lash-line. Underline the outer one third of the lower lid with the same-color red pencil and smudge to blend, once again keeping as close as possible to the lash-line.

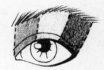

EYE COLOR TIPS
- Stay in shades of one color, adding darker and lighter tones where needed. Smokey grays, browns, and plums are good on most eyes.
- Use lightest shades on lid centers for contour, deeper shades on the sides of the eyes.
- As with your foundation makeup, use a light shade to highlight a feature, a dark shade to disguise it.

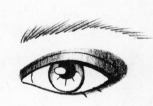

TIPS FOR GORGEOUS EVENING EYES
- Use richly colored eyeshadow at night.
- If you're feeling festive, you might try iridescents or colors that mirror other colors, but avoid using frosted eyeshadows because they accentuate lines and creases that can make the eyes look swollen.

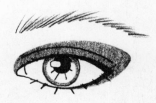

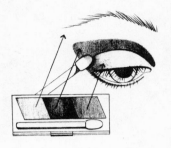

Step 5: Contour Eyes

Create the shape you want with darker and lighter shades of the same basic color of shadow. Contour your eyes to compensate for any problems they may have (see Eye-Care Clinic on page *000*.)

Step 6: Highlight Browbone

Use a lighter shade of shadow under the brow down to the crease.

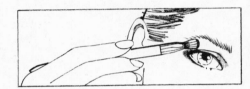

Step 7: Highlight your Eyes

Add a touch of golden brown shadow in the corner of each eye and blend into the rouge on the cheek.

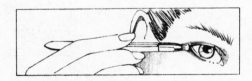

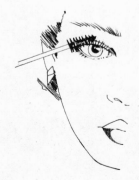

Step 8: Apply Mascara

Mascara the top side and bottom side of the upper lashes, then tip the bottom lashes. Allow to dry, separate lashes with a lash brush, and apply mascara a second time.

Step 9: Apply Eyeliner

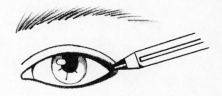

Choose an eyeliner in the same family of colors as your eye shadow—just a shade or two darker. Use an eyeliner pencil for a natural look. Draw the line and then smudge to blend.

Eyebrows

After your eyes, work on your eyebrows. It is important to keep their shape and color natural and soft, but here again you are not limited by nature and can change your entire look by shortening or lengthening your eyebrows. They may need tweezing and reshaping to open up the eye, so keep up with their maintenance, for if your eyebrows are correct, everything else will fall into balance. Always use a soft pencil and draw the eyebrow in the brow with very fine outward strokes beginning in the chair (the thickest part) of the eyebrow itself. For an even softer look, use a soft brush and dab it into a powdered color. Use the center of your eye as your guide when drawing an eyebrow. This is where the arch should be, and from that point you will want to extend the line out toward your temple about half an inch.

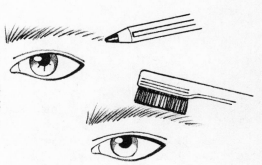

Step 10: Shape and Color Eyebrows

A feather eyebrow is best achieved by filling it in with a pale blonde pencil and then going over it lightly with a smokey-colored eyebrow powder.

Rouge

The next step is rouge. Today you can choose from powders, gels, or creams. Whichever you use, we suggest that in daytime hours you choose a lighter color, and apply the rouge in the shape of an apple on your cheeks and temples. At night, the blush should be darker, to compensate for the artificial light, and applied in the shape of a diagonal on the sides of the cheeks, moving up to the temples, around the face, and down to the tip of your chin. This will give you balanced color all around your face. But remember to use a light touch when applying this and all other cosmetics, so that you don't gild the lily!

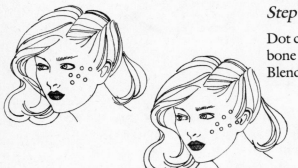

Step 11: Apply Rouge

Dot creme or gel rouge on the apple of the cheekbone for daytime and in the form of a V for night. Blend with a makeup sponge.

or Powdered Blush

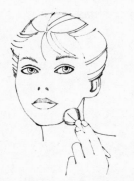

If you're using powdered blush, brush it on in the shape of an apple for daytime, in a V for night, as described above. Add a small amount of blush under the chin and blend to the bone and across the rim of the jaw. This will shadow a double chin.

Lipstick

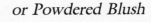

The final touch is your lipstick. Start by outlining your lips with a lip-lining pencil, the tool that allows you the freedom of wearing a different smile. You may want full fashionable lips, small pouty lips, etc., depending on your mood, your dress, or the occasion. Don't be heavy-handed; use a pencil that is close in color to your lipstick—one shade darker is best—or a brown pencil, which works with everything. When outlining your lips, refrain from making a definite line, but rather mark a colored area which will prevent your lipstick from bleeding out. Put a lighter shade of lipstick in the center area of your mouth, and a darker shade on the perimeter. This contouring will make your lips appear extra sexy and luscious. Top it off with a colorless gloss for a perfectly polished you.

    If you are a smoker, the chances are that you have hatch marks on your upper lip. The wax lip pencil will help to fill in those spaces and to some extent cover them. The pencil stains the lips so that their color lasts long after your lipstick is gone. The lip pencil also prevents your lipstick from bleeding into your hatchmarks, creating ugly lines.

Step 12: Apply Lipliner

Use a lipliner pencil one shade darker than your lipstick to define lips and to prevent color from bleeding. Use short, firm strokes and don't make a definite line, but rather a colored area.

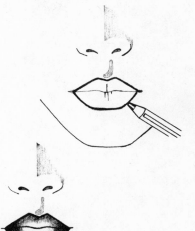

Step 13: Apply Lipstick

Use a darker shade on the perimeter of your mouth and a lighter shade in the center for softer, fuller, more attractive lips.

Roland Patino Answers Questions Frequently Asked:

Q. What color makeup should I wear?
A. Select your foundation by matching it to the color of your neck, not to the back of your hand which is often three shades lighter. Always choose a water-base makeup.

Q. Should I use a liquid foundation, a press-powder foundation, or a cake foundation?
A. Liquid foundation is best. It provides a natural sheen, whereas cake or press powders build up and press into facial creases, making them more noticeable.

Q. What makeup is best for women under forty?
A. Less is best. Always look your age; don't try to look younger than you are.

Q. What makeup is best for women over fifty?
A. Stay current! Don't date yourself with the makeup fashions of a time past when you felt you looked your best. Stay with a natural-finish liquid makeup, and use a natural cream rouge. Also, try to be objective and see yourself as others see you. Adjust to your time in life, and create the look that's best for your age. Put moisturizer on wrinkles to keep them soft and use a light hand when applying makeup to these areas, so it won't settle into the facial creases and accentuate them.

Q. How can I determine what my coloring is so that I can pick the proper eye shadow?

A. Here you have two considerations: your skin tone and the color of your eyes. These will determine the eye-shadow colors that you can wear. For example, let's imagine that you have blue eyes. We don't want to apply blue eye shadow to blue eyes; we want to complement those baby blues, whereas blue shadow will cause them to fade away. Instead, use a color in the brown family, such as violet, mauve, or rose. If your eyes are green, once again, don't use green eye shadow, but rather anything in the bronze or metallic colors, as well as gray, violet, mauve, etc. Brown eyes are truly blessed because they can wear any color, including brown, according to their skin tones. And that brings us to the second determinant of eye-shadow color—skin tone. Not everyone can wear roses, peaches, etc. Be sure your eye shadow does not clash with the rest of you—skin, hair, makeup. It takes some time to figure out what colors are most flattering on you. You can go to a color specialist to find out what your coloring is, or you can read books on this subject, and you can easily purchase a color chart. Through observation, select the color that best suits you.

A Final Word

The whole philosophy of the Figure-8 program is to enhance your natural assets to the fullest, because you deserve to be the best you can be. Makeup is a valuable means of achieving this goal.

STEP 5: CLEANSING, MOISTURIZING, AND MAKEUP

Check the things you currently do, and make a note to incorporate anything you've neglected into your routine.

Each Morning:

Clean your face, using a mild soap and tepid water. Rinse twenty times.

Use eye cream.

Add a collagen cream such as La Prairie where and when you need it.

Put on moisturizer.

Apply makeup (experiment, have fun).

Clean your makeup tools.

Each Evening:
Clean your face.
Remove eye makeup.
Apply eye cream.
Use a collagen cream where and when you need it.
Put on moisturizer.

Weekly:
Maintain eyebrows—tweeze where necessary.
Exfoliate.

Monthly:
Make sure that your makeup is clean.
Use a facial masque—be careful of the skin around your eyes. Don't exfoliate on the day you use a masque.

To Apply Makeup:
Step 1: Conceal imperfections and even out skin tone
Step 2: Cover dark rings and flaws
Step 3: Apply foundation. Highlight, if desired.
Step 4: Apply eye shadow
Step 5: Contour eyes
Step 6: Highlight browbone
Step 7: Highlight eyes
Step 8: Apply mascara
Step 9: Apply eyeliner
Step 10: Shape and color eyebrows
Step 11: Apply rouge or powdered blush
Step 12: Apply lipliner
Step 13: Apply lipstick

---

[1] Sandy Rovner, "Health Talk: Run From the Sun," *Washington Post* (May 6, 1983), B5a.

Step Six:
Environmental Protection

*"Mirror, mirror on the wall,
Who's the fairest of them all?"*

Everybody knows the answer was "Snow White." Trust us, she didn't stay snow white by accident! Snow White didn't go out in the sun and abuse her skin! And we promise you, even after she married her prince and he started taking her to the Riviera in the summer and Aspen in the winter, she wore sun blocks and ski masks. If she hadn't, she'd have had to change her name.

Seriously, damage to the skin from factors in the environment is a chief cause of premature aging. Too much sun in summer and the weather extremes in winter will wrinkle and dry your skin long before your time. Unfortunately, the damage, once done, is considered by most doctors to be irreversible; even a total change of lifestyle may not mitigate it. The good news is that damage to your skin from the environment is largely preventable, since nearly all the possible hazards are under your control. If you take a few simple precautions you can protect your skin from harm, and at the age of fifty, sixty, or even beyond, the mirror on your wall will still tell you that you look more like the princess than the witch.

Learn To Be Sun Sensible

Standards of beauty and physical well-being have changed dramatically in the last half-century or so. Time was when the leisure class sought lily-white complexions. Mammy probably cautioned Scarlett O'Hara not to go out in the sun for fear of her freckling or "looking like a field hand." Ladies of quality throughout the nineteenth century wore long skirts and broad-brimmed hats, and carried parasols, a word which literally means "for the sun."[1] Only farm laborers, sailors, and other people forced to work out of doors had sun-darkened skins.

In the first twenty or so years of our own century, genteel ladies continued to be covered and demure; the cameo complexion was still prized, and bathing beauties at the beach covered practically every inch of skin with bathing costumes guaranteed to drag a swimmer down even without an undertow. Even among black women, a pale complexion was considered a sign of refinement.

But a white skin was no longer limited to the leisure class; the Industrial Revolution had moved many common workers off the farms and into factories where they lost their tans from lack of exposure to the sun.

Then, legend has it that sometime after World War I, the famous designer Coco Chanel came back from a summer cruise sporting a tan, and *voilà!* Tans immediately became fashionable with the French and anyone else who followed French trends.[2] By the 1920s the German nobility had adopted the custom of regular sunbathing. And soon in America, changing mores about how much skin one could appropriately show in public, the rise of a larger leisure class, the advent of airplane travel (so one could jet to tropical climes in winter), and the development of the coasts of California and Florida as vacation areas contributed to a new attitude toward tanning. If you looked like the California girl, it meant you had the leisure to pamper yourself. Hence, a tan became associated with the upper class.

Houston psychiatrist Dr. Milton Altschuler suggests that there also developed, during the latter part of the nineteenth century and the early part of the twentieth century, a mystique linking tanning with good health. Tuberculosis was a prevalent disease during that period, particularly in cool, damp climates. Its victims were pale and pasty; they generally were sent to sunnier, drier climates to effect cures through rest and sun. Actually, it was the rest rather than the sun that brought about the improved health. But those who were cured of TB generally ended up with good tans as well. Thereafter, people began to think of the sun as a life-giving, health-giving entity, and they subjected their bodies to it whenever it was available.

Most of us grew up with the idea that tanned skin was a mark of beauty, class, and good health. It came as a shock about twenty years ago to learn that excessive exposure to sunlight was a chief cause of various skin ailments, including wrinkling, dry skin, and superficial as well as serious cancers. Because the cultural bias toward tanning is so compelling, some people steadfastly refuse to pay attention to warnings and continue compulsively tanning their skins. But Dr. Altschuler cautions that suntans and sunburns are one and the same thing—burns of the skin.

BEAUTIFUL SKIN

A tan is the body's reaction to mild injury; extra amounts of *melanin*, the chemical that gives the skin its tan color, are secreted as a result of injury to those cells which produce skin pigment. Whether you tan or burn, those cells have been injured; either burning or tanning can lead to permanent drying of the skin, loss of elasticity, and cancerous lesions.

Houston dermatologist Dr. Roy Knowles explained to us just how the skin reacts when the sun does its destructive work. The epidermis and dermis fit together like the fingers of two hands interlaced; fingerlike projections from the dermis contain elastic tissue that come close to the outer skin's external surface are vulnerable to ultraviolet rays penetrating through the outer layers of the epidermis. In areas where the epidermis is thin, as it is on the face, there is less protection for the elastic tissue of the dermis, and as exposure gradually changes their chemistry, they become fragmented. Eventually the skin wrinkles because of a lack of elasticity.

If you have repeatedly exposed the skin on your face to burning or tanning, compare it for a moment to the skin on a part of the body that is less often exposed, such as the underside of the breasts or on the buttocks. You'll clearly see the difference; the unexposed skin is softer, smoother, more even in color. It's truly unfortunate that facial skin not only is more often exposed to the elements but is also thinner and therefore more vulnerable to damage.

Dr. Knowles says that if you were to stay indoors from the age of five and never expose yourself to the hazards of the sun, at forty-five you'd have the skin of a five-year-old. A person who limits her exposure to the sun all her life will tend to retain smooth facial tissue for years and even decades longer than those who continue to expose themselves.

One common reaction of the skin to injury from sun exposure is freckling. The sun's rays also cause expansion of the capillaries in the inner layers of the skin. This is what gives you the hot, red look of a sunburn. Repeated sunburns can contribute to the condition known as *rosacea*, permanent dilatation of the blood vessels. Excessive heat can cause broken blood vessels and spider veins.

Other cumulative damage can include irreversible pigmentation or mottling of the skin; cell buildup, creating a thickened, leathery look; and seborrhea keratoses, those brownish, warty growths associated with aging. These occurrences are especially common in people who work or play out of doors—farmers, sailors, or men and women who pursue year-round outdoor sports. The bad thing about cumulative damage is that it may take fifteen to twenty years before you start paying the consequences, but if you're tanning at all, you need to realize you're doing damage.

Sun exposure can also exacerbate skin conditions like herpes, and can bring on allergic reactions, especially in people who are taking diuretics, tetracycline antibiotics, sulfa drugs, and some kinds of hypertension medications. Oral contraceptives plus sun exposure may trigger brown, blotchy pigmentation. Some sensitive people may develop photodermatitis from sun exposure combined with the use of certain colognes, perfumes, deodorants, or soaps.

Yet another danger is damage to the body's immune system. Recent experiments with laboratory animals indicated that excessive exposure to the sun's rays caused alteration in their immune responses. Hence, too much sun exposure may make you susceptible to other diseases besides those of the skin.[3]

Houston pathologist Dr. Doyle Rogers says that his personal observation of thousands of skin-tissue biopsies, correlated with the people they came from, convinced him of the damaging effects of the sun. The sun's ultraviolet rays fray the collagen fibers and fragment the elastic tissues in the dermis, making the tissue lose its tautness and "give," like overstretched elastic. Dr. Rogers notes that because of differences in their hormonal makeup, women tend to get increased pigmentation, splotches, wrinkles, and droopy skin from sun exposure, whereas, statistically, men tend more often to get skin cancers. Of course, women do get cancer and men do wrinkle, so hormones are only a part of the picture. Dr. Rogers cautions all people, men and women, adults and teenagers, to wear hats and protect themselves when going out into the sun. And don't forget to cover babies and small children; they burn more easily than older people.

Genetic makeup and ethnic background also play a significant role in one's predisposition to wrinkling and cancer from sun exposure. There are some few people who, even when exposed to the sun, tend not to wrinkle. This tendency must be credited in some degree to their genetic makeup. Fair-skinned blondes and redheads are more susceptible to damage than brunettes. People of Scottish or Irish descent, or of Scandinavian or mid-European stock will tend to wrinkle earlier and to be more prone to skin cancers than those of Mediterranean or Oriental stock. Certain American Indian groups, for example, Cherokee Indians, tend toward fine wrinkling and cross-hatching. Blacks, on the other hand, are least susceptible to both wrinkling and skin cancers.

These differences in susceptibility to sun damage are due to the skin's pigment cells—known as *melanocytes*—which lie at the base of the epidermis. Melanocytes produce melanin, a brown-black granular substance that gives the skin most of its color and which further protects us from sun damage by absorbing energy from ultraviolet light. All ethnic groups have about the same number of melanocytes, but those of fair-skinned people produce smaller amounts of melanin, made up of small individual granules of pigment, while the melanocytes of Blacks produce large amounts of melanin composed of large individual granules. Orientals and brown-skinned races produce intermediate amounts of melanin and, as you might expect, the individual melanin granules are middle-sized.[4] You can pretty much determine your tendency toward developing skin cancers and wrinkling by where you fall in this ethnic continuum.

We should probably say a few words here about skin cancers, since they can be a threat to life. The two most common types are basal and squamous cell carcinomas; these are readily treatable, grow slowly, and together account for less than 0.1 percent of deaths due to cancer, though squamous cell carcinomas do sometimes spread to other organs. Malignant melanomas, on the other hand, though rarer, are the leading cause of death among all diseases which result from skin disorders. (For a more detailed discussion of skin cancers, see chapter entitled "Alternative Measures.") The incidence of skin cancers of all types is up, but the incidence of melanomas has become frighteningly high—up six hundred percent over the last half century. While a predisposition to melanomas is thought to be genetic in origin, most scientists agree that sun exposure, which stimulates the melanocytes to secrete extra melanin as part of the tanning process, can trigger melanoma and is in some degree responsible for this overwhelming increase in malignancies. If you're a beach or snow bunny, work out of doors, or spend most of your recreation time in outdoor activities, you maximize the risk of developing all types of skin cancers.

It was once widely thought that the sun's two kinds of ultraviolet (UV) rays were tolerated differently by the body. The UV-A rays, those longer rays which strike the earth between sunrise and 10:00 A.M. and 4:00 P.M. to sunset, were thought to be "cooler" and less damaging than the shorter UV-B rays that you get between 10:00 A.M. and 4:00 P.M. However, The American Academy of Dermatology, The Skin Cancer Foundation, and virtually every doctor we have interviewed agrees that the long-wave UV-A rays are potentially extremely hazardous, and scientific studies are confirming that UV-A rays may actually contribute to the increased incidence of cancer. So just avoiding the sun at midday isn't enough. You must protect your skin whenever you're outdoors.

If we can't talk you into staying out of the sun altogether, at least you can practice sensible preventive maintenance. Sunscreen products containing para-aminobenzoic acid (PABA) are a real boon to those who want sun fun without its dangers; PABA is primarily protection from UV-B rays, but some products with higher numbered sun protection factors (SPF's) may protect against UV-A rays as well. SPF's are generally numbered from 2 to 15, and there are even a few products with higher SPF's; the higher the number, the greater the protection.

Despite the wide range of SPF's, there are really only four categories of skin type. Type I is very fair skin which never tans and burns easily; if you're a Type I, use a sunscreen in the range of 15 SPF's or above. Type II skin is fair; while it may tan faintly, it usually burns. If you have Type II skin, get a sunscreen with a range of 8 to 15. Skin Types I and II account for about a third of the population;

such people should never even *try* to tan! Type III skin usually tans, though it may still burn; an SPF rating of 6 to 8 is recommended for Type III skin. Lucky people with type IV skin virtually never burn and always tan, so an SPF range of 2 to 6 is usually sufficient for their protection. All types should start with the highest numbered product in their recommended range early in the season. Just remember that tanning causes long-term damage; no matter what your skin type, we feel it's best to avoid tanning and to stick with sunscreen products that carry the higher SPF ratings.

Some products contain benzophenones, which afford protection from UV-A rays. If you can find them, buy sunscreens with broad-spectrum protection. Also note that sunscreens with an alcohol base allow the skin to breathe more readily than cream products.

Read directions carefully; some products need to be reapplied every thirty minutes. And certainly reapply after swimming or exercise. Don't forget to protect the tops of your feet and your neck.

It still is best to avoid the sun during the really hot part of the day, that is, 10:00 A.M. to 4:00 P.M. For additional protection, use a sunblock on lips and perhaps nose (didn't you always want to look like Ray Bolger in *The Wizard of Oz*?). Sun hats with encircling brims protect the back of your neck as well as your face. Sunglasses minimize glare and keep you from squinting, thereby limiting the tendency toward wrinkles and crow's feet around the eyes. And always moisturize, moisturize, moisturize—both inside and out (drink lots of water!)—after you come in from the sunshine.

Weather Watch for Other Hazards

Wind exposure can exacerbate the sun's damage. Snow and sunlight are also worse than sunlight by itself, because snow reflects the light and maximizes its damaging effects. If you ski or spend much time out of doors in winter, wear a ski mask, goggles or sunglasses, and apply a PABA sunscreen to any exposed areas of your body.

Water, too, can contribute to skin damage from sun exposure. All types of water—salt, fresh, or chlorinated—remove oils and natural acids from the skin, and thus make it more prone to burning. Furthermore, sunbathing beside a pool or on the beach gives you a double dose of the sun's rays, which will be reflected off the water and, at the beach, off the sand as well. And you can even burn underwater, so take care not to stay in too long. *Always* reapply the sunscreen after emerging from the water.

While we're on the subject of water, we should note that recently shaved, waxed, or depilated skin can be injured by the water alone, especially chlorinated water. So shave, wax, or depilate a couple of days before you swim. Also, swimmers who sit in wet bathing suits are more susceptible to fungus or yeast infections, especially in the genital area, under the breasts, or in skin folds—anyplace where air can't circulate well. Always change after swimming and dry off well. If you're susceptible to swimmer's ear, always wear ear plugs, and be sure to put alcohol in your ears after swimming.

Pollution is a year-round problem. If pollutants in the air can eat away at marble statues, don't assume your skin is safe. Worst are compounds containing sulfur; these can be partially changed to sulfuric acid on your skin. Then come auto emissions, industrial chemicals, and household cleaners and detergents. To protect yourself from these common hazards, always wear makeup—a good cover foundation creates a thin layer of protection between your skin and the environment—and get into a nightly beauty routine to remove pollutants at the end of every day.

If you go in for hot saunas, hot towels, or extremely hot water, you may be doing damage to your facial skin that is similar to sun damage. Treat your skin, and your face, gently. Avoid extremes of heat and cold. Going from cold outside air to warm inside air in winter can also cause damage, especially in the form of broken capillaries. One way to avoid this situation is to "decompress" your skin immediately upon coming indoors, splash it with cold water, then cool, then warm, to adjust it slowly to the temperature change.

Another problem in wintertime is the lack of moisture, aggravated by your going from dry, cold, outdoor air to dry, artificially heated indoor air. Use a room humidifier to help put needed moisture into the air and lessen the possibility of overdrying your skin. To further minimize drying, take only short showers in winter, and use only warm, rather than hot, water.

No matter what the season or environment, you have to take responsibility for maintaining your skin's health and your body's balance. Too much sun, wind, heat, cold, or water damage can make you old well before your time. Make a commitment to love yourself. Be your own EPA—"environmental protection agent"—and give your magic mirror something to brag about.

STEP 6: ENVIRONMENTAL PROTECTION CHECKLIST

Check the things you currently do. Make note of any things you have been neglecting and add them to your skin-care routine.

1. Wear a sunblock when outdoors, both summer and winter—by itself for sports, under makeup at other times.

2. Protect face and neck with hats in summer and ski masks in winter, when engaged in winter sports. Buy some fancy new ones, if you need a lift.

3. Wear sunglasses or goggles in summer and winter to protect the fragile skin around the eyes. Get a pair that are ultracomfortable and look great—they're worth the investment.

4. Protect nose and lips with ointment whenever you're going to be in the sun, wind, or cold for very long.

5. Use plenty of moisturizer after being outdoors.

6. Drink lots of water after outdoor work or sports.

7. Protect your skin from wind damage with hats, ski masks, etc., as applicable.

8. Replace skin oils lost when swimming by using moisturizers (or natural vegetable oils).

9. Shave, wax, or depilate a day or more in advance of swimming.

10. Never sit in a wet bathing suit if you can help it.

11. Use earplugs and alcohol in ears if you're susceptible to swimmer's ear.

12. Follow a nightly beauty regimen to cleanse pollutants from your skin.

13. Always wear makeup (when not exercising) to protect your skin from pollution.

14. Avoid exposing your skin to extremely hot water, hot towels, or hot saunas.

15. "Decompress" your facial skin when coming indoors from the cold in winter by splashing with cold, then cool, then warm water.

16. Use room humidifiers in winter to avoid dry skin.

17. Take only short showers in winter for the same reason.

---

[1] John A. Parrish, Barbara A. Gilchrest, and Thomas B. Fitzpatrick, *Between You and Me* (Boston and Toronto: Little, Brown and Company, 1978), p. 96.

[2] Helena Rubenstein, *Helena Rubenstein's Book of the Sun* (New York: Times Books, 1979), p. 3.

[3] Sandy Rovner, "Health Talk: Run From the Sun," *Washington Post* (May 6, 1983), B5a.

[4] John A. Parrish, Barbara A. Gilchrest, Thomas B. Fitzpatrick, *Between You and Me* (Boston, Toronto: Little, Brown and Company, 1978), p. 22.

Step Seven:
Rest and Stress Relief

Among the things we often neglect in the hurry-up hustle of modern living are proper rest and relaxation. The two are really not synonymous, and a sufficiency of both are important to a balanced, healthy body and clear, young-looking skin. In this chapter we'll explain why the body needs rest, and why and how to relax on a regular basis. We'll also show how vital are mental and emotional well-being to true physical fitness, and how mind and body, when in balance, keep each other whole and sound.

To Sleep, Perchance To Dream

Sleep is a universal requirement, and for most people, the optimal amount is between seven and eight hours a night. The human body operates on two cycles: the catabolic, during which tissue is torn down and destroyed; and the anabolic, during which tissue is rebuilt and restored. Since the anabolic cycle takes place while the body is at rest, it should be apparent why good sleep is essential for anyone concerned with healthy, clear skin. Insufficient rest doesn't allow time for proper healing and tissue regeneration. We've known people who claimed to get along on anywhere from three to six hours of sleep a night. And indeed, you can probably survive temporarily, without serious effects, on less than seven to eight hours. But if you deprive your body of the rest it needs for too long, your mirror will begin to show you negative results—a grayish, doughy complexion and, eventually, wrinkles and bags under the eyes.

There's another very good reason why you should get enough sleep—namely, if you don't sleep long enough, you won't dream long enough. Studies have shown that dreaming is a natural and necessary mental function. Everybody dreams; people who believe they don't are simply not remembering their dreams. But whether you remember dreaming or not, the mental activity that goes on during your nightly dream cycles is a significant balancing mechanism; not only is it an important outlet for fantasy and wish-fulfillment, it also seems to have a cleansing effect on the emotions and to stimulate problem solving and creative thinking. People who, during laboratory experiments, are deprived of their dream periods will shortly begin to show signs of anxiety and serious stress. After several days of dream deprivation, they develop symptoms of psychosis; eventually, not being allowed to dream can even result in death.

Normally, you'll experience about four dream periods during a regular eight-hour cycle. The first such dream period is usually brief, while subsequent periods become longer; the longest dream period is usually experienced just prior to waking in the morning. As a consequence, if you curtail too often the amount of sleep you get, you'll be robbing your body and mind of perhaps as much as fifty percent of this highly beneficial activity. So for the sake of a healthy dream life and your health in general, be sure the rest you get is adequate in both quality and quantity. In other words, forty winks really isn't enough sleep for most of us.

Stress, Illness, and Aging

During the last two decades researchers have compiled a huge amount of data on the effects of stress on physical health. One of the things they've discovered is that different people have widely varying emotional responses to the same stressful situation. Some people's responses are counterproductive, aggravating the effects of the stress; other people's responses minimize the stress. Though we're concerned here primarily with the health of the skin, we'd like to examine briefly what constitutes stress, how different individuals may react to it, and what these reactions have to do with illness and the aging process, because we believe several points made by stress researchers have a bearing on the health of the skin.

The most prominent figure in stress research has been endocrinologist Hans Selye.[1] According to Dr. Selye, stress may be defined as "the nonspecific response of the body to any demand made on it." In everyday life you encounter any number of specific experiences that place demands on the body's resources. Examples of demanding experiences might be burning the morning toast, exposure to excessive heat or cold, running to catch a bus, ingesting a large amount of sugar, confronting or being confronted by an authority figure such as a policeman or your employer, being bored by your job, and so forth. To each of these demands, the body may react specifically, for example, by grabbing the toast, shivering in the cold, or running to catch the bus. But it will also have a nonspecific physiological reaction as it automatically attempts to balance itself while meeting the demands of the stressful situation; the reaction is referred to as "nonspecific" because chemical changes occur in the body regardless of the kind of stress situation encountered. We may be aware of this nonspecific reaction as a "rush" of excitement, fear, or anger—or, if the stress situation is one of long duration, we may be unaware of the working of the body's adaptation mechanisms. But whether we are aware of these automatic chemical reactions or not, such physiological adaptation activity is what Selye refers to as the "essence of stress."

Basically, the chemical changes that take place in the body, and especially in the endocrine system, as a reaction to stress are part of the "fight or flight" response—your body automatically prepares you to "fight" the demanding experience or to "flee" from it. Anger, excitement, or fear equips you to deal with an emergency by stimulating the neuroendocrine system to produce hormones that increase the heartbeat, constrict the arteries, and raise the blood pressure, all for the purpose of moving more blood to the brain and the muscles. The blood draws back from the skin, and its clotting ability increases, so that if the body is injured it will lose less blood; this reaction accounts for the white, drained look of the skin in a person who is intensely angry or frightened. The production of white corpuscles increases temporarily, preparing the body to fight infection if it is injured. Sugar is released into the bloodstream so that more fuel becomes available for immediate use, and the body's metabolism increases in order to get that fuel to the cells.

Once upon a time, this "fight or flight" response to stress made a lot of sense. Our ancient ancestors, confronted by a predatory animal, would have made use of the increased flow of energy described above either by engaging the predator in battle or by running away. Unfortunately, our modern social structure forces us to inhibit our natural fear/anger reactions much of the time. For example, if a policeman stops you to give you a ticket, you can neither run away nor hit him in the nose, even though your body's defenses prepare you for those two alternatives. For the sake of social protocol, you're required to override your body's inclinations. And when you're forced to override reactions to stress day after day, the negative effects accumulate, and you develop what is known as "chronic stress." Among the serious side effects of chronic stress is suppression of the immune system; this lowering of the body's defenses can sometimes result in serious illness.

Dr. Selye notes that stressors need not always be damaging or unpleasant. Indeed, we need some stress in our lives to keep the body charged and working properly. Selye uses the examples of a game of chess and a passionate embrace, either of which might precipitate the need for adaptation activity but neither of which would be likely to cause *harmful* effects. And we know that sex, a very pleasurable activity, stresses the body. So does exercise. But these are positive stresses which have positive effects on the body. Unpleasant or disagreeable stress, however, has negative effects and might be referred to more accurately as "distress." At least part of the reason for this distinction is our subjective emotional response to the stressor.

Dr. Selye calls the process by which the body attempts to adapt to stress the "general adaptation syndrome" and describes it as having the following three primary stages:

1. ALARM REACTION, wherein the body demonstrates changes characteristic of exposure to a stressor (the "fight or flight" reaction).

2. STAGE OF RESISTANCE, during which the body attempts to adapt to the stressor and "learn to live with it"; in this period, resistance rises above normal.

3. STAGE OF EXHAUSTION, wherein, after long-continued exposure to the stressor, the body's adaptative energy becomes exhausted. Unless the body is allowed to rest, alarm reactions reappear, the body is no longer able to react, and death occurs.[2]

Research has shown that major illnesses are generally correlated with the number of stress factors in people's lives during the months preceding the onset of the illnesses. Some diseases to which stress is known to be a major contributor are certain types of allergies, infections, migraine and tension headaches, backache, angina, irregular heartbeat, heart attack, hypertension, various digestive ailments, diabetes, arthritis, and cancer.[3] The same stressor may cause different diseases in different individuals largely as a result of factors such as age, sex, genetic makeup, diet, amount of exercise, cultural attitudes, and emotional stability, which predispose one body system over another to susceptibility.

As we've mentioned, a person's emotional attitudes toward a given stressor play an important role in determining the effects of that stress. A situation that may be devastating to one person may be experienced by another with little or no distress reaction. Take, for example, two married women who discover their husbands are having extramarital affairs. If religious or moral convictions or monetary reasons exclude the option of divorce for one of these women, the situation could constitute stress that is both chronic and without means of alleviation. If the marriage is seen by this woman as intolerable and inescapable, it would be possible for the woman to become sufficiently depressed and despairing that serious illness or even death through illness is an acceptable—though perhaps subconscious—solution to her problem. On the other hand, if the second woman views her husband's infidelities as an excuse for her to escape from a marriage that has not been satisfactory, and if she is willing and able to get a divorce, the woman may escape the stressful situation relatively unscathed.

Selye views aging as the cumulative effect of all the stresses to which the body has been exposed during its lifetime; he sees it as paralleling the exhaustion stage of the general adaptation syndrome, with the difference being that, in aging, the effects of stress are no longer reversible.[4]

Since stress can cause severe damage to any of the body's major systems, it would be a little surprising if it didn't have some direct effects on the health of the skin as well. The emotional component of stress, the disruption of the body's hormone balance, and its occasional suppression of the immune system are some obvious factors that have a bearing on the skin's condition. And, since stress seems to accelerate aging, management of the stress in your life is an important way of keeping your skin young. In the rest of this chapter we'd like to examine some specific skin problems to which stress can contribute, as well as some of the ways in which stress can be handled.

How Stress Gets Under Your Skin

According to dermatologist Norman Goldstein, the skin is truly an emotional barometer; if you're in love, it becomes warm; if you feel fear, it turns pale and prickly; if you're angry, it turns hot red or blood-drained white; if you're nervous, it sweats; if you're embarrassed, it flushes. Dr. Goldstein maintains that because the psyche has so much influence on the skin, most skin disorders, from acne to eczema, are triggered by stress. Acne in particular is aggravated by stress because of the overproduction of oil which results from a disrupted hormone balance.[5]

Dr. Hal Boylston, President of the Houston Psychiatric Association, says that when adolescents and adults are anxious, their skin tends to break out in rashes of various kinds, and that, for those who have it, acne is much, much worse.

Houston psychiatrist Milton Altschuler notes that a whole gamut of skin problems can be caused or worsened by mental or emotional problems, including various rashes and eczemas, psoriasis, acne, and factitional dermatitis, caused by picking at the skin and thereby ulcerating or infecting it.

Dr. Ted A. Grossbart, a clinical psychologist affiliated with the Department of Psychiatry at Harvard Medical School and with Beth Israel Hospital in Boston, says that while the causes of skin disorders may vary from heredity to bacteria, viruses, or external causes, there's no doubt that emotional problems can worsen some cases of skin ailments, and may even be responsible for initiating others.[6]

Dr. Grossbart cites a study done in 1978 by Robert Griesemer, a Boston dermatologist, which assessed the role of emotional events in triggering the skin disorders of 4,576 patients. Results of the study demonstrated that the majority of the cases of psoriasis, hives, various types of eczema, and itching were attributable to emotional causes, while over 90% of all cases of rosacea, warts, and neurotic excoriations were similarly emotionally induced. Hyperhydrosis, or extreme sweating, was determined to be 100% emotional in origin.[7]

Outbreaks of genital herpes and vaginitis are two other skin disorders which doctors now believe may frequently have an emotional, stress-related basis. Both may sometimes involve unresolved sexual feelings and insecurities.

According to Dr. Grossbart, the most common emotion at the base of these various disorders seems to be anger; if the anger brings about a conflict, or if the anger cannot be verbally expressed, the person's feelings may cause the skin to rage. The second most common basic emotion in skin disorders is an unfulfilled need for affection or love. If the skin breaks out, it may symbolically be "weeping"; a person may be expressing emotional need through the skin. But Dr. Grossbart notes that this kind of somatic reaction to a psychological problem is ineffective since it doesn't change the situation that caused the problem and generally makes the person with the problem feel worse instead of better.[8] It is, after all, a turning of all the internal negative feelings onto the self.

Even if you aren't suffering from any skin disorders, consider the following: a person under emotional distress is going to show some strain in her face. Habitual muscle contraction in tense circumstances is going to create tension lines on the skin. Dr. Boylston says that some patients who have suffered from traumas or major losses will develop drooping eyelids and folds and lines around the mouth. "Their lives are reflected in their faces." Further, he says that in addition to causing alteration in the body's levels of hormonal secretions, stress puts the whole musculature in a constant state of tension. "These two factors [traumas and major losses] alter body metabolism as well as skeletal structure. People who are stressed move with stiffness and not spontaneity. Chronic pull of the muscles alters posture, so instead of standing straight and looking ahead, they [the people under stress] walk stooped over." In other words, a person under severe stress begins to show the physical configurations associated with aging.

Add to this the fact that stress increases enormously the demand of the body for vitamins B and C (both of which are wrinkle retardants), and you'll surely see that eventually stress is going to cause wrinkles. Unless, of course, you learn to manage it early and keep your responses to it under control.

Stress Management

In our experience, there are three ways to improve the management of stress in your life—by preventing it, by minimizing it, and by learning to handle it. We've already noted that stress will always be with us, so avoiding it altogether is really impossible. But probably some of the distress in your life can be avoided, or at least better handled, if you take time to note what it is and how you can circumvent or minimize it.

Begin by making a list for a week of all the situations, encounters, experiences, and relationships that you find stressful. Some of them will be mini-distresses: you get into a traffic jam that causes a minor delay; your garbage disposal breaks down and you have to call a repairman; you discover your daughter has absconded with your last pair of runless hose; you have a run-in with a testy salesperson; etc. Some of them may be medium distresses: an angry dispute with a close friend or relative; an unexpected outlay of money to replace your son's broken glasses; a little fenderbender on the freeway. Some of them may be major distresses; serious illness of a family member; impending divorce; an unwanted job change or move. Put on the list whatever occurs that distresses you, or any ongoing situation that may be causing you pain. At the end of a week, sit down with your list and rank the stresses according to the degree of distress they caused or are continuing to cause—minimal, moderate, or maximal.

Stresses are situational and vary from person to person; even little stresses will be more taxing at some times than they will be at others. A traffic jam isn't much hassle on your way home from work, but it could seem ruinous on your way to an important meeting. A visit to the divorce court could be a minimal strain if you've been looking forward to it for months.

Next, examine the ways in which you contributed to the stresses or in which you may be responsible for maintaining them. Be honest, but don't berate yourself. Think of ways you might avoid some of these stresses in the future: would getting up fifteen to thirty minutes earlier eliminate the jams of rush-hour traffic? Would billing your son for the glasses make him less careless with the next pair? For stresses that cannot be avoided, think about ways you can minimize their unpleasantness. For example, never go to the doctor's office without taking reading material of your own—he may have canceled his subscription to the magazine you usually read there. If paying the bills or doing the income taxes or defrosting the freezer are on your hit list of most hated jobs, get someone else to do them, if possible—if not, treat yourself to something nice when you do get them done. And for those distresses from which there presently seems no escape, do you have a support network of close friends who will permit you to express your negative feelings during distressing times? Consider actions you might take which would eliminate or better balance the stress in your future.

Once you've become more aware of the stress in your life and you've begun to realize how it affects your health and vitality, you'll want to consider methods of alleviating your stress responses. Our first recommendation is simple and immediate: make a point of doing things just for fun. Have a massage, take a leisurely bath with an expensive bubble compound, go to a movie that you've been wanting to see, have lunch at an outdoor French restaurant and watch the passersby. And get in touch with those you love: hugs or handholding or lovemaking will all make the stresses of life a little easier to bear.

Some of the other methods most commonly used to alter stress responses will require a doctor's or other professional's help; others you can learn easily on your own—all they require for effectiveness is a little discipline on your part in practicing them. We'll provide you with our preferred ways of relaxing and relieving stress at the end of this chapter.

Stress Relievers

1. DRUGS: One remedy often prescribed for stress relief over the past couple of decades has been the use of stress-reducing drugs, such as Valium. As you remember from Step 2, we don't recommend your putting any unnatural chemicals into your body since you can never be sure about their side effects. Furthermore, taking drugs for stress relief, even nonhabitforming drugs (of which Valium is *not* one), isn't going to make the problem that's causing the stress go away. If you're presently taking any of them, please consider some of the other methods of stress relief cited below. Then consult with your doctor about weaning yourself away from the drug habit.

2. PSYCHOTHERAPY: A tried and true method of getting people to face their problems and become aware of reasons for their responses is psychotherapy. Dr. Grossbart has used psychotherapy, combined with hypnosis, relaxation, and imagery, to treat patients referred to him by dermatologists. So far, he has treated over fifty patients, with half of these experiencing total or nearly total skin improvement, and the rest improving significantly.[9]

Anyone with a serious skin problem should see a dermatologist first; psychotherapy as a method of getting to the emotional root of skin disorders could certainly be a useful treatment in addition to regular dermatology care, but the physical side of the ailment should be addressed first for quickest results. Psychotherapy may be helpful in permanently alleviating stress, especially in confronting those problems which are ongoing stress causers. However, psychotherapy can be of long duration, so we suggest that for more immediate relief you try some of the other relaxation methods listed here, even if you are already involved in psychotherapy.

3. GROUP THERAPY: An alternative to traditional psychotherapy is the encounter group, which can range from a single, in-depth visit to an open-ended treatment program going on week after week for as long as the member desires the support. It has several advantages as a stress reliever, one of them being the freedom to speak out among people who are neither friends nor relatives and therefore not personally involved with the individual, and another being that it provides a support network of other people who can help the individual in working out his or her problems. But like psychotherapy, this form of stress relief does not often provide an immediate relaxation technique. So while it may help in coming to terms with long-established problems, we recommend that you try some of the other more immediate paths to relaxation, as well.

4. BIOFEEDBACK: Many dermatologists as well as other doctors have found biofeedback training a quick method for obtaining results in their patients. Initially, such training requires some kind of equipment to which the patient is attached; most instruments measure muscle tension, skin temperature, and brain waves. As the patient observes his body's reactions to stress, he usually finds he can control those reactions. When he does something to relax, the equipment registers a slowing down of his reactions—for example, of his brain waves. If he accelerates his responses, the machine registers the increase. Feedback is instantaneous, and before long, patients learn how to enter a state of peace and tranquillity. Additionally, they find they can learn to control many functions usually assumed to be "involuntary," and to remedy such ailments as high blood pressure, irregular heartbeat, migraine headache, improper circulation, and so forth. Usually, after a few sessions, the patient becomes competent in controlling his physiological reactions anytime he chooses, without being attached to the machine. Dr. Goldstein claims considerable success using biofeedback with patients who have skin disorders.[10] If you feel biofeedback training is for you, consult your physician for information. A simple biofeedback device for home use can be purchased for less than twenty dollars.

5. HYPNOSIS/SELF-HYPNOSIS: Actually, all hypnosis is self-hypnosis, according to Dr. Frank S. Caprio and Joseph R. Berger,[11] since in order to be hypnotized, a subject must *desire* to achieve that condition and *allow* a hypnotist to put her into a relaxed state. Generally, hypnosis/self-hypnosis is undertaken as a means to self-improvement: a person who wants to stop smoking or lose weight or improve memory or heal herself of any number of afflictions may do so under

the disciplined practice of self-hypnosis. Hypnosis works because human beings are suggestible. The so-called hypnotic "trance" is actually a state of intense, relaxed concentration in which the subject's subconscious is open to positive suggestions—either those she makes to herself or those made to her by a hypnotist.

Hypnosis is gaining popularity with doctors as a useful adjunct to standard treatment; it has been applied successfully to the treatment of high blood pressure, arrythmia, circulatory control, pain control, mental and emotional problems, headaches, cancer, and many other illnesses. As early as the 1950s, dermatologist Michael J. Scott used hypnosis successfully in treating over forty-five types of dermatoses, including pruritis, hyperhydrosis and hypohydrosis, various kinds of acne, eczemas, lupus erythematosis, rosacea, psoriasis, seborrheic dermatitis, venereal diseases, etc.[12]

If you're interested in pursuing the practice of hypnosis, you may do so through the assistance of a reputable professional hypnotist or a doctor who uses the technique. Alternatively, any number of books currently on the market explain the basics of the technique, and tapes are available that, when played on a regular basis, will help you attain a relaxed state of openness to suggestion; they offer self-improvement techniques in a whole range of areas, from weight-loss and quitting smoking to improved memory, physical healing, and happier sex. We offer some self-hypnosis techniques in Step 8 for the improvement of self-image and the development of youthening attitudes.

The intense relaxation of the hypnotic state is a terrific stress reliever, especially when invoked on a regular basis. When self-hypnosis is undertaken for self-improvement, however, it may be pursued for a period of time and then stopped, or at least practiced only irregularly, once the desired results have been achieved. But since stress and distress are always with us, we recommend that you practice a relaxation technique on a daily basis, not just when you want to achieve some specific result. The relaxation techniques described at the end of this chapter can be modified for use in self-hypnosis; Step 8 will explain how to move from deep relaxation to positive suggestibility, imaging, and affirmation.

6. AEROBICS/STRENUOUS EXERCISE: We've already discussed the benefits of exercise in Step 3, so we'd just like to note a couple of further points here. First, physical exercise allows the body to discharge the built-up tension that results from stressful encounters; in this way it functions to assuage the body's need for fight or flight. Running, swimming, cycling, jumping rope, dancing—all are good negative energy dischargers, and will have many positive physical effects besides. These emotional side effects of exercise are just one of the many good reasons to pursue a vigorous aerobics program. But we urge you, in addition, to practice at least one other relaxation technique regularly.

7. YOGA: This ancient discipline is tailor-made for those interested in good health, youth, and facial improvement. A major advantage of practicing yoga is that a set of "asanas" or postures generally includes a period of deep relaxation and concentrated visualization, both of which we recommend for improvement of body/mind wholeness; we have combined the yoga concept of "one pointedness" with our own positive imaging technique in Step 8. If you are interested in learning more about yoga, there are probably classes being taught in your area; there are also several good self-teaching books available. Though yoga requires discipline, commitment, and time, your efforts will be well-rewarded. However, since yoga isn't for everybody, and since we want you to start relaxing right away, we offer some other simple relaxation techniques below.

While all of the techniques for stress relief described above may offer advantages, none of them encourages relaxation *simply for the sake of relaxation*. In biofeedback and hypnosis, relaxation is a means to an end; in aerobics and yoga, it is a by-product of disciplined practice. We certainly do not intend to disparage any of these techniques—if you are already a regular jogger or yogin, or if you regularly use biofeedback or self-hypnosis techniques, you have doubtless learned to relax, as well as to motivate yourself. But if you aren't practicing these techniques on a daily basis, you're missing some distinct advantages of relaxation for its own sake.

8. MEDITATION: Herbert Benson, in his book *The Relaxation Response,*[13] advocates a method of relaxing based on historical meditative techniques. He found four things common to all meditation practices: 1) a quiet environment to prevent distractions; 2) a mental device, either an image to hold in mind or a chant, known as a *mantra.* Any sound or prayer or word will work, such as the word "one," or "love," or "relax," or even a nonsense syllable; the object of the *mantra* is to provide a focus for the mind; 3) a passive attitude—the purpose of the technique is not to *make* anything happen, but to relax, let go, and *let* whatever happens, happen; 4) a comfortable position, usually sitting in a chair with the feet flat on the floor; this is preferable to lying down because you don't want to go to sleep.

The technique for meditating, or as Dr. Benson refers to it, for evoking the "relaxation response," is generally to sit comfortably in a chair in a quiet place and breathe naturally through the nose; relax all your muscles; breathe in, then out, and on the outbreath, mentally or orally say the word or phrase you have decided to use as a *mantra,* or concentrate on the mental image you have chosen. Continue focusing on the *mantra* for ten to twenty minutes, and try to remain passive throughout. Practice this technique twice a day; within a few days you'll begin to notice that you can attain a peaceful, relaxed state very readily, and that you are beginning to feel more capable of coping with your tensions and distresses.

Dr. Benson cites studies at Thorndike Memorial Laboratory of Harvard about the physiological effects of meditation. The relaxation response causes your whole body to slow down—you breathe more slowly, pump less blood, develop a relaxed brain-wave pattern, and use less cellular energy, allowing your body to rest and heal. This slowed functioning is called hypometabolism.

There may well be other physiological benefits to meditation that haven't been discovered in the lab. The Association for Research and Enlightenment in Virginia Beach, for example, often publishes materials suggesting that healing of the endocrine glands takes place during meditation. If this is true, it can do much to repair your adaptative mechanisms.

Dr. Benson notes that sleep is another hypometabolic state; both sleep and meditation tend to reduce oxygen consumption. However, during sleep, oxygen use decreases slowly, until after four or five hours it's about eight percent lower than when you are awake, at which point it levels off. In meditation, on the other hand, the decrease occurs almost immediately, within the first three minutes, and averages ten to twenty percent lower than in normal wakefulness. He notes that during meditation a few people feel ecstatic, though most will simply feel very calm and relaxed; a few have no subjective reactions to meditation. According to his tests, the same physiological changes occur during meditation, regardless of the individual's subjective response.

After several days you'll probably begin to notice some other benefits. Meditators report a decreased dependency on alcohol, tranquilizers, cigarettes, sleeping pills, coffee, and other stimulants and depressants. They have also reported decreases in anxiety, worry, nervousness, fear, and tenseness, and increases in energy, creativity, calmness, patience, health, stamina, positive attitudes, happiness, contentment, joy in living, problem-solving ability, and attention span.

We sometimes find it helpful to combine meditation with the technique described below.

9. PROGRESSIVE RELAXATION: This is the name applied by Edmond Jacobson to his technique for relaxing the body in stages.[14] The technique is simple and requires only a few minutes of quiet. Sit in a comfortable chair, hands resting in your lap, feet flat on the floor. Become aware of your breathing, and with each outflow of breath, mentally tell yourself to "relax." Repeat this step eight or ten times. Next, become aware of your body parts, beginning with the parts of your head. Are your eyes staring, even though they're closed? If so, gently give them the order to relax. Is your tongue tense? Tell it to relax. Become aware of your scalp; tell it to relax. Concentrate on your face, tense it, then tell it to relax. Notice the muscles of your jaws; clench your teeth and tell your jaws to relax. Move to

your neck muscles and do the same. As you feel all the tension drain out of your head, feel the relaxation begin to wash over the rest of your body. Progress downward to shoulders, arms, hands, fingers, chest, abdomen, thighs, calves, feet, and toes, progressively concentrating on tensing and then giving the command to relax to each set of muscles as you go. By the time you reach your feet, the tension will have completely left your body. Remain seated for a few minutes, keeping your mind clear of any intrusive thoughts. Then lightly open your eyes and become aware of how refreshed and relaxed you feel.

Progressive relaxation is really a variety of meditation; if practiced faithfully for twenty minutes twice a day, the same physiological benefits accrue. The primary difference is the emphasis of the first technique on a mantra as a focusing device. We have found the mantra helpful, but not essential. Since the purpose of these exercises is to learn to relax, we suggest you practice whichever form seems easiest to you at the time. Some people start with progressive relaxation, then begin repeating a mantra as soon as they feel relaxed. Do whatever works.

Dr. Benson notes a further proviso: don't try to meditate for two hours after a meal, since digestion seems to interfere with your ability to relax deeply. Any other time you can work it in is fine; if you're a commuter, do it on a train or bus or any time you aren't driving; if you're a student, beween classes in empty classrooms; if you stay home, meditate after everyone else goes off in the morning and before they come back in the afternoon; and if you work, take a decompression break instead of a coffee break.[15]

If you have trouble keeping your mind empty of distracting thoughts, don't be disturbed; just gently nudge it back to the focusing device or to a state of emptiness. You'll probably have days when it seems more difficult for you to relax, but don't be discouraged. Just keep on practicing—twice every day for twenty minutes—and be confident that the physiological benefits are occurring, getting your body and mind in balance and working for each other to keep you healthy, relaxed—and younger for longer.

STEP 7: STRESS RELIEF CHECKLIST

1. If you don't presently incorporate *any* relaxation techniques in your daily activities, set aside two daily periods when you can get off by yourself and meditate. After about a week, you'll be able to relax quickly and you'll find the stresses you encounter have become less threatening.

2. At the end of every day, for one week, make a list of all the stresses you have experienced. At the end of the week, rate them as major, moderate, or minor.

Consider how you may be responsible for causing or maintaining the stresses in your life. Then consider how you can eliminate or minimize the same or similar stresses in the future.

3. Make a list of the things you've done for fun during the day. If you haven't done anything just for fun, list at least four things you'd like to do, and make time to actually do them during the next week. See a movie, go to the zoo, have lunch at an unusual restaurant, take a bubble bath, etc.

4. Consciously remember every day to a) smile at three people you don't know; b) hug some friends or relatives; and c) stroke a pet if you have one. These actions of reaching out and touching can function as "warm fuzzies" and are wonderful stress relievers.

5. Allow yourself at least seven to eight hours of sleep a night. Go to bed in a calm, relaxed mood to get the greatest benefit from your time there.

6. Suggested readings:
Herbert Benson, *The Relaxation Response* (New York: Avon, 1975).
Norman Goldstein, *The Skin You Live In* (New York: Hart, 1978).
Walter McQuade and Ann Aikman, *Stress* (New York: Bantam, 1974).
Hans Selye, *The Stress of Life* (New York: McGraw-Hill, 1956) and *Stress Without Distress* (New York: Signet, 1974).
O. Carl Simonton, Stephanie Matthews-Simonton and James L. Creighton, *Getting Well Again* (New York: Bantam, 1978).

---

[1] Hans Selye, *The Stress of Life* (New York: McGraw-Hill, 1956); *Stress Without Distress* (New York: Signet, 1974).

[2] Hans Selye, *Stress Without Distress* (New York: Signet, 1974), pp. 26–27.

[3] For a full discussion of the causal relationship between stress and these illnesses, see Walter McQuade and Ann Aikman, *Stress* (New York: Bantam, 1974).

[4] Hans Selye, *Stress Without Distress* (New York: Signet, 1974), p. 93.

[5] Norman Goldstein, *The Skin You Live In* (New York: Hart Publishing Co., 1978), pp. 35, 48, 196.

[6] Ted A. Grossbart, "Bringing Peace to Embattled Skin," *Psychology Today* (February 1982), p. 55.

[7] Ibid., p. 58.

[8] William Gottlieb, "Your Emotions and Your Health: A Woman's Guide," *Spring* (April 1983), p. 42.

[9] Ibid., p. 42.

[10] Norman Goldstein, *The Skin You Live In* (New York: Hart Publishing Co., 1978), pp. 191–193.

[11] Frank S. Caprio and Joseph R. Berger, *Helping Yourself with Self-Hypnosis* (Englewood Cliffs, New Jersey: Prentice-Hall, 1963), pp. 16–17.

[12] Michael J. Scott, *Hypnosis in Skin and Allergic Diseases* (Springfield, Illinois: Charles C. Thomas, Publisher, 1960).

[13] Herbert Benson, *The Relaxation Response* (New York: Avon, 1976), pp. 159–161.

[14] Dr. Jacobson's "progressive relaxation" technique has been adapted for use with cancer patients by oncologists O. Carl Simonton and Stephanie Matthews-Simonton and is described fully in their book with James L. Creighton, *Getting Well Again* (New York: Bantam, 1978), pp. 138–140.

[15] Herbert Benson, *The Relaxation Response* (New York: Avon, 1975), pp. 166–168.

Step Eight:
Positive Imaging

It is known that as long as cells maintain their ability to divide, they can repair damage and filter out defects; only when cell division begins to decrease does the body—that is, the cell population as a whole—show signs of aging. Aging is the result of the nondividing cell's limitations: a weakened ability to repair damage and a concomitant buildup of waste products in the cell that it is unable to eliminate. Scientists project that if sufficient talents and resources can be dedicated to research, by the year 2000 we'll have answers to the questions of 1) exactly what causes cell division to cease, and 2) what can be done to deter it.

By now it should be apparent that we believe cellular deterioration can be slowed, provided we give each cell its optimal environment. Aging, at least at the rate it occurs in this country, is neither natural nor inevitable. So far, we've provided you with information on all the conscious actions you can take to retain youth and a healthy skin indefinitely: eat a nutritious, poison-free diet, rich in vitamins, minerals, and RNA; get plenty of physical and sexual exercise to keep your circulation, respiration, bone structure, muscles, nerves, and glands in tip-top condition, and to help keep your skin taut, smooth, and moist; clean, moisturize, protect, and be aware of your skin and its needs on a daily basis; and learn how to handle stress through rest and mental quieting. But even the very best *conscious* actions may not accomplish your goals if your *unconscious* remains unconvinced that you can attain them; and if rejuvenation or aging reversal is your goal, your own unconscious may be the biggest adversary you'll have to overcome.

Getting Your Subsconscious on Your Side

Do we age merely because we think we have to? The Bible is filled with stories of our progenitors who lived to ages well beyond the norm, and while we'll admit such claims can't be substantiated, they are still instructive. Remember Methuselah, reputed in Genesis 5:27 to have lived 969 yerars? And how about Abraham, who sired a child in his nineties? And maybe we should give some credit to Sarah, his wife, who gave birth to that child as a nonagenarian (giving birth is not considered an easy matter these days for any woman over forty or so). Moses is said to have gone to his reward with his vision unimpaired, still vigorous and healthy in both mind and body.

Emile Coué, the French pharmacist/psychologist, offered an affirmation for self-improvement in the 1920s that ultimately became a common household slogan: "Every day in every way I am getting better and better." The efficacy of such positive affirmations in pursuit of any of life's goals is attested to today by the many proponents of the José Silva system of "mind control," which maintains you can accomplish any positive thing to which you set your *full* mind—both conscious and unconscious.

A positive mental attitude is a tremendously potent force in attaining and maintaining health, vitality, and youth. In fact, more and more doctors are beginning to encourage their patients to use the faculties of the mind to facilitate the healing process, and when they do, they often find patients attaining amazing cures in what had been diagnosed as incurable or even terminal illnesses. We've already discussed in the previous chapter how our thoughts and feelings—both conscious and unconscious—can affect the immune system, the endocrine system, and thus the body as a whole. It is also our contention that we age, at least in part, because we think we have to. But, since there's no longer any doubt that the mind has a real, physical influence on the body, there's no reason not to get it working for you in your personal skin care/youthening program.

Why wait until A.D. 2000 for the scientists to come up with an explanation of the aging process and a treatment to reverse it? You have within you the magic mechanism to reverse the aging process *now*! In fact, Step 8 may just be the most important part of the Figure 8 program; it's a step we call "positive imaging."

Your "Self" versus Your "Self-Image"

It's no accident that the method of positive thinking known as "psycho-cybernetics" was developed by a plastic surgeon, Maxwell Maltz.[1] As a cosmetic surgeon, he was impressed by the dramatic personality changes which often accompanied the correction of a facial defect. It was as if by altering the external appearance he had somehow changed the person's inner motivations as well. Shy, retiring people became courageous and self-confident; formerly "dull" people became bright and successful; hardened criminals became model prisoners, and, later, responsible citizens.

Equally striking to Maltz were those cases where plastic surgery made tremendous changes in appearance—but the patients themselves denied seeing any difference at all! Neither the insistence of family and friends that they were beautiful nor confronting them with before and after pictures did anything to change their minds. It was as if they suffered from some internal psychic wound, the scars of which could never be removed by the plastic surgeon's art alone.

Finally, he was struck by the numbers of people, especially women in the range of thirty-five to forty-five, who, although they were perfectly nice-looking and in some cases really attractive, erroneously believed they were due for plastic surgery. It was as if, simply by reaching a given age, they were convinced they were "old."

As a consequence of these observations, Dr. Maltz became interested in the psychology of self-esteem and its effect on personality and behavior. He realized the "self-image" was the common element in all these cases: how a person thinks of himself or herself, how the person *believes* he or she appears is what matters, rather than the actual face and figure presented to the world. If the self-image is intact, the person feels confident, secure, and happy; if the self-image isn't healthy, the person becomes fearful, insecure, and anxiety-ridden.

From this realization, he began developing a treatment program whereby he could help people counter their negative self-images, and hence lead more successful lives. That program, which he called psycho-cybernetics, maintains that the "subconscious mind," consisting of the brain and nervous system, is actually what he calls a "servo-mechanism," which can be used and directed by the consciousness for the purpose of goal attainment. This is not to say that a person *is* a machine; rather, as Dr. Maltz reiterates, each person *has* a machine which he or she can use to attain goals, if he or she so chooses. This machine functions automatically, depending upon the goals the individual establishes for himself or herself; if the goals are positive, it will function for the attainment of success, whereas if they are negative, it will function for the accomplishment of failure instead.

It is the individual's self-image—and the attitudes, beliefs, and emotions it generates—that defines the limits for the attainment of goals. If we see ourselves as worthy, valuable, and adequate, the subconscious will operate to grant us success in our goals; if we see ourselves as unworthy, inadequate, or valueless, the subconscious will achieve what we believe we deserve—failure.

Based on this premise, Dr. Maltz maintains that positive thinking can't work if it isn't consistent with the individual's self-image; until the self-image is positive, attempts at positive thinking will meet with too much internal resistance. The first step in his program is therefore a reshaping of the self-image, in order to convince the subconscious that success is what you really want and deserve. As Dr. Maltz points out, changing the self-image doesn't mean transforming the self; it merely means truly believing that you are a valuable person just the way you are.

This idea is the reason why, in the introduction to this book, we asked you to go to your mirror on a regular basis and tell yourself you are a worthy person, deserving of health, life, and beauty, and we asked you to begin professing self-love. Changing your self-image means changing the mental picture you have of yourself, so that you can unleash and realize your potential. In order to bring about the changes in your face and health we've outlined earlier in this book, we want you to continue to make this self-love talk a regular part of your daily routine, because practicing self-acceptance and self-love can lead to self-fulfillment.

If one posits, as proponents of psycho-cybernetics do, that the brain and nervous system function as a machine, then it would seem you have not only the right but the *obligation* to take charge and direct the workings of that machine. If you owned an electric lawn mower, you wouldn't turn it on and let it run off across the lawn by itself. Nor would you use it to chop up all the flowers and shrubs in your flower beds. So why let the subconscious ramble off by itself without your guiding and directing it? Or why use it (albeit unwittingly) to accomplish negative goals? Instead, give it regular guidance in appropriate and positive paths. The technique for positive imaging outlined below combines the best techniques of various schools of positive thinking and self-hypnosis with an approach to improving your self-image that is patterned after the concepts of psycho-cybernetics.

The Power of the Imagination

Positive imaging is a technique commonly used in motivational psychology. We mentioned in Step 7 that it has recently been incorporated into various kinds of medical treatment programs. It has been applied to relieving stress in patients with heart disease and high blood pressure, to cancer therapy, and to skin problems; it has even been used for female breast augmentation as an alternative to plastic surgery. Psycho-cybernetics, mental-control techniques, and hypnosis/self-hypnosis all make use of the human imaging faculty to some degree.

The imagination is a very powerful tool, because the mind creates according to the images it holds. We know that the body is under the control of the subconscious, which creates conditions in the body according to what we believe to be true. When we feed our subconscious negative thoughts, suggestions, and images, we create negative physical conditions. We mentioned in the previous chapter that patients with skin problems frequently develop symbolic conditions, that is, ailments that symbolically express emotions they are unable to communicate verbally. When the suggestion is made to them in hypnotic therapy that they should imagine their conditions as clearing, the conditions frequently go away, especially when the source of the emotions which caused the conditions can be identified and the emotions can be experienced more directly.

It would appear also that the subconscious takes words and phrases literally that we speak metaphorically. Clinical psychologist Leslie M. Lecron labels this phenomenon "organ language" and explains that when we use such phrases as, "That's a pain in the neck," or, "That's a headache," we open ourselves to exactly those disorders. Used often, a phrase like, "I can't stand any more of that," may perceptibly weaken our legs or ankles to the point where we become susceptible to sprains or knee injuries. This is because the ever-literal subconscious translates the metaphor into a physical condition. Lecron has found that many patients with skin disorders referred to him for therapy have incurred their conditions through use of organ language; he cites the case of one young lady whose skin erupted in a severe case of neurodermatitis because she thought of herself as "irritated" by her life situation and "itching" to make significant changes.[2]

The point is that our negative thoughts and feelings, verbal or symbolic, communicate negative goals to our subconscious and cause it to set up negative conditions in our bodies. We contend that aging is one of these conditions, and can be countered by our taking charge of all our mental activities. If we want beautiful, clear, healthy skin, if we want skin that's young and wrinkle-free, we have to be aware and *in control* of our thoughts and the images we create with our minds, to be sure the messages we communicate to the subconscious are positive.

How To Accentuate the Positive

The purpose of Step 8 of the Figure-8 program is to define and focus on your own ideal self-image, which includes your physical face and body, and to maintain or bring back youthful looks and attitudes. We have found that the best way to control the mind's image-making capacity is twofold: to practice positive imaging during meditation, and to make positive suggestions to all your senses at other periods throughout the day to reinforce your positive imaging. There are actually five things we suggest you do for rapid accomplishment of your goals.

In the last chapter, we encouraged you to start meditating for twenty minutes twice a day. The best time to practice positive imaging is after you have relaxed fully and started reaping the benefits of the meditative process. You can, of course, set aside a separate time, but we find it more convenient to combine the two processes.

1. Picture yourself in a natural setting of your own choice. It can be either a spot from memory or an imagined place. Make an effort to concentrate on the details of the place and attempt to experience it with all your senses. One of the authors uses a spot in a national forest in New Mexico where her family has gone picnicking. It is secluded and very green, with birds chirping and twittering and a little brook trickling nearby. The musky smell of earth and the scent of pines are very distinct; there's a fallen log near the water where she pictures herself sitting; dragonflies flutter by, and the sun glimmers on the water. Choose a place you can evoke in similar or greater detail.

Picture yourself in the natural setting. As you breathe in, picture yourself drawing the life-force energy from your surroundings into your body and having it fill you with light. Let the light flow through your body, from nostrils to lungs, then downward through your legs and feet and outward through arms and hands. Then as you exhale, picture the light flooding your head with energy. Now visualize yourself as you want to be—relaxed, peaceful, filled with happiness and love for everyone, and radiating the beauty and youth that come from successful, balanced living. As you watch yourself you notice that you are younger and healthier than you have been in a long time. You are so relaxed that you can see any tension lines in your face smooth out. Your face is becoming beautiful and ageless—your body is young, graceful, and vital, reflecting your balanced life-style and your joy in living. Try to hold this image of yourself for a few minutes. Then, as you finish your meditative exercise, give yourself the verbal suggestion that you are youthening, growing younger every day.

Focused visualization requires concentrated effort; in yoga it is known as "one pointedness." At first you may find it difficult to hold on to an image. Remember, never criticize or berate yourself if you have trouble at times either meditating or imaging. Sometimes the mind will wander; when it does, just nudge it back to the picture of yourself you are trying to retain, and continue to practice. And don't be discouraged; eventually you'll be able to succeed at positive imaging.

2. To reinforce the visual images of your meditation exercise, make a poster for your wall—bedroom, bathroom, or wherever—just put it in a place where you'll see it several times a day. Make a large figure 8 on it, that is, two circles balanced, one on the other. The figure 8 is a symbol of balance; for you, it will stand for the balances you are striving to attain: of the mental and physical, of your inner and outer selves, and of yourself within your environment. And, of course, it represents the balanced body image you are developing. Since the circle is representative of perfection, wholeness, integration, and unity, the double circle is also symbolic of these things, twofold. And certainly you are working to achieve unity of body, mind, and spirit and of wholeness and integration in attempting this youthening program, and you know by now you can attain that unity through the keys of balance, awareness, and positive attitude. Turned on its side, the same figure becomes a symbol of infinity, an idea which is also applicable to the path you are now following, for your potential is infinite; you *can* attain anything to which you set your whole mind. When you create a poster with the figure 8 on it, you impress all these symbolic meanings on the subconscious and reinforce them each time you look at the poster.

In one circle on your poster, put a picture of yourself, preferably taken at the age you feel was your optimum. If you believe you were at your best at thirty-two, put a picture of yourself from that period in one of the circles. In the other, write the goal you want to attain and the date by which you want to attain it—for example, a healthier, younger you by October 31.

3. Repetition of the goal you seek is very important, so make positive affirmations aloud several times a day—on waking, on retiring, and especially every time you look in the mirror. Some people are visual learners; some are auditory learners; and some are both. We therefore want to encourage you to get both faculties in operation. If you're now used to telling yourself you are worthy and loveable, you can vary your affirmations with some verbal suggestions that are more specifically directed toward the youthening process, such as the following:

"You, _____(state your name), are a young, vital, vigorous person. You are attaining health, beauty, and permanent youthfulness, and you're looking younger every day."

If you're in a public place and don't want to appear exhibitionistic, just affirm silently while smiling at your reflection, "You're getting better every day," or "You're getting younger all the time." Just be sure there are *no negatives* in the affirmations.

4. To reinforce these verbal affirmations, you may want to make a tape on which you repeat the affirmation of your choice for ten to twenty minutes. This is a particularly good thing to go to sleep with at night. You can put yourself in

a restful state, just as you would if you were going to meditate, but lying down preparatory to going to sleep. As soon as you are fully relaxed, turn on the tape and listen to yourself making these positive affirmations. This procedure will help convince your subconscious that you really want to be younger and healthier.

5. Learn to control your thoughts and the metaphors you use. Never say to anyone, even yourself, "I guess I'm getting old," or "I'm too old to do that," or any other negatives. Become aware of the words you choose and choose *only* words which are positive in their implications.

Dr. Maltz counsels in *Psycho-Cybernetics* that a minimum of twenty-one days will be required to change a self-image. He says that after plastic surgery, it takes about twenty-one days for a patient to become accustomed to a new face; after amputation of a limb, a patient will feel a "ghost" limb for about three weeks; he therefore believes it takes about three weeks for an old mental image to fade and a new one to form. We, too, believe that twenty-one days are necessary to effect any changes in mental attitudes and, consequently, any changes in physical appearance. So we want to give you the following warning: Don't become discouraged; give yourself a full three weeks to begin observing changes in your appearance. If you follow all aspects of the Figure-8 program religiously, you cannot fail to get results in that time. This is not to say that you'll have accomplished all you want to in three weeks, but if you really have communicated your desire for change to your subconscious, you *will* begin to see results.

Furthermore, authorities agree that when imagination and willpower are in conflict, the imagination will win. Sometimes we try to accomplish our goals by sheer willpower alone; then we spend time worrying and picturing all the things that can go wrong. But worrying means you are misusing your imaging faculty and sending it negatives instead of positives. So don't pit your imagination and will against each other; get them working together by following all parts of Step 8 and then letting the subconscious do its job, while you relax and go about your other business.

On the other hand, do expect results; creating an atmosphere of positive expectancy helps get you moving and acting in ways that bring about the desired result. So actively hope, believe, expect, and anticipate.

Using Positive Imaging for Other Goals

The positive imaging exercises we've outlined above are, of course, a form of self-hypnosis. They will work equally well in the attainment of other goals, for example, as an aid in breaking any negative habits you might want to put an end to as part of your personal youthening program. Just visualize yourself in the peaceful, natural setting of your choice, and hear yourself say, "I am going to break this habit, beginning *now.*" Picture yourself experiencing a sense of well-being and joy as a result of being free of the negative habit. Hold that image of yourself for a few minutes. Then pat yourself on the back and give yourself a hug for being so good to yourself.

Make a poster that graphically shows the habit and your new attitude toward it. For example, if you're trying to give up smoking, you might cut a picture of a cigarette smoker out of a magazine and paste it on your poster—then put a big red X through it. Or to keep your sense of humor and perspective, paint a Groucho mustache and glasses on the smoker first. Remember that habits are hard to break, and that it does take about three weeks to change a mental attitude. You may be rid of the habit before that time, but don't criticize yourself if the desire for it persists a while.

Reinforce your imaging with positive affirmations: "I am breaking this habit to improve my health, to give myself a longer life and youth, and to make my skin the very best and prettiest it can be. Because I'm worth it!" Motivation is very important in habit-breaking; if you have other motives (for example, your doctor has told you to cut out smoking, or alcohol, or starches, or heavy meats, or whatever it is you want to eliminate from your life-style), include those other motives in your affirmation as well.

In attempting to break a habit, by all means make a relaxation-affirmation tape to play as you go off to sleep at night. Or invest in a tape specifically geared toward the elimination of the habit you want to be rid of; several companies around the country now market tapes on various kinds of self-improvement through hypnosis.

It's best to work on only one thing at a time; otherwise you'll tend to weaken your forces. Also, be specific about the goal you want to accomplish, but keep only the result in mind. All authorities on positive thinking agree that the means of attainment are best left to the subconscious. Trust your subconscious to work for you once you've set it in motion with positive images and suggestions; it knows better than the conscious mind *how* to accomplish what you seek.

Some Advice for Beautiful Thinking

Although this book, and the whole Figure-8 Program, is about skin care and the process by which you can stay young longer, it's obvious there are elements of beauty that are more than skin-deep. They radiate from within, generated by an attitude of love and self-assurance. Ageless people in every era are people at peace with themselves and with others who still have important goals to pursue and joys to experience. Once you've set your foot on the path to youthening, the following ideas for staying ageless and maintaining positive attitudes may help you to get where you're going quicker and to stay there longer.

Think about others, but don't neglect your own needs in the process.

Once you've put your subconscious to work, let it do its job in peace, and turn your conscious mind outward so that you can better fulfill yourself through helping others. But, as in everything else, remember to maintain a healthy balance—don't be so self-sacrificing that you neglect your own needs. When you're giving out positive strokes to others, be sure you give yourself a few in the process. You have to love yourself before you can love others, and loving yourself means meeting your own needs; you'll have more energy to spread around in the end.

Practice generosity of spirit.

Since you aren't going to listen to negatives about yourself, especially *from* yourself, don't listen to and don't repeat negatives about other people either. When friends start to gossip, tell them you've given up gossip "for Lent" or "for Passover"—and then pass over the gossip.

Pursue happiness actively.

"A merry heart doeth good like a medicine," said the Proverbialist. The body functions better when we're happy, so it's in our best interest to stay happy as much of the time as possible. Don't look at the cloud instead of the silver lining, or the hole instead of the bagel. If you've reached what our culture calls middle-age, don't think of your cup as half-empty; think of it as half-full.

Happiness cannot be achieved if it is contingent upon some external event—it's a mental attitude that comes from engaging in an activity you find important and fulfilling day after day, regardless of occasional setbacks and disappointments. The kind of happiness we're talking about isn't the momentary pleasure you feel when you get a raise or your husband gives you a lovely gift, although these "uppers" are wonderful and important. The kind of happiness we want you to focus on is the deep contentment you feel from an exciting job, a loving relationship, and deep-down self-satisfaction—these are the ongoing, fulfilling things that give you the emotional strength to deal with any problems you may have to face from time to time.

The pursuit of happiness may mean the pursuit of a goal that's meaningful to you. Notice we didn't say you need to attain the goal to be happy; it's the pursuit of the goal that's significant. And since laughter is good medicine for anything that ails you, look for the humor in your life and experiences and try to give yourself a few good laughs every day.

Judge yourself against your own standards, not somebody else's.

If you use someone else's criteria for judging yourself, you'll invariably fall short in your own estimation. We don't play the piano like Van Cliburn, but it doesn't bother us since we play well enough to please ourselves. Barbra Streisand doesn't sing like Beverly Sills, but we doubt she loses any sleep over the differences in their styles. You are *you*, and nobody else's abilities or talents diminish you in any way.

The only way out is through.

At a seminar in Hawaii several years ago, Dr. Aoki, the Head of the Religion Department at the University of Hawaii, suggested this as the key to dealing with life's problems. Each and every one of us has to choose between facing our problems right away, or collecting leftover baggage, year after year, to carry along the way. Work your problems out on the spot, whenever possible, so you won't have to carry unnecessary burdens.

Learn to forgive and forget.

Forgiveness is one of the most difficult virtues to practice—and one of the most abused. Often someone will assert he or she has forgiven another for an injury or slight, and will then proceed to hold a grudge and bring the situation up again and again, or, worse, walk around in silent suffering, nursing an open wound. If you're really willing to forgive, you have to be willing to forget, and never reopen old wounds or old subjects. Remember, grudges are heavy, can cause backaches, and will eventually give you an old-age stoop.

One way of practicing real forgiveness is the following affirmation, sometimes called "The Prayer of Loving Indifference": "I forgive you, I bless you, and I love you. May that occur which will bring harmony between us." Recited frequently while imaging the person with whom you've had a problem, this affirmation is guaranteed to bring you more peace of mind.

Another way of resolving old grudges, recommended by writer and minister Catherine Ponder, is to develop an affirmation of *mutual* forgiveness (since grudges are often held by both parties to an unpleasantness): "I forgive you, love you, and bless you, and what is more, *you* forgive *me*." It's amazing what good things begin to happen when you are willing to forgive; and when you send others the signal to forgive *you*, they most often do.

The Simontons, in their book *Getting Well Again*, recommend the following technique, suggested by Emmett Fox's *Sermon on the Mount*, as a means of overcoming grudges and resentments: While in the meditation/relaxation mode, picture good things happening to the person you resent. Think about your reactions to the unpleasant experiences you've had with the person and try to see them from the person's point of view. Try to reinterpret the experience and the person's behavior from a more understanding point of view. Carry your more relaxed attitude with you as you come out of meditation.[3]

And finally, learn to forgive yourself. Guilt for past mistakes doesn't alter those mistakes and only makes you feel less worthy in your own eyes. Guilt and regret erode self-esteem and are therefore to be avoided. So, don't be afraid to try anything, but be forgiving of yourself if you miss your goal. Instead of upbraiding yourself, put yourself on your mental screen and say firmly, "You have no need to feel guilty." Then, instead of expressing annoyance at yourself, take your hand and pat kisses on your cheeks while saying, "Kiss, kiss." This may seem silly, but the habit reminds you to love yourself first, for then you'll know how to love others.

Don't hang on to unhealthy, negative relationships.

If a relationship isn't based on mutual esteem and mutual supportiveness, it very likely isn't the kind you're going to want in your newly balanced life. Balance in a relationship means give and take; if one side is mostly give and the other is mostly take, somebody's needs are probably not being met. A popular slogan on posters and other items runs, "If you love something, let it go. If it comes back, it is yours to keep; if it doesn't, it never was." If this saying applies to any of your relationships, consider letting go, or asserting your need for release.

Express love often.

It doesn't matter whether the relationship is between lovers, friends, siblings, or parents and children—mutual love should be expressed regularly and frequently, either verbally or through affectionate touching, or through just smiling and listening to others. You can express love even to people you don't know; make it a point to smile at strangers at least three times a day.

Take responsibility for the world around you.

This doesn't mean you have to feel guilty for it if it isn't pleasant. What it means is that if you find something in your life unpleasant, change it. You have the power, so use it. Remember that no problem is insoluble once you've harnessed your subconscious mental powers. In fact, it sometimes helps to look at life as a series of problem-solving exercises and challenges. Accepting the challenges can be fun, and you'll have a firm sense of accomplishment and control with each challenge successfully met and overcome.

Live in the present moment.

A lot of people live in the past, fretting about the things they've done or the things they've suffered, or worrying that life will never be as good as it used to be. Unfortunately, our memories of the past are often colored by hindsight—we see what has happened to us and believe things would be different if we had taken other paths. Or maybe we develop a nostalgia for bygone days, the simpler, less demanding times of our youth, or the romantic period of early marriage, or the recognition and esteem we enjoyed in school or in a job or when our children were growing up. But living in the past is for old people, and old is the last thing you want to be.

So don't play old negative tapes. Let past mistakes remain in the past. Don't blame yourself for your errors and don't pity yourself for the slights and injustices (either real or presumed) of others. All these do for you is evoke negative feelings, anxieties, and hostilities.

One way to handle old negatives is the following: when an unpleasant or unhappy scene from the past comes to mind, instead of dwelling on it and tasting its bitterness all over again, create a mental movie screen in your mind, replay the scene on it, and change the ending. We've all had nightmares from which we've awakened in fear, and psychologists tell us the way to handle such dreams is to slip back to a state of semisleep and control the ending of the dream so it becomes favorable. When you think about it, past negatives have only about as much relationship to the present moment as bad dreams, so take charge of these unpleasant memories and give them new, more favorable outcomes. If you had bitter words with someone, picture yourself and that person together again, this time reasoning amicably. If someone refused to listen, replay the scene so that this time the other person reacts positively and lends you an ear. If you failed at a task in the past, picture yourself succeeding in similar circumstances.

Another way to handle old negatives is to consciously set them aside and play a positive tape instead. When you're tempted to dwell on failure, conjure up your past successes. When you're tempted to blame someone else for your present woes, try thinking of the good things that that person may have done.

On the other hand, instead of living in the past, some people live "for the future," thinking they'll be happy *when* they have a better job, or *when* they find someone to love them, or *when* they retire. Their happiness is always contingent on something in the future rather than in the present.

Both those who live in the past and those who live for the future are going to miss a large measure of life's pleasure because they're living in the wrong time frame. *Now* is the moment we need to pay attention to.

Set goals for your future that are meaningful for you.

Living in the present moment doesn't mean you shouldn't look forward to the future with eagerness and expectancy. We recently heard an octogenarian on television discussing that he was going to be "when he grew up." People grow old when they no longer have activities that make them happy or that give them an interest in what the future will bring. Whatever you may have accomplished up to now isn't all you can accomplish, provided you find something to do that helps fulfill your potential and makes your future meaningful. Maybe you'd like to go back to school and learn another vocation. Finding a job that is more fun than work will help you live longer and more joyfully. Or maybe you'd like a creative avocation—learn to paint, write, or play a musical instrument. Grandma Moses *started* painting when she was over 70. Find things to do that will fulfill your physical, emotional, mental, and spiritual needs. And when you've accomplished the goals you've set for yourself, establish other goals farther in the future; looking forward to the future with joy and expectancy will help keep you glowing and growing, with no end to the beautiful potential that is the essence of perpetual youth.

STEP EIGHT:
POSITIVE IMAGING CHECKLIST

1. Incorporate positive imaging techniques into your daily meditation.

2. Make posters for your wall which depict the goals you want to accomplish.

3. Acquire (or manufacture your own) self-hypnosis tapes related to the goals you want to accomplish.

4. Make positive affirmations related to the goals you want to accomplish.

5. Regularly imagine good things coming into your life.

6. Give yourself positive strokes every time you look in the mirror.

7. Get control of your thoughts; consciously allow no negatives to intrude into your thinking or conversation.

8. Give yourself at least three weeks to accomplish changes you want to make.

9. Work on only one thing at a time.

10. Look for things to laugh about, and give yourself a few good laughs every day.

11. Consciously try to become your own best friend.

12. Choose activities that will give *you* personal satisfaction.

13. Suggested readings:
Maxwell Maltz, *Psycho-Cybernetics* (New York: Bantam, 1970).
José Silva and Philip Miele, *The Silva Mind Control Method* (New York: Pocket Books, 1977).
Shakti Gawain, *Creative Visualization* (Mill Valley, CA: Whatever Publishing, 1978).
Frank S. Caprio and Joseph R. Berger, *Helping Yourself With Self-Hypnosis* (Englewood Cliffs, NJ: Prentice-Hall, 1963).
Leslie M. Lecron, *Self-Hypnotism: The Technique and Its Use in Daily Living* (Englewood Cliffs, NJ: Prentice-Hall, 1964).

---

[1] Maxwell Maltz, *Psycho-Cybernetics* (New York: Bantam, 1970).

[2] Leslie M. Lecron, *Self-Hypnotism: The Technique and Its Use in Daily Living* (Englewood Cliffs, N.J.: Prentice Hall, 1964), p. 84.

[3] O. Carl Simonton, Stephanie Matthews-Simonton, and James L. Creighton, *Getting Well Again* (New York: Bantam, 1978), pp. 177–178.

Alternative Measures

In general, we believe that the natural approach to skin health, body beauty, and youthening is the best approach. But you may have special problems and concerns not completely covered in the preceding pages. If you have acne, eczema, skin cancer, or any other type of skin ailment, you should be under a doctor's care and should follow his prescribed treatment plan, in addition to the Figure-8 program. You may also want to know the latest innovations in treatment for scarring, broken veins, excess pigmentation, and other cosmetic problems. And you may want to consider plastic surgery for certain conditions. Improving yourself is not vanity, but a necessary part of self-actualization. This chapter is for those who, when they truly believe artificial measures are warranted, would like to know the consensus of the medical community concerning treatment of skin problems.

The Whys and Wherefores of Plastic Surgery

A great deal can be done with modern aesthetic surgery. You can change the shape of a nose or chin, improve a neck, brow, or jawline, pin back ears, reshape breasts, and delete sags from hips, thighs, tummies, and arms. The doctors we consulted all emphasized that every patient is different; as a consequence, it is difficult to generalize about what can be done or when it should be done, since the requirements and degrees of success will differ from person to person.

The procedure you're most likely to be considering is face-lift surgery (rhytidectomy). The purpose of this surgery is to make you look younger, but as we've tried to emphasize throughout this book, how quickly you age is a result of your genetic tendencies and your life-style. Dr. Melvin Spira, Chief of Staff of Plastic Surgery at Baylor College of Medicine, therefore issues the following warning: If a person looks older than her chronological age, she may get very dramatic initial results from face-lift surgery. The removal of excess skin will make an immediate improvement in her looks. But she won't hold the results as long as will a person who has similar surgery but looks younger than her chronological age. In other words, if you aged fast before surgery, you'll age fast after surgery. A plastic surgeon can turn back the clock, but he can't stop it from running.

When should you have a face-lift? There is some controversy about this question. Dr. Spira believes the "minilift," which offers little nips and tucks at an early age, is ineffective. Other doctors feel that early minor face-lift surgery may be warranted for certain patients, depending on their motives. Houston plastic surgeon Dr. Thomas Biggs, however, says that some young candidates for regular face-lift surgery are women with fatty necks whose jawlines could thereby be improved. Dr. Spira recommends face-lift surgery only when there is a great deal of redundant or excess skin, so that a real difference will be apparent in the "before" and "after" pictures.

What can you realistically expect from plastic surgery? Dr. Spira notes first what *cannot* be done: You cannot change the basic configuration of the face; a person with high cheek bones before surgery will have high cheekbones after surgery. Also, plastic surgery will not rejuvenate the elastic tissue of the skin or replace its resiliency.

However, there are two major conditions which can be improved with either plastic surgery or surgery and allied treatment. They are 1) redundant or excess skin; and 2) wrinkling, i.e., fine lines, cross hatching, crow's feet, forehead furrows, etc.

Dr. Spira says the very best candidate for face-lift surgery is the person with a "gullet neck" or "turkey-gobbler neck," that is, a person with an excess of skin in the front and on the side of the neck. This kind of redundancy is easy to correct, leading to improvement of the neck and lower jawline. Several procedures are generally combined in this surgery. An incision is made just underneath the chin, the excess fat is removed, and the muscle is brought together to smooth out the neck. In addition, the surgeon makes incisions around the ears and draws up the excess facial skin, as in the classical face-lift.

Fine lines around the eyelids and vertical lines on the lips can be partially effaced or made less noticeable through plastic surgery. Dr. Spira notes that the two most common eye problems are crow's feet at the sides of the eye and bags under the eyes. Eyelid surgery, called "blepharoplasty," is usually quite successful because the skin of the eyelid and around the eyes is very thin and heals well; as a general rule, the thinner the skin, the less the scarring. Dr. Biggs notes that in eye surgery, it is possible for the surgeon to remove excess fat, skin and muscle. He can move, rather than remove, droopy skin on the upper lid. Dr. Biggs generally makes a patient's eyes the focal point of face surgery because, aesthetically and practically, they are a person's point of contact with others and with the world around her.

Lines around the lips, known as "fish mouth," can be improved during face-lift surgery or freshened with chemical peels, about which we'll have more to say in a moment.

Lines in the forehead are a common problem for which women sometimes seek surgery. Dr. Spira notes that rarely do they occur as a result of excess skin. Most of the time, forehead lines are "use lines," the transverse grooves in the forehead which derive from raising the eyebrows or overwidening the eyes and lifting the forehead, or "frown lines" between the brows at the base of the nose. Dr. Spira suggests four general ways of dealing with these lines.

The first is to make an incision in the forehead at the hairline or, more popular now, over the top of the scalp; turn the forehead down; cut the muscle that is in part responsible for the horizontal grooves or wrinkles; lift the forehead up, pulling it up a little higher than it was before and thereby ironing out the wrinkles to some extent.

Another approach is direct excision, actually cutting out very deep forehead wrinkles; this procedure is reserved for only a few cases.

Forehead lines can also be improved through chemical peeling or through the newer therapy of collagen injection, which we'll discuss at length shortly.

What are the negative aspects of plastic surgery? As with any surgery, the extreme negative is that a patient can die on the operating table. This is a very, very rare occurrence in cosmetic plastic surgery, but any time general anesthesia is used, it becomes a possibility. A good bit of aesthetic surgery, however, is done under a local anesthetic; the doctor can recommend which is the better procedure. Sometimes paralysis occurs due to damage or traumatization of nerves; usually, however, nerves do regenerate. Other possible negatives are bleeding under the skin, loss of integrity of the skin, thick scarring (this seldom occurs on the face because facial skin is thin and heals well), permanent discoloration, and permanent numbness. Dr. Spira suggests, therefore, that all patients become familiar with what he calls ARB: *alternative* treatment plans to the surgery, the *risks* involved in the surgery, and the realistic *benefits* which can be expected from the surgery.

Interestingly, Dr. Spira notes that there is not as much pain with plastic surgery as there is with some other, simpler procedures. The reason for this is that during a face-lift, the skin is elevated off the underlying muscle. In the process, it is temporarily denervated, and the patient experiences numbness, but little pain.

If you believe you are a candidate for plastic surgery, we suggest you shop very carefully for a good doctor. Before you put your face or body in the hands of a plastic surgeon, it is best to know some of his patients and thereby know the fruits of his labor.

Peels, Dermabrasion, and Injections

As we mentioned above, chemical peels are sometimes recommended to eliminate fine lines, as well as imbedded wrinkles, scars, and other facial flaws. Chemical peels may be light (*chemabrasion*) or deep (*chemosurgery*), depending on the flaws which need to be corrected.

A chemical peel requires that a strong chemical be applied to the skin to, in effect, burn it. The outer layers of epidermis peel off, and fresher, younger-looking skin rises to the surface to replace the older, lined skin, thereby erasing lines and wrinkles.

Dr. Spira told us the story of an elderly female patient he and his associates had recently seen at Ben Taub Hospital in Houston, who had been the victim of a gas-oven explosion. Her face had second degree burns from what was referred to as a "heat flash fire." As her face healed, everyone began to realize her wrinkles were gone; the flash fire had functioned like a skin peel.

Similarly, we are told that in days of old, sultans would force their concubines to run in front of lighted torches held by the court eunuchs, in order to give them a face peel. (Life wasn't always good in the good old days.)

We aren't suggesting you should stick your head in an oven or hold a torch to your face. But treatment that burns the skin's outer layers does have a high rate of success in removing wrinkles.

According to Houston dermatologist Dr. Roy Knowles, the negative side to chemical peels is that they are somewhat painful. Furthermore, phenol peels are potentially toxic to the heart and the kidneys, so this procedure has to be done in the hospital under carefully monitored conditions. And an unfortunate possible side effect is that the stronger peels can result in changes in pigmentation that are harder to cover up than the original wrinkles.

Dermabrasion is a technique which planes the skin with a high-speed sander. It, too, can be used to remove fine wrinkles as well as to improve the texture of the skin.

Drawbacks of dermabrasion include the following: it can be painful; there is a possibility of permanent damage if the sanding instrument abrades too deeply; and pigmentation of the newly abraded skin may not match the rest of the skin.

Every physician we consulted was, in general, negative about silicone injections for cosmetic purposes. Silicone is not absorbed, and tends to wander. It can harden, and may cause numerous complications such as nerve damage and unsightly lumps. An advantage, however, is that silicone injections are permanent; there's no need for repeat treatments as there is with collagen. Dr. Spira also mentioned to us that silicone is useful in the treatment of Romberg's Atrophy, an atrophy of the subcutaneous tissue of one side of the face.

Collagen injections, however, are another matter. There are two types of collagen, or Zyderm, which is the trade name for artificial collagen, on the market. Zyderm I has about 35 percent pure collagen in it and 65 percent water, whereas Zyderm II has about 60 percent collagen, and the rest is water. Since collagen is a natural body protein that has been hydrolyzed to make it hypoallergenic, injections are usually well tolerated.

While the results are not permanent, collagen injections give sufficient improvement, in many cases, to warrant their rather high cost and possible complications, which include pain, allergic reactions, and scarring. It is necessary to do a sensitivity test first, to minimize the probability of such complications. The normal procedure is then to overcorrect, or inject more collagen than is actually necessary to puff out the area; as noted, collagen injections are thirty-five to sixty-five percent water, which will be absorbed rather quickly, leaving the proper amount of fullness. If the area to be treated doesn't puff out well, the person being treated may not be a good candidate for the collagen injection.

The length of effectiveness of a collagen injection will vary with the individual. Generally, a person will require a reinjection anywhere from six months to two years after the original treatment, although Dr. Spira knows of people who, more than three years after the original treatment, have still not needed reinjections. Nevertheless, since the treatment only lasts a year or two in most women, it is in essence a maintenance therapy and has to be repeated on a regular basis. Most people go to the dentist twice a year to take care of their teeth; people who opt for collagen injections will similarly need to go to their physicians once or twice a year to take care of their wrinkles. If you are willing to maintain your wrinkle-free face over the years through repeated injections, you could be a candidate for this procedure.

Acne Management

Dr. John Wolf, Chief of Staff of Dermatology at Baylor College of Medicine, maintains that acne is often caused by changes in hormone levels accompanied by plugged pores. The acne which occurs in puberty or as an accompaniment to use or stoppage of the birth-control pill results when the body's androgen hormones stimulate the sebaceous glands to produce excess oil. Pores can be plugged from overgrowth of the lining of the hair follicle, excess sebum, or greasy facial products. Inside those clogged pores, various problems may develop: external bacteria can break down the oil into fatty acids and create papules; white blood cells can collect and form pustules; breakdown of the follicle under the skin can create cysts. Closed pores or pores with tiny openings develop whiteheads; blackheads, on the other hand, are open pores containing oxidized oil.

Of the several ways to unclog pores, some can be pursued at home, while others require a medical setting. Home remedies include the use of granular soaps or a Buf-Puf to help remove surface layers or use of drying soaps that cause peeling and thereby open pores. Extractors, which press around the pore and empty its contents, should be used only by your physician; never squeeze the papules, pustules, or blackheads yourself. Other treatments currently favored for acne management are 1) topically applied antibiotics like erythromycin or tetracycline; 2) topically applied peeling agents that dry, peel, and help unplug pores, the strongest of which is Retin A, a form of vitamin A acid; 3) orally administered vitamin A in a form called Accutane, which was approved for use in 1982.

According to Dr. Knowles, vitamin A acid taken by mouth limits the ability of the sebaceous glands to produce excess oil and eliminates many of the bacteria that infect the oil glands and cause the lumps and scarring of severe cystic acne. Treatment runs sixteen weeks; improvement usually continues even after treatment is discontinued. A side effect is drying of the skin, lips, mucous membranes, and eyes; nose bleeds may occur and artificial tears may be required. Accutane should only be taken under a doctor's supervision, and you must be a safe candidate for the treatment. It is used only in the treatment of severe cystic acne, as the side effects can be extremely unpleasant.

Dr. Wolf warns that vitamin A taken orally in large doses can be toxic; explorers of the North Pole sometimes died of vitamin A toxicity from eating excessive amounts of polar-bear liver.* So do *not* undertake to treat yourself with vitamin A.

The doctors we consulted listed the following possible measures for treatment of acne scarring:

1. Dermabrasion, to sand scars away with an abrasive instrument.

2. Chemical peeling, to remove the scar tissue and improve skin color match (sometimes combined with dermabrasion).

---

* Polar bear liver is the only known *natural* source of such high amounts of vitamin A that, in normal quantities, it causes such toxicity; you're not likely to overdose on beef or chicken liver.

3. Collagen injections, to puff up the scars.

4. Surgical removal—the scars can be punched out with a dermal punch. The holes are then filled in with collagen or fibrin and the spots are dermabraded.

5. Facelift—sometimes recommended for patients who are over thirty as a means of smoothing out the pits of acne scarring. Dr. Spira says that patients who have heavy scarring, deep pits, sinus tracks, and residual cysts may do well to consider plastic surgery. If the acne scarring involves the nasal-labial folds and the anterior part of the cheeks, this portion of the skin can sometimes be completely removed; skin that is in back or in front of the ear can be moved forward.

If you have serious acne scarring that spoils your self-image, consult your dermatologist about whether you may be a candidate for one of these procedures. Help is possible, and you're worth the effort.

Erasing Discoloration

Some people experience the distress of pigmentary changes on their face and hands. In older skin, excess pigmentation may be due to thinning of the skin or excessive sun exposure. Known as "liver spots" because of their liverlike color, such changes can be unsightly. Some of the more common treatments are bleaching, chemical peeling, dermabrasion, or freezing with liquid nitrogen (cryosurgery). Another form of unwanted pigmentation in older skin is keratoses, brownish rough patches, which are actually benign lesions. These are commonly treated with burning or freezing compounds. However, one of the authors had more success with castor oil; after having had some of these lesions frozen twice to no avail, she began applying castor oil topically twice a day. The lesions disappeared in a week. Castor oil is also reputed to be effective in treating warts—but then, so is rubbing them with an old dish rag and burying it in the back yard at midnight! In any case, treatment of skin lesions with castor oil is rarely supported by the medical community.

Another common pigmentary change is melasma, known also as the "mask of pregnancy"; it appears during pregnancy or the use of some kinds of birth control pills. Usually a result of the combination of sun exposure and an increase in estrogen levels, melasma can be treated with bleaching creams and the daily use of a sunscreen. When estrogen levels return to normal, it often fades naturally.

Birthmarks are another type of pigmentary problem. According to Dr. Wolf, raised, vascular, lumpy birthmarks often shrink and go away by middle childhood.

Flat, port-wine birthmarks don't go away; treatment with lasers is currently the only available therapy.

Rosacea, or chronic flushing, for which there is no known cause, may result in permanent capillary damage and spider veins. It is in part aggravated by anything that produces flushing, such as stress, physical activity, sunlight, infection, vitamin deficiency, endocrine abnormality, and extremely hot or cold beverages. Alcohol or hot liquids can cause vasodilatation of the blood vessels; eventually the capillaries rupture and remain open. Spider veins can be closed with laser beam therapy or with electric desiccation needles, a procedure wherein the blood vessel is given a burst of electric current through a tiny platinum needle inserted into it. Treatment for spider veins is often successful on the face, but is much less so on the legs, though exercise can be helpful (maybe you should jog over to the doctor's office?).

Laser-beam therapy has been found useful in treatment of warts, blood vessel malformations, port wine birthmarks, and tattoos, but Dr. Wolf feels that it's much more expensive and not better enough than other therapies to make it cost-effective in treating most skin problems at present.

Skin Cancer Treatment

Houston pathologist Dr. Doyle Rogers was our chief informant on the subject of skin cancers. Most skin cancers are what are known as basal cell carcinomas; they rarely spread unless neglected, because they grow very slowly and are completely treatable. They are typically nonpigmented, elevated, white, pearly nodules with a central indentation.

Another type of skin cancer is squamous carcinoma; this type of cancer is generally a nonpigmented nodule, fairly well circumscribed, with a roughened, possibly keratotic or mottled surface. These can destroy cells locally, and they can kill if they metastasize and get into the bloodstream.

People get into trouble with skin cancers because they ignore them, so be sure to have any mass that is harder than the surrounding skin examined by a physician.

Dr. Wolf says skin cancers may be readily removable by curetage or excision and suturing, or they can be treated with X-ray therapy. Almost all can be cured if treated early.

Melanomas, the most serious type of skin cancer, account for less than one in a thousand skin cancer cases, although their incidence has been on the rise in recent years (see Step 6). These may be genetic in origin, but are very likely also stimulated by sun exposure. They are frequently multi-colored, containing red, white, or blue areas, or several shades of brown to black, with irregular surfaces and borders. They generally grow rapidly and bleed easily. They are dangerous malignancies.

Melanomas are treatable if caught early, before they have penetrated deeply, but frequently are not caught early enough.

Since one of the greatest contributors to skin cancer is sun exposure, all the doctors we consulted agreed: Once you've had a skin cancer, *don't go back in the sun.* You obviously have a predisposition to skin cancer and are at high risk.

Secrets
of Internationally
Recognized Beauties

Beauty is an elusive quality. Each culture has its own standards of beauty; each generation seeks its own "look," its own style. Yet in all times and places we know a beautiful woman when we see one.

The women quoted below are recognized throughout the world for their beauty. We asked each of them to share with us one beauty secret.

Lynn Sakowitz Wyatt (Mrs. Oscar Wyatt)—
international beauty and wife of the chairman of the board of Coastal Corp.

"I drink six to eight glasses of Evian mineral water each and every day. I also spray it on my face before and after makeup. And even though I have a water well on my grounds, you can still see the Evian trucks delivering my favorite."

B. A. Bentsen (Mrs. Lloyd Bentsen Jr.)—
international beauty and wife of U.S. Senator Lloyd Bentsen, Jr.

"I believe that when spending time outdoors, women should wear both moisturizer and sun block to protect their skin from the ultraviolet rays of the sun. Today we have so many wonderful protective blocks to choose from, each performing on the level we desire, that fashion no longer has to compensate for the sun with hats, gloves, and parasols, as it did at the turn of the century."

Winifred Hirsch (Mrs. Maurice Hirsch)—
international beauty from Houston

"Protect your skin from the sun's harmful rays, and remember that you can't get beauty out of a jar. It begins with the right attitude toward life. Eat a balanced diet and get lots of sleep, seven to eight hours a day keep the lines and wrinkles away. I also believe in the importance of exercise. Choose an exercise you like and get plenty of it."

Rosemarie Stack (Mrs. Robert Stack)—
international beauty

"I feel that women should learn to wear their faces. When talking, avoid frowning, wrinkling your forehead, and pulling down the sides of your mouth. So many women overuse their faces, when they would do better to use their personalities."

Adriana Longoria Banks—
international beauty and wife of Samuel Banks and daughter of business tycoon Eduardo Longoria

"My secret is that beauty is in the eyes of the beholder. I think it was beautifully depicted in the story 'The Enchanted Cottage' in which two physically ugly people fall in love and find themselves shunned by society. They move away from the world and day by day they find that they grow more beautiful in their love for one another. In time, they decide to return to society with their newfound beauty, and lo and behold, people still turn from them in disgust. The message is quite profound, really, and it is to always remember beauty is in the eyes of the beholder."

Marjorie Reed—
international beauty from New York and author of *Marjorie Reed's The Party Book* and *Entertaining All Year Round*

"I truly believe that the passion for living is reflected in your body and in your skin."

Warner Roberts (Mrs. Bob Roberts)—
television personality and hostess for the Warner Roberts Show in Houston, Texas

"Everything in life is attitude, and if you have a beautiful, positive attitude, it produces a beautiful, positive person."

Nellie Connally (Mrs. John Connally)—
the wife of former governor of Texas, secretary of the Navy under Kennedy and secretary of the Treasury under Nixon

"I use soap and water and a good moisturizer on my face. However, I believe true beauty comes from within and shows somehow on every face."

Carolyn Hunt Schoellkopf
(wife of Buddy Schoellkopf and daughter of H. L. Hunt)—
gourmet cook, author, and hotel tycoon

"Recently a new acquaintance told me that she had heard that I eat a little pumpkin every day. Of course, I don't, but I try not to let a day pass without consuming a food containing vitamin A, as all yellow vegetables have not only vitamin A but vitamins B, C, D, E, and all the other vitamins and minerals that I understand are recommended as necessary to maintain good health.

"As a child, I was fortunate to have been served balanced meals of nutritious, fresh foods, grown in our home garden. As an adult, I have maintained my interest in gardening, cooking, and nutrition.

"Few of us are bestowed with the features and shapes considered beautiful by our culture, but the vitality of good health has a glow and beauty of its own. Exercise, sufficient rest and other factors are necessary, but I think that the old saying is true: 'We are what we eat is to our physical health as we are what we think is to our souls.' "

Neile McQueen (Mrs. A. Toffel)—
actress and dancer on both stage and screen

"As a dancer and actress, I understand the importance of exercise, diet, and a good attitude on life."

Gail Bentsen (Mrs. Lloyd Bentsen III
and daughter-in-law of U.S. Senator Lloyd Bentsen, Jr.)—
international beauty

"The security and contentment of both a loving husband and a happy marriage are the very best makeup base known to man, for they create within one a true natural glow."

Joan Schnitzer—
international beauty

"When I need a quick pick-me-up and I want my skin to look wonderful for a special evening, I get an ice cube and I run it over my face. I don't know what it does, but my makeup stays on better and my skin looks better that evening."

Maxine Mesinger (Mrs. Emil Mesinger)—
international Houston beauty and famous gossip columnist

"My skin is very sensitive, so I use Nutroderm to cleanse and Clinique products for other facial treatments, as well as Max Factor Number 1 as a makeup base."

Debra Paget—
star of stage, screen, and television

"People should do everything they can to improve their physical appearance, but should also seek to bring out the uniqueness and inner beauty that God has given all of us. As for beauty tips, no sun, it is your greatest enemy. Always remember to wear a base, and sunblocks. Remember, a warm loving smile can attract more people than skillfully applied makeup."

Mary Ann Mobley (wife of television personality Gary Collins)—
international California beauty, past Miss America, and star of movies, stage, and television

"I think vitamins are the most important part of any beauty routine because having good skin has to come from the inside out. I specifically believe in vitamins E, C, B_6, selenium, and beta carotene. I think selenium and vitamins E and C help keep elasticity in the skin. Also, when my skin gets dry, I clean it and put a layer of Vaseline on, and tissue off the excess. You can do this with your entire body, too."

Jane Dudley (wife of Guilford Dudley, the retired ambassador to Denmark)—
international beauty from Tennessee

"I think that eating a balanced diet, exercising properly, and getting an appropriate amount of sleep are the basis for my beauty regimen."

SECRETS OF INTERNATIONALLY RECOGNIZED BEAUTIES

Joan Benny (daughter of famous comedians Jack Benny and Mary Livingston)—
international beauty from California

"I'm certainly not a 'beauty,' but I have found that I can appear to be beautiful. I do the normal things in the way of body and skin care—night cream, monthly facials, exercise, etc., and although there is no one kind of face-cream color or makeup, style of hair, kind of diet, or set of exercises that works for everyone, I have a secret that I believe *can* work for everyone. *Attitude!* It is how you feel about yourself. Attitude is contagious. If you feel unattractive, in subtler, subconscious ways, your posture, your walk, your facial expressions, how you use your hands—that feeling communicates itself to others. They will see you as you see *you*. When I go out I think beautiful. I hold my head up high and tell myself I'm the most beautiful, glamorous, chic woman at the party—and pray Jacqueline Bisset isn't there!"

Margaret, Duchess of Argyle—
international beauty from Scotland

"I have no great beauty secret, but I believe that whatever your regime, you must keep to it very consistently."

Gene Tierney—
international Houston beauty and star of stage, screen, and television

"I never use soap on my skin, and that's one of my beauty secrets."

C. Z. Guest (Mrs. Winston F. C. Guest)—
international beauty, author of *C. Z. Guest's First Garden* (Putnam's) and *Garden Planner and Datebook* (Crown), and writer of a syndicated garden column

"I am an outdoors person, and spend a great deal of my time in my garden, and with my horses and dogs. I am also blond, with a very delicate, fair skin. As a result, I use a sunblock with a moisture cream underneath. I started looking after my skin at a very early age—even before my debut in Boston—which I feel is essential. One final word: Protect yourself in the sun, for if you could see the damage sun does to the leaves of a plant, you would never venture out unprotected."

Princess Mary Obolensky—
international beauty residing in England and Houston

"For good skin care, I believe in keeping the skin clean with Estée Lauder's Prescriptive Program, twice a day diligently, and using a strong sunblock when in the sun. I also had dermabrasion done by Dr. Ivo Pitanquy several years ago, which helped my skin immeasurably."

Margie McConn—
wife of former Houston Mayor James McConn

"My magic secret for good skin care has been to use soap and water once a day to cleanse my skin. I then use a moisturizing skin-conditioner before applying my makeup, to prevent dryness. Also, in the evening before retiring, I use an eye cream. I hope my secret works as well for someone else as it has for me."

Eva Gabor—
international beauty and famous movie star

"Today there is no such thing as an ugly woman. If your hair is not gorgeous, buy an Eva Gabor wig; if your eyelashes are not long enough, buy a good mascara. But the truth of the matter is that beauty comes from within!"

Louise Cooley (Mrs. Denton Cooley)—
international beauty and wife of famous Houston heart surgeon, Dr. Denton Cooley

"I use La Prairie products because they are rich in collagen and I find them most beneficial to the skin."

Alexandra Marshall—
international beauty

"My favorite beauty line: 'It's hard work being so glamorous. The older I get, the harder I work, the longer it takes, the shorter it lasts, and the less it means.'"

Paula Douglass (Mrs. Sam Douglass)—
international beauty and wife of the chairman of Equus Corporation

"There are some things I feel are essential to having good, clear skin: lots of exercise (aerobic), Phisoderm and H_2O (*cold* aftersplash to close pores), and plenty of rest. Most important is a healthy attitude towards oneself; if you feel good about your life, it will show in your glow."

SECRETS OF INTERNATIONALLY RECOGNIZED BEAUTIES

Marie Curran (Mrs. Michael Curran)—
former Miss Montana and wife of the chairman of the board and president of Curran Goldrus and president of the National Pipeline Contractors Association

"I believe in protecting the skin from the sun by using a sunblock and moisturizer in both summer and winter."

JoAnne Herring (Mrs. Robert Herring)—
international socialite, consul general of the Republic of Pakistan and Kingdom of Morocco and international liaison for multinational companies, and TV personality

"I wear a leotard when I swim or snorkel, and a ski mask when I snow-ski. I believe in staying out of the sun, and as a result, my children refer to me as a pink panther in the summer and the abominable snowman in the winter."

Lollie Lowe (Mrs. Richard Neville Jack)—
president of M. David Lowe Personnel in Houston, Texas

"As the years have passed from my college days to a life complicated by the rituals regarding a 'personal image,' I've had to add several items to my makeup repertoire. They are *crème couvrante* and a lightweight skin-tone cream, which I have become adept at using to conceal and minimize the lines and shadows that additional birthdays inevitably bring to us all."

Laurie Sands (granddaughter of H. L. Hunt)—
Dallas socialite

"I use aloe vera on my skin for everything from sunburn to scratches. My grandfather was one of the first to use aloe vera in his cosmetics, the HLH products."

Betsy Bloomingdale (Mrs. Alfred Bloomingdale)—
international beauty

"Everything in moderation. Discipline is the key to life."

Joanna Carson—
socialite and international beauty

"I don't believe in facials or facial manipulation. I wash my face with soap and water and Buf-Puf three times a week. I believe in all sorts of exercise to keep the glow, and enjoy mostly brisk walking and swimming. I never go to bed with makeup on my face and started to put eye cream around my eyes at age twenty-one."

Victoria McMahon (Mrs. Ed McMahon)—
international beauty

"I studied nutrition, and I am under the care of a nutritionist. I follow her diet and advice as much as possible, and eight to ten glasses of water a day are a must. I cleanse my face at night and, most importantly, I use three creams alternatively. They are Tova 9, Vera Brown Products and Pigments Products. I know that eight hours of sleep are necessary, though with my life-style, it is sometimes difficult to get. Ed and I feel that exercise is so important that we have added an exercise room to our home."

Diane Von Fürstenberg—
chairman of the board, Diane Von Fürstenberg Studio

"Drink a lot of water and stand on your head, as good circulation feeds the skin. Go on a shopping spree alone, and have fun by yourself."

Mary Greenwood—
international beauty and Houston socialite and fundraiser

"The Lord blessed me with good health, a lot of strength, and the desire to be happy. In addition, I take vitamin B_{12} shots regularly for a more supple skin."

Paige Rense—
editor of *Architectural Digest*

"My friend, the makeup artist Antonio Dubois, gave me a beauty tip for traveling that helps me look rested when I'm not at all. I just call room service for a dish of yogurt, unflavored. Instead of eating it, I slather it on my face and lie down flat on the floor, for ten or fifteen minutes. Hot rollers, a hot bath, eye drops, blusher and a quick change into something with white near the face, and no matter how tired I may be, I'm ready to face whoever and whatever."

Eileen Eastham (Mrs. Gerald Eastham)—international beauty, tennis champion, and wife of oil tycoon and chairman of the board of Big E Drilling

"I use La Prairie products for my beauty regime. First I wash and rinse my face thoroughly. Then I smooth the PH balancer all over my entire face. Next I use wrinkle cream, followed by day cream and makeup."

Nina Brown (Mrs. Joseph Brown)—
artist, illustrator, and daughter of steel tycoon Samuel Proler, the inventor of steel prolerizing

"My beauty secret is to combine love and work in my life. I enjoy being productive, and I take time to smell the flowers. I meditate twice a day, and I really do follow the *Beautiful Skin* beauty regime."

Madelyn Renée—
opera star

"Being on the stage with heavy makeup and hot lights, I am well aware of the need for a good skin-care program. I cleanse and rinse my face thoroughly several times a day, apply moisturizer lightly to a damp face and wear very little makeup in my personal life. I always moisturize before going to bed to revitalize my skin."

Laura Sakowitz (Mrs. Robert Sakowitz)—
wife of the chairman of the board of Sakowitz Department Stores

"I follow a beauty regime of washing my face thoroughly and moisturizing both morning and evening. I drink lots of water, eat a balanced diet, and get plenty of exercise. I feel that balance and moderation in all things leads to harmony in my life and that my happy marriage is the best foundation for my glowing skin."

Viscountess Harriet de Rosière (wife of Viscount Paul de Rosière)—
writer for *Town and Country* Magazine

"I swim in sea water, when on a yacht, and leave the sea water on my skin and hair for as long as possible. It makes my skin tighten and my hair wave."

Barbara Hines (wife of prominent investment builder Gerald D. Hines)—
international beauty

"When the mirror tells you that you've done your best, fill your heart with love and your head with positive thoughts, and forget about yourself. For true beauty is genuine animation and warmth of personality."

Louise Shepard (wife of Rear Admiral and former astronaut Alan B. Shepard)—
international beauty

"My beauty secret is joy and not the kind you buy in a bottle but the kind that is within you, that comes from understanding, contentment, and happiness with yourself and is automatically reflected in such things as your smile, the quickness of your responses, the sparkle of your eye, and your general radiance. The nice thing about beauty such as this is that you can pass it on to others."

Margaret Love (wife of Benton Love, chairman of the board and chief executive officer of Texas Commerce Bancshares, Inc.)—
international beauty

"I find that reclining on a slant board is like having a mini-facial, as it gets the circulation going. I enjoy doing my exercises on a slant board while watching David Hartman on 'Good Morning America,' and in that way manage to get three things done at once."

Brenda Duncan (wife of John Duncan, Private Investor)—
international beauty

"A wonderful marriage filled with love and happiness is the best treatment for anyone's skin, as it puts a glow in your cheeks, a gleam in your eyes, and a smile on your lips."

Barbara Hurwitz (wife of Charles Hurwitz, chairman of the board and chief executive officer for MCO Holdings, Inc.; chairman of the board of Federated Development Company; and president and chief executive officer of United Financial Group, Inc.)—
international beauty

My beauty secret includes a busy schedule, yet adequate rest (I need my eight hours), a positive mental attitude, and most importantly, a close, loving family.

Bibliography

Abelove, Lauren. "Diet and Weight Loss," *The Classic Aerobic Woman*, booklet and tape. AER-AER, 5-1000 (London, England).

Abrahamson, Dr. E. M., M.D., and A. W. Pezet. *Body, Mind, and Sugar* (New York: Pyramid Books, 1976).

Alexander, Dale. *Dry Skin and Common Sense* (West Hartford, Connecticut: Witkower Press, 1978).

American Medical Association. *The AMA Book of Skin and Hair Care* (Philadelphia and New York: J. B. Lippincott Company, 1976).

Arpel, Adrien. *Adrien Arpel's 3-Week Crash Makeover/Shapeover Beauty Program* (New York: Pocket Books, 1982).

——. *How To Look 10 Years Younger* (New York: Warner Books, 1981).

Atkins, Dr. Robert C., M.D. *Dr. Atkins Diet Revolution* (New York: David McKay Co., 1972).

——. *Dr. Atkin's Nutrition Breakthrough* (New York: Perigord Press, 1981).

August, Bonnie. *Complete Bonnie August Dress Thin System* (New York: Rawson, Wade Publishers, 1981).

Bailey, Covert. *Fit or Fat?* (Boston: Houghton Mifflin Co., 1977).

Baker, Oleda, and Bill Gale. *29 Forever* (New York: Berkley Publishing Corporation, 1977); excerpt rpt. in *Cosmopolitan* (special beauty edition, summer, 1979): pp. 74–79.

Benson, Herbert, M.D., with Miriam Z. Klipper. *The Relaxation Response* (New York: Avon, 1975).

Birkinshaw, Elsye. *Turn Off Your Age* (Santa Barbara, California: Woodbridge Press Publishing Co., 1980).

Body Forum, The. 2, 3 (April 1977).

BIBLIOGRAPHY

————. 2, 6 (July 1977).

————. 3, 3 (April 1978).

————. 3, 5 (June 1978).

————. 3, 9 (October 1978).

————. 4, 2 (February, 1979).

Brinkley, Christie. *Christie Brinkley's Outdoor Beauty and Fitness Book* (New York: Simon and Schuster, 1983).

Brody, Jane. *Jane Brody's Nutrition Book* (New York: Bantam, 1981).

————. *Jane Brody's Guide to Personal Health* (New York: Avon, 1983).

Brothers, Joyce, Ph.D. *Better Than Ever* (New York: Simon and Schuster, 1975).

Burtis, C. E. *The Fountain of Youth* (New York: Arco, 1964).

Caprio, Frank S., M.D., and Joseph R. Berger. *Helping Yourself with Self-Hypnosis* (Englewood Cliffs, New Jersey: Prentice-Hall, Inc., 1963).

Chase, Deborah. *The Medically Based No-Nonsense Beauty Book* (New York: Pocket Books, 1974).

Cheraskin, E., M.D., D.M.D., and W. M. Ringsdorf, Jr., D.M.D., M.S., with Arline Brecher. *Psychodietetics* (Toronto, New York, and London: Bantam, 1974).

Clark, Linda, M. A. *Face Improvement Through Exercise and Nutrition* (New Canaan, Connecticut: Keats Publishing, Inc., 1973).

————. *Stay Young Longer.* (New York: Jove/HBJ, 1977.)

Cooper, Kenneth H., M.D., M.P.H. *Aerobics* (Philadelphia and New York: J. B. Lippincott Co., 1968).

————. *The Aerobics Program for Total Well-Being* (New York: M. Evans and Company, Inc., 1982).

————. *The Aerobics Way* (New York: Bantam, 1977).

Cooper, Mildred, and Kenneth H. Cooper, M.D., M.P.H. *Aerobics for Women* (New York: Bantam, 1972).

Davis, Adelle. *Let's Eat Right To Keep Fit* (New York: Signet, 1970).

————. *Let's Stay Healthy: A Guide to Lifelong Nutrition* (New York: Harcourt Brace Jovanovich, Inc., 1981).

Dickinson, Peter. *The Fires of Autumn: Sexual Activity in the Middle and Later Years* (New York: Drake Publishers, 1974).

Dufty, William. *Sugar Blues* (New York: Warner Books, 1975).

Elting, Dr. L. Melvin, M.D., and Dr. Seymour Isenberg, M.D. *You Can Be Fat Free Forever* (New York and Baltimore: Penguin Books, Inc., 1974).

Evans, Linda. *Beauty and Exercise* (New York: Wallaby Books, 1983).

Fisher, Seymour. *Understanding the Female Orgasm* (New York: Basic Books, 1973).

Fixx, James F. *The Complete Book of Running* (New York: Random House, 1977).

Flandermeyer, Kenneth L. *Clear Skin* (Boston: Little, Brown and Company, 1979).

Fonda, Jane. *Jane Fonda's Workout Book* (New York: Simon and Schuster, 1981).

Ford, Eileen. *Beauty Now and Forever: Secrets of Beauty After 35* (New York: Simon and Schuster, 1977).

BIBLIOGRAPHY

Fox, Dr. Edward L., Dr. Donald K. Mathews, and Jeffrey N. Bairstow. *I.T.: Interval Training for Lifetime Fitness* (New York: Dial Press, 1974).

Frank, Dr. Benjamin S., with Philip Miele. *Dr. Frank's No-Aging Diet* (New York: Dial Press, 1976).

Frank, Dr. Benjamin S., M.D. *Nucleic Acid Therapy in Aging and Degenerative Disease* (New York: Psychological Library, 1969).

Fredericks, Carlton, Ph.D. *Eating Right for You* (New York: Grosset and Dunlap, 1972).
———. *Psycho-Nutrition* (New York: Grosset and Dunlap, 1976).

Gawain, Shakti. *Creative Visualization* (Mill Valley, California: Whatever Publishing, 1978).

Goldstein, Norman, M.D., F.A.C.P. Dermatology, with Robert B. Stone. *The Skin You Live In* (New York: Hart Publishing Company, Inc., 1978).

Gottlieb, William. "Your Emotions and Your Health: A Woman's Guide," *Spring* (April, 1983), 49–48.

Gross, Joy. *30-Day Way to a Born-Again Body* (New York: Rawson, Wade Publishers, Inc., 1979).

Grossbart, Dr. Ted A., Ph.D. "Bringing Peace to Embattled Skin," *Psychology Today* (February, 1982):55–60.

Hayes-Steinert, Jan. *Your Face After 30* (New York: A and W Publishers, 1978).

Heiman, Julia, and Leslie LoPiccolo. *Becoming Orgasmic: A Sexual Growth Program for Women* (Englewood Cliffs, New Jersey: Prentice-Hall, 1976).

Hensel, Carol. *Carol Hensel's Exercise and Dance* (Cleveland, Ohio: Mirus Music Inc., 1982).

Hittleman, Richard L. *The Yoga Way to Figure and Facial Beauty* (New York: Avon Books, 1970).

Hoehn, Gustave H., M.D. *Acne Can Be Cured* (New York: Arco, 1978).

Hoffer, Abram. *Nutrients to Age Without Senility* (New Canaan, Connecticut: Keats Publishing, 1980).

Isenberg, Dr. Seymour, M.D., and Dr. L. Melvin Elting, M.D. *The 9-Day Wonder Diet* (New York: Dell, 1978).

Jody, Ruth, with Vicki Linder. *Facelift Without Surgery* (Philadelphia and New York: J. B. Lippincott Co., 1979).

Kassorla, Dr. Irene. *Nice Girls Do* (New York: Stratford Press, 1980; Playboy Press, 1982).

Kline-Graber, Georgia, and Benjamin Graber. *Woman's Orgasm: A Guide to Sexual Satisfaction* (Indianapolis: Bobbs-Merrill, 1975).

Kolata, Gina. "Dietary Dogma Disproved," *Science* (29 April 1983):487–488.

Kraus, Barbara. *Calories and Carbohydrates* (New York: Signet, 1981).

Kuntzleman, Charles T., and the Editors of *Consumer Guide, Rating the Exercises* (New York: William Morrow and Company, Inc., 1978).

Ladas, Alice Kahn, Beverly Whipple, and John D. Perry. *The G-Spot and Other Recent Discoveries About Human Sexuality* (New York: Dell, 1983).

Lappé, Frances Moore. *Diet for a Small Planet* (New York: Ballantine Books, 1971).

Lecron, Leslie M. *Self-Hypnotism: The Technique and Its Use in Daily Living* (Englewood Cliffs, New Jersey: Prentice-Hall, 1964).

Leonard, Jon N., Jack L. Hofer, and Nathan Pritikin. *Live Longer Now* (New York: Charter, 1974).

Lesser, Michael. *Nutrition and Vitamin Therapy* (New York: Grove Press, 1980).

Levinson, Daniel J., with Charlotte N. Darrow, Edward B. Klein, Maria H. Levinson, and Braxton McKee. *The Seasons of a Man's Life* (New York: Alfred A. Knopf, 1978).

Livingston, Lida, and Constance Schrader. *Wrinkles: How To Prevent Them; How To Erase Them* (Englewood Cliffs, New Jersey: Prentice-Hall, Inc., 1978).

Lowe, Carl, James W. Nechas, and the Editors of *Prevention Magazine. Whole Body Healing* (Emmaus, Pennsylvania: Rodale Press, 1983).

Lubowe, Irwin I., M.D., F.A.C.A., with Harry L. Ober. *The Modern Guide to Skin Care and Beauty* (New York: E. P. Dutton and Company, Inc., 1973).

Lubowe, Irwin I., M.D., with Barbara Huss. *A Teen-Age Guide to Healthy Skin and Hair* (New York: E. P. Dutton, 1979).

MacLeod, William N., and Gael S. MacLeod. *Mind Over Weight* (Englewood Cliffs, New Jersey: Prentice-Hall, 1981).

Maltz, Maxwell. *Psycho-Cybernetics* (New York: Essandess, 1968).

Mannerberg, Don, M.D., and June Roth. *Aerobic Nutrition* (New York: Hawthorn/ Dutton, 1981).

Masters, William H., M.D., and Virginia E. Johnson. *Human Sexual Response* (Toronto, New York, and London: Bantam, 1980).

McCary, James Leslie, Ph.D. *Human Sexuality* (New York: Van Nostrand Reinhold Co., 1967).

McQuade, Walter, and Ann Aikman. *Stress* (New York: Bantam, 1974).

Morrison, Dr. M., D.C. *How To Radically Improve Your Skin* (New York: Parker Publishing Co., 1981).

Natural Way to a Healthy Skin, The (Emmaus, Pennsylvania: Rodale Press, 1972).

Nourse, Alan Edward. *Clear Skin, Healthy Skin* (New York: Franklin Watts, 1976).

Null, Gary, and Stephen L. Null. *Handbook of Skin and Hair* (New York: Pyramid Books, 1976).

Parrish, John Albert, M.D., Barbara A. Gilchrest, M.D., Thomas B. Fitzpatrick, M.D. *Between You and Me* (Boston, Toronto: Little, Brown and Company, 1978).

Pearson, Durk, and Sandy Shaw. *Life Extension: A Practical Scientific Approach* (New York: Warner Books, 1982).

Ponder, Catherine. *The Healing Secret of the Ages* (West Nyack, New York: Parker Publishing Company, 1967).

—————. *Open Your Mind to Prosperity* (Unity Village, Missouri: Unity Books, 1971).

Pritikin, Nathan. *Pritikin Permanent Weight Loss Manual* (New York: Grosset and Dunlap, 1981).

————, with Patrick M. McGrady, Jr. *The Pritikin Program for Diet and Exercise* (New York: Bantam, 1979).

Reuben, David M., M.D. *The Save Your Life Diet* (New York: Random House, 1975).

Roseboro, Elas. "Poise and Personality," a course in makeup and social graces (University of Houston, Houston, Texas, 1963).

Ross, Milton S. *Skin Health and Beauty* (New York: Funk and Wagnall's, 1969).

Rovner, Sandy. "Healthtalk: Run from the Sun," *Washington Post* (May 6, 1983):B5a.

————. "Psychosomatic: The New Meaning," *Washington Post Health* (April 3, 1985): p. 11.

Rubinstein, Helena, *Helena Rubenstein's Book of the Sun* (New York: Times Books, 1979).

Saffron, M. J. *The 15-Minute-a-Day Natural Face Lift* (Englewood Cliffs, New Jersey: Prentice-Hall, 1979).

————. *Youthlift: How To Firm Your Neck, Chin, and Shoulders, with Minutes-a-Day Exercises* (New York: Warner Books, 1981).

Sassoon, Beverly. *Beauty for Always* (New York: Avon Books, 1982).

Sassoon, Vidal and Beverly Sassoon. *One Year of Beauty and Health* (New York: Simon and Schuster, 1976).

Sattilaro, Anthony J., M.D., with Tom Monte. *Recalled by Life* (New York: Avon, 1982).

Scott, Dr. Michael J., M.D. *Hypnosis in Skin and Allergic Diseases* (Springfield, Illinois: Thomas, 1960).

Selye, Hans, M.D. *The Stress of Life* (New York: McGraw-Hill, 1956).

————. *Stress Without Distress* (New York: Signet, 1974).

Sheehan, Dr. George. *Running and Being: The Total Experience* (New York: Warner Books, 1978).

Shelmire, J. Bedford. *The Art of Being Beautiful* (New York: St. Martin's Press, 1975).

————. *The Art of Looking Younger* (New York: St. Martin's Press, 1973).

Silva, José, and Philip Miele. *The Silva Mind Control Method* (New York: Pocket Books, 1977).

Simonton, O. Carl, M.D., Stephanie Matthews-Simonton, James L. Creighton. *Getting Well Again* (New York: Bantam, 1978).

Slim amd Trim: A Guide for Women Over 35 (West Palm Beach, Florida, et al.: Globe Communications Corporation, 1983).

Smith, Cameron L. *Skin Care for Men and Women Outdoors* (Mountain View, California: World Publishing, 1980).

Somers, Susan. *Beauty after 40* (New York: Dial Press, 1982).

Starr, Bernard D., Ph.D., and Marcella Bakur Weiner, Ed.D., *The Starr-Weiner Report on Sex and Sexuality in the Mature Years* (New York: McGraw-Hill, 1981).

Steinhart, Lawrence. *Beauty Through Health* (New York: Arbor House, 1974).

Sternberg, James H. *Great Skin at Any Age* (New York: St. Martin's Press, 1982).

Stewart, Pat, ed. *U.S. Fitness Book* (New York: Simon and Schuster, 1979).

Stinnet, J. Dwight. *Nutrition and the Immune Response* (Boca Raton, Florida: CRC Press, 1983).

Sullivan, Connie. "Hair and Nutrition," *The Classic Aerobic Woman*, booklet and tape. AER-AER, 5-1000 (London, England).

Szekely, Edmond Bordeaux. *The Golden Door Book of Beauty and Health* (Los Angeles: W. Ritchie Press, 1967).

Taylor, Robert B. *Doctor Taylor's Guide to Healthy Skin for All Ages* (New Rochelle, New York: Arlington House Publishers, 1974).

Thomas, Ilene. *Spot Aerobics* (Arlington, Texas: Upstart Music Co., 1982).

Tremblay, Suzanne. *The Professional Skin Care Manual* (Englewood Cliffs, New Jersey: Prentice-Hall, 1978).

Valmy, Christine. *Esthetics* (New York: Keystone Publishing, 1979).

———. "Skin and Makeup," *The Classic Aerobic Woman*, booklet and tape. AER-AER, 5-1000 (London, England).

Vander, Arthur J. *Nutrition, Stress, and Toxic Chemicals* (Ann Arbor: University of Michigan Press, 1981).

The Editors of *Vogue. Stay Young* (New York: St. Martin's Press, 1981).

Whittlesey, Marietta. *Killer Salt* (New York: Avon Books, 1977).

Williams, Roger J. *Nutrition Against Disease: Environmental Prevention* (New York: Pitman Publishing Corporation, 1971).

Zizmor, Jonathan. *Dr. Zizmor's Skin Care Book* (New York: Holt, Rinehart and Winston, 1977).

———. *Super Skin Deep* (New York: Crowell, 1976).

ABOUT THE AUTHORS

Gail M. Gross has spent the past seven years researching the science of skin care. As a former schoolteacher for the Houston Independent School District, she did undergraduate work at the University of Houston and graduate work at Sam Houston University. Mrs. Gross now lectures on the subject of skin care for major department stores, modeling agencies, health spas, universities, and other organizations. She is currently a skin-care consultant for Continental Airlines and writes a beauty column for *Style Magazine*. She has achieved distinction as one of the few American women to be a member of Lloyd's of London, and has been an active entrepreneur as Vice President of both Gross Interiors and Gross Investment Builders. She is currently on the Board of Directors of Harwell Movie Production Company and is listed in *Who-Houston*. Her writing career began in high school, where she was voted most talented girl in her high school and she earned recognition for her writing, which was featured in the Houston Baptist College Yearbook of 1979. In the same year she continued on, winning national competitions for her poem "The Brace" and her satirical one-act play, "The Passover, pass over," which was later performed by the Maybee Theater in Houston. Mrs. Gross has become a regular on the Warner Roberts daytime TV show, answering questions on health and beauty, and she is currently working on her second book on skin care for women over forty. Mrs. Gross is highly visible in social and civic affairs in Houston, Texas, where she has served on the board of directors of twelve major organizations. As a student of Elena Nikolaidi, long considered the greatest living Greek mezzo-soprano, Mrs. Gross' love of opera led her to chair the Houston Grand Opera Ball of 1982. In 1983 she was elected one of the "Top 10 Best-Dressed Women in Houston." Mrs. Gross is the wife of Jenard Gross, a major real estate developer and Chairman of the Board of United Savings of Texas, and the mother of a 20-year-old daughter, Dawn, and a 17-year-old son, Shawn.

Honora M. Finkelstein has been a writer, researcher, editor, and lecturer for over twenty years. She began her professional career as an officer in the United States Navy, where she edited publications for the Office of Naval Intelligence; she later became the editor of the Center for Management Studies at the Johnson Space Center. She has taught writing and other subjects at several universities, including the University of Houston, where she was elected a member of Phi Kappa Phi Honor Society and received her Ph.D. in English in 1976, and Houston Baptist University, where she was voted "Faculty Woman of the Year for 1979" by the Association of Women Students. She has been an entrepreneur in small press publishing and editorial consulting, and has published in such diverse fields as business technology, consumer protection, Jungian psychology, language usage, and British drama. Her interests in holistic health, psychology, and nutrition are ongoing; she is currently a practitioner of Reiki healing and dream therapy and is working on a book on natural healing. Mrs. Finkelstein resides in Reston, Virginia, with her husband, Jay Finkelstein, a senior space systems engineer with the U.S. Navy, and her four children, Aileen, 20; Kathleen, 18; Bridget, 14; and Michael, 4.

Directions

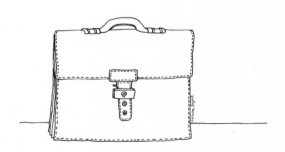

Houghton Mifflin Company
Boston
Dallas
Geneva, Illinois
Hopewell, New Jersey
Palo Alto
London

Thomas D. Bachhuber / University of Maryland

Richard K. Harwood / University of Virginia

Directions:
A guide to career planning

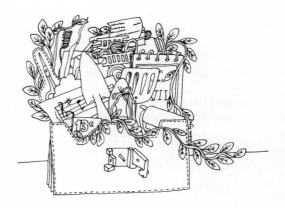

Printed in the U.S.A.

Library of Congress Catalog Card Number: 77-78015

ISBN: 0-395-25385-3

Contents

Preface

The acceptance of the career development movement has led to the publication of an abundance of related materials. Everywhere one turns there are publications dealing with aspects of career development — "T-groups for career growth," an accountability model for justification, a sure-fire way to get *the* job of your life, and so on. Why, then, another book about career planning?

We believe there are several reasons why *Directions* is a uniquely helpful resource. First, while the vast bulk of literature focuses on only one particular facet of career development — career explorations, decision-making, the interview process — this book comprehensively presents the total career development process as we perceive it (see the career development model before page 1) from the point of nondirection to the point of attaining a career position consistent with one's interests, abilities, and aspirations.

Our career development model illustrates in graphic form the steps involved in any person's career development. Additionally, the model unifies the book and relates all the chapters to one another by providing topical guidelines for each chapter. We have tried to present the process of career development, often viewed as both complex and ambiguous, as an understandable and rational program.

Directions is "self-help" in approach and is intended to be a classroom text and resource that can be used according to individual career development needs. The contents are designed to initiate activities and exercises, stimulate career planning, and provide assistance in the accomplishment of the steps of career development.

This book incorporates the concepts of academic planning (course selection, choice of a major or program of study, community college, four-year college, and graduate or professional school selection) within the context of overall career planning. This important decision-making process is usually not discussed in career development literature.

Directions contains exercises, activities, references, and general information that apply to all post-high school students who want or need help in answering the common questions: "Who am I?"; "Where am I going?"; and "How do I get there?"

The authors would like to express their sincere appreciation to James Childress for his cartoons which appear throughout the book. Although we knew Jim only briefly before his death this spring, 1977, his efforts and concern for our project were outstanding. Thanks also to Arlen Twedt, Counselor at Des Moines Area Community College, for his help in the cartoons.

We thank our wives—Leslie and Tinny—for their support, cooperation, and understanding.

Also, a brief word for our children — Libby and Emmy, and Robert, Katy, and Betsy — with the hopes that their futures will be happy, healthy, and influenced by wherever their aspirations take them.

The reviewers, whose help we would like to acknowledge, were: Linda Fowler, Education Commission of the States; J. Donald Mault, Bucks County Community College; Cecil Nichols, Miami-Dade Community College; and Michael Rooney, Meramec Community College.

T.D.B.
R.K.H.

Directions

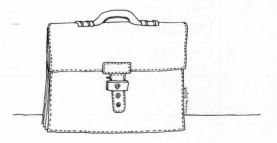

Career development model — Chapter 1

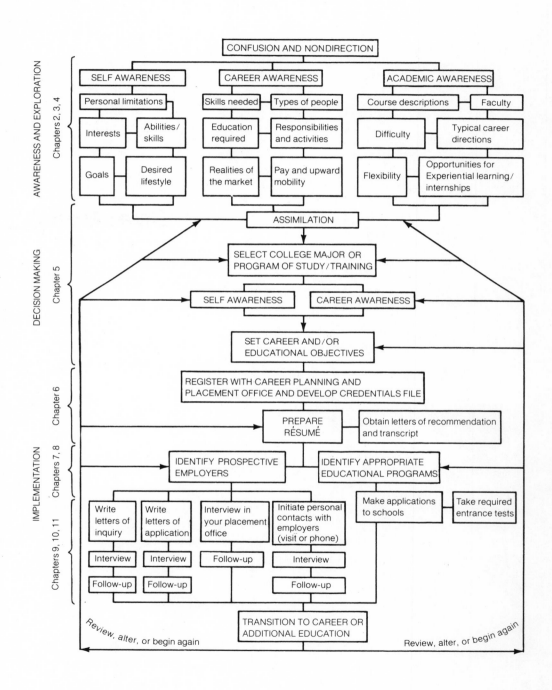

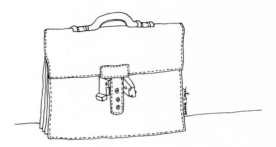

1 Introduction

Career development, life and work planning, and career counseling are all "in" phrases that touch nearly all of us at every education level these days. Unfortunately, as with most "in" phrases, people use them to mean different things.

Definitions

Regarding the comprehensive term *career development*, the word *development* is fairly self-explanatory — it is a process that is sequential, progressive, and usually involves some kind of "growing" on the part of the individual. *Career* is also a fairly understandable term, but it can mean different things to different people. Depending upon your own values, needs, and lifestyle, it can refer to an eight-hour work day that you want to forget or an experience that completely envelops (and provides meaning to) your life. *Career* can also mean a set of skills and interests within a desired lifestyle that remain fairly stable but can be utilized in a series of changing and developing "work settings."* So it seems rather

*Paraphrased by permission of the author and publisher from Peter H. Jacobus, "Liberal Arts: Education and Employability," Pennsylvania Department of Education, Harrisburg, 1973.

odd, then, that when you combine the two, the result is a multimeaning term that includes such limited concepts as placement, career education, and "job finding," to name a few.

For our purposes, *career development* is defined as the sum of the above definitions — simply, a developing, progressing process whereby an individual proceeds from a point of having no career direction to that of attaining a career consistent with his or her interests, abilities, and aspirations. We don't even pretend to get caught up in the psychological jargon that is so much a part of traditional vocational development theories. For our purposes here, we believe that would do more harm than good.

In this context, then, life and work planning (by students) and career counseling (by trained career counselors) are means by which you can progress within this career development process. So much for definitions and "in" phrases.

A model for career development

The model for career development at the beginning of this chapter helps to illustrate this explanation. Take a look at it. Our purpose is to help you progress through any or all of the steps shown in the model. It is our belief that an individual who wants to enter a career happily and successfully will proceed, in most cases, from an awareness of himself or herself, an awareness of programs of study or training (academic awareness), and an awareness of the world of careers — assimilating the three, setting career and educational objectives, and then proceeding to attain those objectives through a systematic job-search strategy.

The contents, activities, and exercises in this book are sequentially compatible with each step in the model. However, they should not be viewed as a final answer or as the solution to all your career-related problems, but rather as *one* means of assistance that we believe can be helpful in your own life and career development.

Take a good look at the career development model and determine where you are in regard to your career-related concerns. Where do they fit into the model? See a career counselor or career planning or placement staff member if you are having difficulty with this initial task. If you encounter difficulties as you proceed through the book or have questions about its content, take these concerns to a career counselor or to an individual in your college or university career planning and placement service. Although this book is intended as a self-help tool, other people can assist you to use it effectively.

With the day of "education for education's sake" quickly departing the campus scene and a major goal of a college education being a viable life career, we believe the emphasis on career development is here to stay. The tight employment market, the oversupply of professionals in many career fields, and the ever-rising costs of a college education necessitate this change. Surveys, too, demonstrate that you, as students, are concerned with your career development. A recent survey by the National Association of

Student Personnel Administrators shows that job placement is the number one concern for a large national sampling of college students. In essence, then, this is the reason for this book — your concern with your career development. You would have quit reading this introduction long before this point if, indeed, you were not concerned.

A need for convincing?

One final word before we begin looking at your own career development process. The fact that you are concerned about who you are and where you are going is encouraging to us. Unfortunately, however, it alone is not sufficient for you to continue with this book and thereby gain assistance in answering these difficult questions. What else is necessary? Some of our colleagues say that although college students are concerned about their career development, they don't have the commitment to hassle with the process that will give them these answers. Students need to be hooked into this process. They need to be convinced that career development is important enough to warrant some time and energy that might otherwise be spent socially, athletically, extracurricularly, or even curricularly.

We don't like to think that we have to hook you into this process — the importance it can play in your life would seem to be a sufficient stimulus. If not, then we'll stoop (just for a minute) to trying to convince you of its importance, and in so doing, encourage you to read the following statements by students and workers alike.* They tell it like it is, and their feelings, fears, joys, anxieties, and wishes illustrate the need for some early planning. Read them carefully and imagine yourself in their situations. It will help you feel some of their sadness and confusion at not being where they want to be — to experience some of their joy at doing what they want to do and knowing that it contributes to a happier life. There is no better way to begin this book and, in so doing, to begin to plan and influence your own life and career.

> I think most of us are looking for a calling, not a job. Most of us, like the assembly line worker, have jobs that are too small for our spirit. Jobs are not big enough for people. (p. xxix)

> I was out of college, an English Lit. major. I looked around for copywriting jobs. The people they wanted had majored in journalism. Okay, the first myth that blew up in my face is that a college education will get you a job. (p. 57)

*From *Working: People Talk about What They Do All Day and How They Feel about What They Do,* by Studs Terkel. Copyright © 1972, 1974 by Studs Terkel. Reprinted by permission of Pantheon Books, a Division of Random House, Inc.

I don't know what I'd like to do. That's what hurts the most. That's why I can't quit the job. I really don't know what talents I have. And, I don't know where to go to find out. I've been fostered so long by school and didn't have time to think about it. (p. 60)

My job as a reservationist was very routine, computerized. I hated it with a passion. Getting sick in the morning, going to work feeling, "Oh, my God! I've got to go to work." (p. 82)

I can't relax. 'Cause when you ask a guy who's fifty-eight years old, "What does a press agent do?", you force me to look back and see what a wasted life I've had. My hopes, my aspirations — what I did with them. What being a press agent does to you. What have I wound up with? Rooms full of clippings. (p. 127)

I consider myself one of the lucky ones because I really enjoy what I do. I love my occupation. But I've spent most of my life working at jobs I hated. I've worked at boring office jobs. I never felt they were demeaning, but they exhausted my energy and spirit. I do think most people work at jobs that mechanize them and depersonalize them. (p. 217)

I'll look at the watch pin on my coverall and see what time . . . you would look at your watch and it would be nine twenty. And you look at your watch again and it's twenty-five minutes of ten. It seems like you worked forever. And it's been roughly fifteen minutes. You want quittin' time so bad. (p. 237)

I usually say I am an accountant. Most people think it's somebody who sits there with a green eyeshade and his sleeves rolled up with a garter, poring over books, adding things — with glasses. (Laughs.) I suppose a certified public accountant has status. It doesn't mean much to me. Do I like the job or don't I? That's important. (p. 351)

I have a couple of friends there. We get together and talk once in a while. At first you're afraid to say anything 'cause you think the guy really loves it. You don't want to say, "I hate it." But then you hear the guy say, "Boy! If it weren't for the money I'd quit right now." (p. 355)

I'd like to go back to college and get a master's or Ph.D. and become a college teacher. The only problem is I don't think I have the smarts for it. When I was in high school I thought I'd be an engineer. So I took math, chemistry, physics, and got my D's. I thought of being a history major. Then I said, "What will I do with a degree in history?" I thought of poli sci. I thought most about going into law. I still think about that. I chose accounting for a very poor reason. I eliminated everything else. Even after I passed my test as a CPA I was saying all along, "I don't want to be an accountant." (Laughs.) I'm young enough. After June I can look around. As for salary, I'm well ahead of my contemporaries. I'm well ahead of those in teaching and slightly ahead of those in engineering. But that isn't it. . . . (p. 355)

"Ever talk about your day's work with your wife?"
"No. She has enough problems of her own." (p. 364)

I'm a couple of days away, I'm very lonesome for this place. When I'm on vacation, I can't wait to go, but two or three days away, I start to get fidgety. I can't stand around and do nothin'. I have to be busy at all times. I look forward to comin' to work. It's a great feelin'. I enjoy it somethin' terrible. (p. 380)

People imagine a waitress couldn't possibly think or have any kind of aspiration other than to serve food. When somebody says to me, "You're great, how come you're *just* a waitress?" *Just* a waitress! I'd say, "Why, don't you deserve to be served by me?" It's implying that he's not worthy, not that I'm not worthy. It makes me irate. I don't feel lowly at all. I myself feel sure. I don't want to change the job. I love it. (p. 391)

All those examples may have overstated our point, but we feel they say a lot and are worthy, a lot of discussion in themselves. All of them are taken directly from *Working* by Studs Terkel. The book is about people and what they say about their work. You may want to explore further by actually reading the book or some of its profiles. *Working* is discussed again in Chapter 4, "Career Awareness," where profiles of people in their careers are also reprinted.

Let's get started. Take a look at the model for career development at the beginning of this chapter, determine where you are, check the table of contents, and begin by exploring the corresponding section of this book. Don't forget to seek out help whenever you develop concerns (write to us, if you like). Best of luck, success, and patience as you progress through this book — as well as through your own career development.

Career development model — Chapter 2

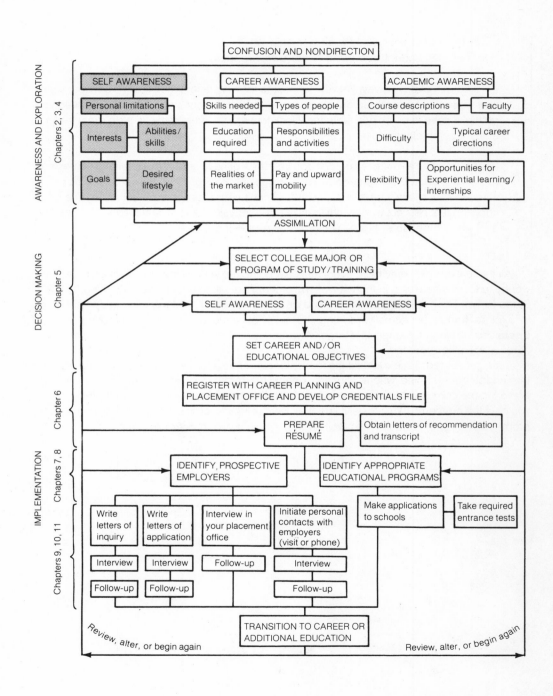

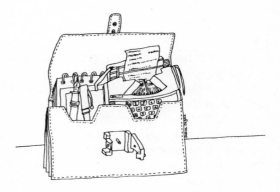

2 Self-awareness

Introduction

Self-awareness is a psychological-sounding term, but when we use it in this book, it means nothing more than knowing yourself — your abilities, skills, interests, goals, lifestyle, and limitations and your similarity to people in different careers. We feel that this is a logical starting point in the sequential steps of your career development. The following questions and activities are intended to "evidence" some of these self-awareness attributes. When you are aware of and have drawn some conclusions about these attributes, they can help you get a better idea of your own particular career direction.

Reading this chapter of *Directions* is not the only method of accomplishing this task. Discussing your interests with a career counselor or using different interest inventories (Strong-Campbell, Kuder, Hall, and others) can also help you get to know yourself better. These inventories must be used carefully, however; not to make decisions for you, but rather as a *single piece of information* in helping you determine a career direction. These inventories give information concerning your interest in doing things and tell you how your interests compare with those of people in different careers. As mentioned previously, these are only a couple of aspects of *self-awareness*. Abilities, limitations, lifestyle, and goals are other important considerations. These can be clarified through other tests or inventories (ACTs, SATs, achievement tests, personality tests, aptitude tests), of course, but due to limitations in these instruments, this information can just as effectively be gathered by answering and drawing conclusions from some of the questions we pose in this section.

One final point before going to the questions and exercises. A relatively new approach to getting at this *self-awareness* has been developed by an educator named John Holland. His *Self Directed Search* (1974) is highly recommended and can be used along with this section. In this approach, you participate in exercises where your reported interests, "feelings," and abilities are tied to broad career fields, which can be classified as realistic, artistic, social, investigative, enterprising, and conventional. There is nothing magical (as sometimes appears in some of the tests and inventories we mentioned) about this tie-in. You can easily see how your answers correspond to the different careers. If self-awareness is your immediate task, we recommend you read the *Self Directed Search* (ask your placement director or career counselor) as well as complete the exercises in this section.

Self-awareness inventory

Daydreams

1. List approximately five careers you've thought, imagined, fantasized, or daydreamed about. Also list in *one or two words* the *major factor* that you found (find) attractive. For example:

lawyer — status
counselor — helping others
plumber — money
computer programmer — working with numbers
forest ranger — being outdoors

Career   *Point(s) of attraction*

_____   _____

_____   _____

_____   _____

_____   _____

_____   _____

"No-way" careers

2. List approximately five careers or jobs that you have always detested or now find totally inconsistent with a potential career direction for you. Also list in one or two words the major reason for this. For example:

doctor — being near sick people
teacher — maintaining discipline

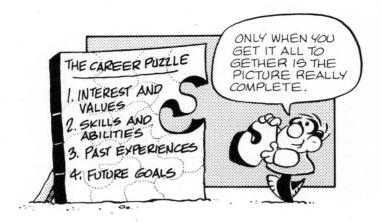

farmer — no vacations
writer — lack of security
career soldier — away from home

Career   *Point(s) of aversion*

_____   _____

_____   _____

_____   _____

_____   _____

_____   _____

_____   _____

Describe briefly in one or two statements, themes or conclusions you can draw from the previous questions. For example, a person who completed the previous section by giving the responses listed in the examples might conclude: "I am interested in a career that will give me status and money, enable me to help others, be outdoors, and work with numbers. I would not want a career in which I was constantly around sick people, was responsible for disciplining others, didn't have guaranteed security, was away from home a lot, or had no free time for vacations."

_____

_____

_____

Likes

3. List about ten activities that are a part of your life and that you enjoy doing. Jot them down as they come to your mind, but after you complete the list, go back and put an * by the *three* you value the most. For example:

talk to people   succeed in class
plan activities   lead groups
read by myself   go to plays

_____   _____

_____   _____

_____   _____

_____   _____

_____   _____

Dislikes

4. List about ten activities that really turn you off and that you may or may not have to contend with in your daily life. As in question 3, go back and star the three worst. For example:

study economics   go to dances
keep my room clean   give speeches

_____   _____

_____   _____

_____   _____

_____   _____

Discuss briefly with a couple of short statements the common themes or conclusions you can draw from questions 3 and 4.

_____

_____

_____

Types of people

5. Think of a few people you either like or admire and then determine what it is about them that makes you feel that way. Do the same thing for people you dislike. List them below. Examples might include

likes the same things I do   personable
funny   honorable
authoritarian   spineless
too technical   rude

Things I like in people   *Things I don't like in people*

_____   _____

_____   _____

_____   _____

_____   _____

_____   _____

What themes or conclusions can you draw? _____

_____

_____

_____

Achievements and abilities

6. List five achievements you've accomplished during the past years that you feel are important. Don't worry about whether or not they were large or small or if they were formally recognized.

Under each achievement, indicate what abilities or traits enabled you to accomplish this task. For example:

Achievement — lost ten pounds
Abilities/traits — self-discipline

Achievement — B in Solid Geometry
Abilities/traits — perseverance, self-discipline

Achievement — captain of track team
Abilities/traits — hard work, popularity

Achievement   _____

Abilities/traits   _____

Achievement   _____

Abilities/traits	_____
Achievement	_____
Abilities/traits	_____
Achievement	_____
Abilities/traits	_____
Achievement	_____
Abilities/traits	_____

7. Rate yourself on the following abilities, traits, and skills as to how you would compare with other college students — either on your campus or as a whole. Circle the appropriate number.

		Comparison		
Ability/skill/trait	*Low*	*Average*		*High*
Writing	1	2	3	4	5
Teaching	1	2	3	4	5
Working outdoors	1	2	3	4	5
Managing	1	2	3	4	5
Math	1	2	3	4	5
Socializing	1	2	3	4	5
Solving problems	1	2	3	4	5
Science	1	2	3	4	5
Foreign languages	1	2	3	4	5
Mechanical	1	2	3	4	5
Athletic	1	2	3	4	5
Leadership	1	2	3	4	5
The fine arts	1	2	3	4	5
Poise	1	2	3	4	5
Confidence	1	2	3	4	5

	Comparison				
Ability/skill/trait	*Low*		*Average*		*High*
Practical	1	2	3	4	5
Adventuresome	1	2	3	4	5
Energetic	1	2	3	4	5
Sales	1	2	3	4	5
Patient	1	2	3	4	5
Persuader	1	2	3	4	5
Efficient	1	2	3	4	5
Sociable	1	2	3	4	5
Serious	1	2	3	4	5
Objective	1	2	3	4	5
Friendly	1	2	3	4	5
Thoughtful	1	2	3	4	5
Cooperative	1	2	3	4	5
Secure	1	2	3	4	5
Data oriented	1	2	3	4	5
People oriented	1	2	3	4	5
Thing oriented	1	2	3	4	5

8. Your SAT or ACT scores:
SAT Verbal: Score _____ ; Percentile _____
SAT Quantitative: Score _____; Percentile _____
ACT Scores: English _____ ; Math _____ ; Social Studies _____ ;
Science _____
Your typical high school grades: Math _____ ; English _____;
Social Studies _____ ; Science _____ ; Business _____ ;
Industrial Arts _____ ; Home Economics _____ ; Other _____
Your typical college grades or what you expect them to be: Math _____;
English _____; Social Studies _____; Science _____;
Mechanical Design _____; Business _____; Other _____

Using your answers to questions 6, 7, and 8, briefly draw conclusions or point out dominant themes. For example: "I have achieved some successes because I am a hard worker, can discipline myself, and am popular with my classmates. Compared with my fellow students I am athletic, energetic, sociable, and poised. I am more data-oriented than people-oriented. I am not particularly adventuresome or serious. My SAT (ACT) scores were better than average; however, I did better in the math (quantitative) area than in the English (verbal) area. In high school I did well in math, science, business, and industrial arts and not so well in English and social studies. I expect my college grades to follow this pattern."

_____

_____

_____

_____

_____

Career values
9. The following list of "career satisfactions" are typical of those that most people value in different careers. Pick out three that seem important to you and three you could care less about.

help society
help people
have power
make a lot of money
work outdoors
travel
have a lot of leisure time
work alone
influence people
work with people with similar interests

security
variety of work
independence
recognition
nice office
specific tasks
responsibility
vacation time
moral fulfillment

Important to me

_____

_____

_____

Not important to me

_____

_____

_____

Conclusions? _____

_____

_____

I want to work with people*

10. When most people are asked the question, "What kind of career do you want?" their first response is often "Well, I know I want to work with people." While that response may sound nice, it really brings us no closer to identifying a career direction. After all, politicians, teachers, counselors, entertainers, service station attendants, and undertakers all "work with people." However, the kinds of interactions and relationships they have with those people are very different. To help you clarify what *you* mean by "I want to work with people," complete the following exercise by checking the categories which best apply to you.

I want to . . .	*Sample occupations*
_____Influence the attitudes, ideas of others	Politician Salesperson Public relations specialist
_____Gather information from people by talking with them	Reporter Writer Research investigator
_____Help people with their personal problems	Counselor Social worker
_____Instruct, mentor other people	Teacher
_____Supervise others in their work	Supervisor Office manager Foreman (woman)
_____Manage the work of others, be responsible for their output, even though not in direct contact with them	City manager Business executive
_____Confront others, present them with difficult decisions	Credit collector Lawyer

*Adapted from *Path: A Career Workbook for Liberal Arts Students,* by Howard E. Figler, copyright © 1975, by permission of the publisher, The Carroll Press, Cranston, R.I.

_____Investigate people through contact with other people	Detective Credit investigator
_____Provide service to others	Travel agent Cafeteria manager Insurance agent Social security representative
_____Mediate between contending parties	Labor negotiator
_____Organize others, bring people together in cooperative efforts	Community organizer Community leader
_____Make decisions about others	Business executive School administrator
_____Socialize with people on a regular basis	Diplomat (foreign service) Entertainer
_____Understand people and study their behavior	Psychologist Film maker Criminologist

Previous work experience

11. List five jobs — either full- or part-time — you have had. In one or two words, state what you liked and disliked about each experience.

Job	*Like*	*Dislike*
_____	_____	_____
_____	_____	_____
_____	_____	_____
_____	_____	_____
_____	_____	_____

Primary "thing(s)" you liked _____

Primary "thing(s)" you disliked _____

_____

Summary
12. Go back to the conclusion part of each section and copy or summarize your responses.

Daydreams _____

_____

_____

Likes and dislikes _____

_____

_____

Types of people _____

_____

_____

Achievements and abilities _____

_____

_____

Career values _____

_____

_____

"People" exercise _____

_____

_____

Previous work experience _____

_____

_____

Career clusters

As we implied in the introduction to this chapter, one way you can view careers and your relationship to them is from an "adjustive orientation" perspective (Holland 1962). In other words, how do you (including your personality, heredity, and culture) "fit" with the types of activities, challenges, and characteristics of different careers? Holland divides careers into six clusters according to the "occupational environment" created by its make-up.

Read the following descriptions and the corresponding career listings for each cluster. Using your information from the summary section, determine what cluster or parts of a cluster are consistent with you.*

A word of caution: All of these clusters include *bold,* descriptive words, and in many cases you may find yourself offended by one of them — especially if you feel you might fit with that cluster. Remember that these clusters are *generalizations* about careers and people. As we are concerned with you *as an individual,* we recommend you *not* reject a cluster because one or two words turn you off. Forget the words and look at the cluster as a *whole.* Also, in regard to the six cluster titles, these are *general* descriptive words and not meant to infer that you are or have to be *conventional,* or *realistic,* or *social,* and so forth to find happiness in a career listed under a particular label. The labels are there to help you organize your thinking — not to pigeonhole you.

Realistic

People with this orientation enjoy activities requiring physical strength or skill, aggressive action, and motor coordination. They prefer dealing with concrete, well-defined problems as opposed to abstract, intangible ones. In a sense, they prefer to "act out," rather than "think through," problems. At times they avoid situations that require verbal and interpersonal skills because they lack such skills compared to others. They conceive of themselves as positive people with generally middle-of-the-road political and economic values. People having this orientation are often typified by their physical strength and skills, their concrete, practical way of dealing with life problems, and their lack of emphasis on social skills and sensitivities.

The "realistic" person succeeds in his or her environment by pursuing goals and tasks that include the objective, concrete evaluation and manipulation of things, tools, and machines and by usually avoiding goals, values, and tasks that require intense, abstract thinking.

The "realistic" person prefers, is trained for, or works at the following careers:

*The career descriptions are paraphrased from John I. Holland, "A Theory of Vocational Choice," *Journal of Counseling Psychology* 6 (1959): 35–45; "Some Explorations of a Theory of Vocational Choices: I. One and Two Year Longitudinal Studies," *Psychological Monographs,* vol. 76, no. 26 (whole no. 545) (1962); *The Psychology of Vocational Choice,* Blaisdell Press, Waltham, Mass., 1966; *Making Vocational Choices: A Theory of Careers,* Prentice-Hall, Englewood Cliffs, N.J., 1973, pp. 14–18. All material paraphrased by permission of the author and the publishers. The career listings are augmented by permission from "Vocational Decision Making Series" (unpublished) by Brian M. Austin, Wake Forest University.

Laborers and Skilled Workers:
  Baker
  Construction worker
  Lineman (woman), carpenter, plumber
  Electronic technician (TV station, laboratory)
  Soda fountain clerk
  Inspector of construction, livestock, machines
  Draftsman (woman)
  Watch repairer
  Mechanic (automobile, airplane)
  Radio operator
  Repair worker (TV and radio, piano, furniture)
  Teamster

Agriculture and Livestock Workers:
  Farmer
  Rancher
  Hunter-trapper

Natural Resource Conservationists:
  Forest ranger
  Fish and wildlife specialist
  Soil expert

Engineers:
  Chemical
  Electrical
  Mechanical
  Civil
  Industrial
  Metallurgical
  Marine

College Faculty:
  Engineering and engineering physics
  Mining
  Vocational agriculture
  Industrial arts

Miscellaneous:
  Weather observer
  Detective, FBI agent
  Mail carrier

Police officer, fire fighter
Laboratory technician (not medical technologist or tester)
Surveyor

Investigative

People with this orientation appear to be task-oriented and generally prefer to "think through" rather than to "act out" problems. They have marked needs to organize and understand the world. They enjoy ambiguous work tasks and "thinking" activities and may possess somewhat unconventional values and attitudes. They at times avoid interpersonal problems that require close, interpersonal relationships with groups of people or with new people from day to day.

The "investigative" person copes with the social and physical environment mainly through the use of intelligence: she or he typically solves problems primarily through the use of ideas, words, and symbols rather than through physical and social skills.

The "investigative" person is characterized by such adjectives as analytical, rational, independent, abstract, cognitive, and perceptive.

Physical and Biological Scientists:
Astronomer
Atomic scientist
Chemist
Geologist
Meteorologist
Physicist
Biologist
Botanist
Naturalist
Zoologist

Related Scientists:
Agronomist
Archeologist
Chiropractor
Computer designer and programmer
Dentist
Surgeon
Optometrist
Pathologist
Scientific research worker
Statistician/mathematician
Veterinarian

Medical technologist
Medical researcher
Experimental psychologist

Science Writers:
Writer of scientific articles
Editor of scientific journal
Science-fiction writer

College Faculty:
Physical and biological sciences
Research science
Experimental psychology
Mathematics
Philosophy
Premedical
Computer design and programming
Astrophysics

Social

People with this orientation prefer teaching or therapeutic roles, which may reflect a desire for socializing in a structured setting. They possess verbal and interpersonal skills. They are also characterized as socially oriented people. Their chief values are humanistic and/or religious. They usually avoid situations requiring intense intellectual problem solving, physical skills, or highly ordered activities, since they prefer to deal with problems through feelings and interpersonal relationships with others.

The "social" person uses social skills and an interest in other people as primary activities and motivations in day-to-day living. The "social" person is typified by social skills and the need for social interactions; characteristics include sociability, social presence, and capacity for status. He or she is concerned with the welfare of the disadvantaged: the poor, uneducated, sick, unstable, young, and aged. In problem solving, there is a reliance on emotions and feelings rather than on intellectual resources alone.

The "social" person usually selects careers in the following:

Religious Workers:
Minister
Priest
Rabbi
Foreign missionary (including medical missionary)
Chaplain in armed forces

Social Science:
- Elementary school teacher
- Guidance counselor, therapist (marriage or vocational counselor, speech therapist, psychiatrist, clinical psychologist)
- High school teacher
- Juvenile delinquency expert
- Nurse
- Playground director
- Social service director
- Doctor
- Student personnel worker
- Recreation leader
- Salvation Army officer
- School principal and superintendent of education, schools, etc.
- Social worker
- YMCA secretary, Boy Scout official, director of welfare agency

College Faculty:
- Theology
- Premedical
- Home economics, dietetics
- Education
- Sociology
- Psychology (except experimental)
- Nursing
- Speech therapy
- Audiology

Miscellaneous:
- Bartender
- Host (hotel, motel)
- Employment interviewer
- Judge
- Public health officer
- Truant officer (education)

Conventional

People in this cluster prefer structured verbal and numerical activities. They achieve many of their goals by avoiding conflict and anxiety aroused by ambiguous situations or problems involving interpersonal relationships and physical skills. Their subordination of personal needs appears to make them generally effective in well-structured tasks.

The "conventional" person selects goals, tasks, and values that are usually sanctioned by custom and society. Accordingly, his or her approach to problems is practical, consistent, and at times lacks spontaneity. His or her personal traits are consistent with this orientation. He or she is well-controlled, neat, sociable, somewhat inflexible, and persevering.

The "conventional" person usually prefers such careers as the following:

Financial Workers:
    Investment broker
    Accountant,(certified public accountant, actuary, auditor, bookkeeper)
    Bank employee
    Budget reviewer, financial analyst
    Teller
    Cost estimator, cost engineer
    Credit investigator
    Rate analyst
    Secretary-treasurer of firm
    Tax expert, internal revenue agent

Office Workers:
    Clerk (post office, payroll, shipping and receiving, etc.)
    Duplicating machine operator
    Office manager
    Secretary and assistant (administrative, executive, legal, etc.)
    Receptionist

College Faculty:
    Accounting
    Banking
    Business (not administration or management)
    Commerce and finance
    Economics

Miscellaneous:
    Timekeeper
    Efficiency expert
    Estimator (book publishing)
    Quality control supervisor
    Records supervisor
    Real estate appraiser
    Statistician (except where theoretical or nonapplied statistician is specified)
    Proofreader
    Library assistant
    Supply officer

Enterprising

People in this cluster prefer to use their verbal skills in situations that provide opportunities for influencing, selling, or leading others. They conceive of themselves as leaders. They avoid well-defined language or work situations requiring long periods of intellectual effort. They differ from people in the conventional orientation in their need for verbal tasks and related skills, their sociability, and their greater concern with status and leadership.

The "enterprising" person selects goals and values and tasks through which she or he can express adventurous, dominant, enthusiastic, energetic, and impulsive qualities. The "enterprising" person is also characterized by persuasive, verbal, extroverted, self-accepting, self-confident, and oral-aggressive attributes.

The "enterprising" cluster includes the following careers:

Sales Personnel:
   Salesperson
   Manufacturer's representative
   Store clerk
   Auctioneer (of products)
   Seller of real estate, insurance, stocks and bonds, etc.

Owners and Managers of a Business, Including:
   Contractor
   Importer
   Investment, finance business, speculator
   Publisher (newspaper, book)
   Business or sports promoter
   Advertiser
   Optician
   Travel consultant
   Business executive and manager (not secretary-treasurer)
   Sales manager, sales engineer
   Foreman (woman) supervisor of production and other people (not machines)
   Directors (of research and development laboratories, etc.; not office manager)
   Lawyers (attorney, counsel or private, or corporation; not judges)

College Faculty:
   Business administration and management
   International relations (foreign service programs)
   Political science and government
   Prelaw, law
   History
   Chief student personnel workers, college administrators

Miscellaneous:
   Ship pilot

Politician (congressional lobbyist, political campaign manager, state governor)
Radio or TV program director, announcer, producer
College president
Diplomat, foreign service officer, United Nations officer
Personnel manager
Labor relations specialist
Insurance claims adjustor
Industrial psychologist

Artistic

In general, people of this orientation prefer dealing with environmental problems through self-expression in artistic media. They usually avoid problems requiring intense inter-personal interaction, a high degree of structuring, or physical skills. They differ from investigative people in that they appear to have a greater need for individualistic expression.

The "artistic" person "accomplishes" in the environment by using feelings, emotions, and imagination to create art forms or products. For the "artistic" person, problem solving involves expressing his or her imagination and taste through the conception and execution of art.

Similarly, she or he relies principally on subjective impressions and fantasies for interpretations of and solutions to environmental problems. The "artistic" person is characterized further by his or her complexity of outlook, independence of judgment, and originality.

The "artistic" person generally pursues the following career directions:

Artists:
Writer, editor (novelist, journalist, newspaper reporter, advertising copywriter)
Artist, designer, decorator (portrait artist, furniture or clothing designer, window decorator, interior decorator, advertising layout artist)
Theatrical artist (actor, stage director)
Musician (arranger, composer)

College Faculty:
Dancing
English
Theater, dramatics
Art
Music
Journalism
Speech (general)
Literature

Miscellaneous:

Art and music critic
Art dealer
Cartoonist
Humorist
Linguist, translator, interpreter

Remember that these paragraphs represent the thinking of one individual and that it is difficult to make generalizations about large groups of people in similar careers. When we do, some people are bound to be offended. To help establish some *beginning* thoughts as to a career direction, however, we feel that the previous exercise can be helpful.

Conclusion

13. Apply the information in the summary section (question 12) to the previous career and people descriptions. Which cluster *seems* to be most consistent with you? (For example: Social) _____

Related careers that appear applicable (For example: guidance counselor, social worker, education faculty member): _____

_____

_____

Parts of different clusters that are applicable to you (For example: Like the "realistic" person, I am emotionally stable and like to work with concrete problems. Like the "conventional" person, I am neat, sociable, and try to approach a problem from a practical point of view): _____

_____

_____

Related careers to these cluster parts (For example: Realistic — carpenter, forest ranger, FBI agent. Conventional — Internal Revenue agent, economics professor, statistician):

_____

_____

Remember also, this exercise does not tell you what career is for you. It simply gives you a piece of information that, it is hoped, will help you to begin to establish a career direction. As these are very tentative directions, the next step of our career development process (model) is to explore these directions — gathering information that will either confirm or revise this beginning step.

Career development model — Chapter 3

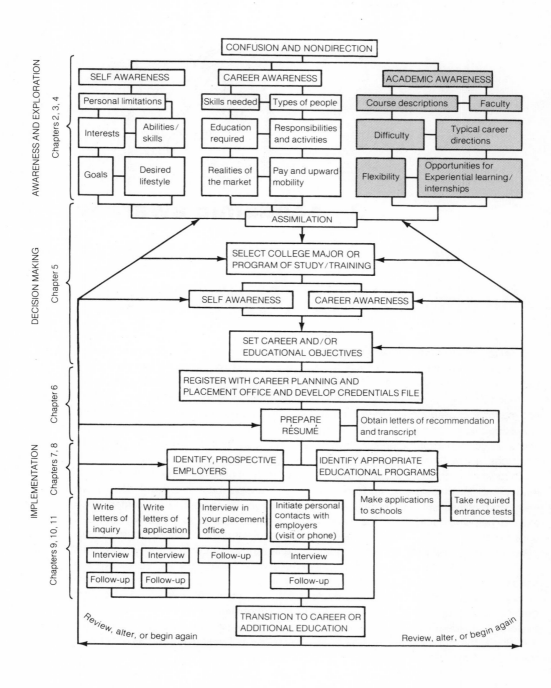

CONFUSION AND NONDIRECTION

AWARENESS AND EXPLORATION — Chapters 2, 3, 4

SELF AWARENESS
- Personal limitations
- Interests
- Abilities / skills
- Goals
- Desired lifestyle

CAREER AWARENESS
- Skills needed
- Types of people
- Education required
- Responsibilities and activities
- Realities of the market
- Pay and upward mobility

ACADEMIC AWARENESS
- Course descriptions
- Faculty
- Difficulty
- Typical career directions
- Flexibility
- Opportunities for Experiential learning / internships

ASSIMILATION

DECISION MAKING — Chapter 5

SELECT COLLEGE MAJOR OR PROGRAM OF STUDY / TRAINING

SELF AWARENESS | CAREER AWARENESS

SET CAREER AND / OR EDUCATIONAL OBJECTIVES

Chapter 6

REGISTER WITH CAREER PLANNING AND PLACEMENT OFFICE AND DEVELOP CREDENTIALS FILE

IMPLEMENTATION — Chapters 7, 8

PREPARE RÉSUMÉ | Obtain letters of recommendation and transcript

IDENTIFY, PROSPECTIVE EMPLOYERS | IDENTIFY APPROPRIATE EDUCATIONAL PROGRAMS

Chapters 9, 10, 11

- Write letters of inquiry
- Write letters of application
- Interview in your placement office
- Initiate personal contacts with employers (visit or phone)
- Make applications to schools
- Take required entrance tests

Interview | Interview | Follow-up | Interview

Follow-up | Follow-up | | Follow-up

TRANSITION TO CAREER OR ADDITIONAL EDUCATION

Review, alter, or begin again   Review, alter, or begin again

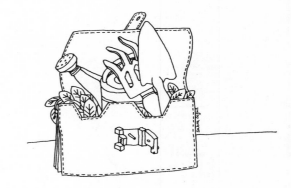

3 Academic awareness

In order to progress from an awareness of yourself and possible career directions gained in Chapter 2, an exploration of these directions as well as the types of preparation necessary for them is essential. This chapter, "Academic Awareness," and Chapter 4, "Career Awareness," will help you to do just that. After you explore preliminary careers and methods of preparing for them, you will be able to answer the key question of whether or not specific fields warrant your consideration and additional exploration. This exploration is a critical part of the career development process, as it is the basis for the future decisions you will make.

In looking specifically at areas of study and preparation at four-year colleges, community and junior colleges, and universities, it is always best to explore descriptive materials that the institutions provide. These can give you up-to-date, specific information that can help you decide which field of study or training is best for you. Most colleges and universities provide catalogs, course description books, booklets describing their major areas of study, and possibly even audio-cassette tapes that contain this information.

This type of exploration can be a point of departure, but you are also encouraged to speak to students, faculty, and staff at your own institution. They can give you personal insight into programs of study and provide information that is valuable and possibly not obtainable through catalog materials. As a final suggestion, check out the college or university's placement operation and ask to see a copy of their survey of graduates. This will tell you the kinds of jobs held by graduates in different majors and areas of study or training and may tell you where they are located.

Whatever your source(s) of information (and we recommend as many different sources as possible), the following questions suggest areas in which you can seek answers. With well-founded answers here, you are on your way to choosing the right program of study for you and, ultimately, gaining a sense of career direction.

1. What is the make-up of this area of study or training? How many courses are offered and what are the opportunities for supporting areas of study and experiential learning? Am I interested in their content?

2. What are the methods of learning in this program: lecture, involvements, experiential, and so forth? What is the average class size? What is the student/faculty ratio?

3. What will my skills and competencies be when I finish this program, and what can I do with them?

4. What kinds of career fields do graduates of this program typically enter and how much difficulty did they have getting that initial position?

5. What are the students like in this field of study or training, and how do my interests compare with theirs?

6. How does the level of difficulty of the program compare with my own abilities and commitment to hard work?

Typical four-year college majors and their related career directions*

Despite our emphasis that the choice of a college major does not *directly* determine one's career choice, it nonetheless has some important bearing. Furthermore, finding the right area of study and gaining applicable "real world" experiences, rather than pursuing an unrelated area of study, can make the entrance to a specific career field considerably easier. Still, the following discussion of college majors and typical career directions is written with a certain amount of caution. You should not infer that curricular choice equals career choice. This point will be emphasized when we discuss the value of a liberal arts education later in this chapter.

Generally speaking, the majority of students in a particular academic program will pursue a beginning career typically and historically related to the discipline in which they major. Thus, the following career *directions* listed by college majors will be of most use to students who are pursuing traditional academic areas.

This does not mean that you must choose a program of study on the basis of career goals. Personal fulfillment, individual interest, and "education for education's sake" are

*From Ralph K. Roberts, "A Guide to Majors and Careers at Virginia Tech.," mimeographed, Blacksburg, Va., 1974. Used by permission.

all viable bases for making this decision. You need to be aware, however, of the potential limitations for postgraduate direction (career, graduate or professional school, et al.) if your choice of a program of study does not take into account planning for the future.

Again, the compilation of majors and careers on the following pages doesn't imply in any way that a history major can only become an historian for a museum or a philosophy major can only teach philosophy, nor does it mean that a business major cannot find a meaningful career in an area other than those mentioned under business. A college education develops skills in communication, problem analysis and synthesis, cooperation, organization, and leadership, to name a few — all of which are applicable to innumerable and varied employment settings. We will discuss this later.

It needs to be emphasized, however, that liberal arts skills and academic learning alone will not guarantee employability. The addition of part-time experience as well as experiential learning (e.g., internships, independent studies, interims, extracurricular activities, volunteer activities, summer and part-time jobs) along with strong supporting courses are necessary to increase your hireability following graduation.

Art

The art graduate has a number of career opportunities, some of which relate directly to the profession, while others incorporate art skills and other competencies. Examples include the following:

Professional artist
Preparation for advanced study in fine or commercial art
Teaching in primary and secondary schools
Curatorial positions, directing, or teaching in museums and galleries
Employment in city recreational departments
Self-employment in setting up community workshops and art classes
Freelance illustration in advertising and commercial art; layout for printers
Directing art programs in nursing homes, hospitals, and veteran's facilities
Employment with a number of government agencies, such as the Bureau of Printing and
    Engraving
Employment with firms that require a liberal arts degree
Directing art programs in large resort hotels
Art librarian (additional study necessary)
Sales representative for art supply firms
Owner or manager of craft and art shops
Directing art programs for United States military bases
Teaching adult education art courses
Publishing, editing, and so forth, of art magazine
Writing books and articles on art
Portrait sculpture or painting
Art critic — newspapers

Art restoration (additional study necessary)
Employment as visiting lecturer — schools, clubs
Employment as artist-in-residence — schools, museums, and so forth
Interior design consulting — offices, restaurants, homes, and others
Graphic design
Fabric design
Greeting card design

Outlook   As in all fine arts areas, employment depends on numerous variables. Your own personal commitment and skills, the effectiveness of your portfolio, your ability to meet people and sell yourself, as well as a certain amount of luck, all contribute to your job search.

The career field of arts administration, which combines art and business management, has a very high demand for qualified graduates.

Business administration and economics
General business

The degree holder in general business may begin careers in any one of numerous positions. Often, the initial position will be in a management training program that will prepare the individual for a specific position in the firm. Following the initial training phase, the individual may be placed in marketing, production, financial analysis, personnel, or another area — depending on his or her interests and abilities. The specific position generally depends on the organization's needs as well as the individual's preference.

Outlook   As long as business enterprise continues to exist in the world, there will be a demand for students in business administration as well as for students who have business-related skills. The current employment outlook for business majors is positive. Although employment opportunities will always be related to the health of the general economy, the major in business administration should not be as severely affected as the individual with a highly specialized degree.

Accounting

Undergraduate degree recipients enter public accounting, private business, industry, or government organizations. Within any of these organizations the graduate may pursue a career in auditing, taxes, or management services. In public accounting the graduate will be providing services to third parties in the form of audited financial statements, tax returns, or various kinds of consulting services. In private industry the accounting graduate will be employed as an internal auditor, accounting supervisor, accounting manager, and in the case of smaller companies, as a controller. A number of individuals may also accept employment with the Internal Revenue Service, the General Accounting Office, or as auditors for other branches of the government.

Outlook Public accounting is enjoying a period of unprecedented growth. Career opportunities ranging from work with the largest public accounting firms to employment with local practitioners are available for qualified accounting graduates. Careers in government service are also open to students in this program. These opportunities range from work with the General Accounting Office through employment with local offices of the Internal Revenue Service. Starting salaries in government are traditionally among the highest paid to accounting graduates.

Economics

As in most fields, job opportunities for economists will depend on economic conditions in the nation. If the nation's economy continues to expand during the 1970s, as business and government leaders predict, there will be increasing opportunities for individuals with economics training. Recent statistics indicate the following distribution with respect to employment of economists: educational institutions, about one-fourth; industry and business, about one-half; and federal government, about one-fifth. Of the remainder, most were employed in private research agencies, and a few were self-employed.

Outlook As stated, the demand for graduates with economics training will depend on the economic health of the nation during the 1970s. As of this date, most predictions are for healthy economic growth, which should indicate a strong market for students with economics training. With respect to earnings, salaries will vary with the type of work performed and with the institution employing the individual. Recent statistics indicate that the median salary for those employed in the field of economics was third in fifteen scientific and technical fields surveyed. Relating specifically to the undergraduate degree, opportunities in banking, general business and industry, and government are also appropriate career directions.

Computer science

Graduates with experience and competency in computer science can expect to be sought by large- and moderate-sized companies, governmental agencies, and many service institutions. As the cost of computer availability continues to decrease, smaller businesses and local governments will increase their demand for computer scientists. Representative job titles for computer science graduates include:

Business applications programmer	Data processor
Computer applications specialist	Information systems analyst
Computer programmer	Scientific applications programmer
Computer programmer/analyst	Systems engineer
Computer scientist	Systems programmer
Computer systems analyst	

Outlook The demand for graduates with computer science training at all levels is quite high and shows no signs of diminishing. With the increasing penetration of the market-place by minicomputers (small, self-contained processors) a growing demand for graduates with a systems perspective is expected. Also, knowledge of data processing and computer utilization can be an asset to almost any career field and is therefore a highly marketable skill for college graduates regardless of their career plans.

Marketing

Graduates earning a degree with an emphasis in marketing have an unlimited number of job opportunities awaiting them on graduation. As industries continue to expand both in the United States and abroad, there is a need for more marketing personnel. Positions are available in many areas of marketing management, such as:

New product development	Sales management
Packaging	Public relations
Marketing research	International marketing
Sales forecasting	Technical sales
Industrial procurement	Pricing
Transportation management	Sales promotion
Advertising agency operation	Media management

Outlook The employment outlook for marketing graduates at all levels continues to be extremely bright. Beginning positions usually include experience in the sales end of marketing, with increasing expertise in marketing and economic analysis needed for advanced positions.

General management

Most students will enter employment in a position related to the production process so that they can fully understand the nature of a company's product or service. Opportunities will follow for them to utilize this knowledge in a more specialized field, such as personnel administration, operations management, or sales management. Increasing numbers of students with management skills are entering public employment at the federal, state, and local levels, as well as in the field of education.

Outlook The employment outlook for graduates interested in management continues to be good. However, the employment outlook is and continues to be related to the health of the economy and will increase or decrease with variations in the business cycle. Demand is strongest for those students who combine a management concentration with knowledge in a technical field, such as engineering or computer science.

Finance and insurance

Finance and insurance are service industries, the fastest growing sector of the labor force. The qualified graduate in a finance and insurance undergraduate area can expect to find the labor market wide open. There is a need for fresh talent in every area of the financial world. The rapid expansion of business and government provides many oportunities for advancement. Many positions are available in the fields of finance and insurance such as:

Controller	Life insurance underwriter
Financial analyst	Property and liability underwriter
Securities analyst	Claims supervisor
Stockbroker	Actuary
Loan officer	Branch manager
Credit manager	Budget officer

Outlook   The future job outlook at the B.A. and M.B.A. or M.S. levels remains very favorable. The job openings listed in the *Wall Street Journal* and in the metropolitan newspapers are extensive. Campus interviewers are unable to meet as many prospects as they would like. Employer requests for qualified individuals far exceed the available supply in finance and insurance.

Public administration

Holders of the bachelor's degree in public administration are employed in a wide variety of jobs on all levels of government as well as in private industry. The most recent earnings figures, as reported in the *Occupational Outlook Handbook, 1972–1973,* listed starting salaries in 1970 for outstanding bachelor's degree holders as about $8,100; however, experienced employees of the federal government earned considerably more. Representative listings of job titles include:

Local	*State*	*Federal*
City manager	Police administration	Civil service
City planner	Public health	Economic and fiscal
Traffic engineer	Highway engineering	specialist
Finance officers	Social insurance	Budget officer
Personnel	Labor relations	Program planning and
Budget officer	Civil engineering	formulation
Accounting	Architectural planning	Investigation
	Recreation officer	Information-gathering
	Budget and fiscal officer	Personnel
		Public assistance
		Economic analyst
		Law enforcement and
		police administration

Outlook   The employment opportunities for public administration graduates are expected to increase rapidly throughout the 1970s. The number of public administration graduates employed in administrative positions will, probably, grow due to an increasing recognition of the value of specialized training in the planning and development of new governmental programs and in the analysis of policy alternatives. College graduates who hold a master's degree in public administration can qualify for a large variety of research and administrative positions not only in government but also in various nonprofit research or civic organizations. An advanced degree in public administration is also useful in obtaining a position with an agency of the federal government that has foreign affairs as its primary emphasis. Holders of the bachelor's degree in public administration may qualify as trainees in research work, in public relations, or in a wide variety of staff positions such as a budget analyst, personnel administrator, and field investigator not only in government but also in industry. Related fields in which public administration training is extremely useful include law, journalism, foreign affairs, personnel, international relations, economics, accounting, and business administration.

Biology
Biology
Many students take special training in the allied health professions and receive advanced degrees in physical therapy, medical technology, occupational therapy, dental hygienics, nursing, and others.

Many industrial firms hire individuals with biology degrees for technical and sales work. Particularly prominent among these companies are pharmaceutical, chemical, drug, and private research firms. Some employment is available in government agencies.

Outlook   Employment for those in the allied health professions is particularly good. There is currently a scarcity of medical technologists, physical therapists, and others in this field.

Employment in the sales field for B.A. degree recipients in biology is also particularly positive. However, technical positions often require additional training. It is advisable for those who are keenly interested in a career in research and teaching to pursue advanced graduate work. The opportunities are greater for those who have earned an M.S. or Ph.D.

Opportunities to teach biology at the secondary level are somewhat limited at this time. However, opportunities still exist for those who are highly motivated in this field. Other career directions include:

Biologist

Research assistant

Science library assistant

Dental or medical assistant or
technologist

Pharmaceutical sales worker

Biological aide (state and
federal government)

Technical aide

Naturalist aide or guide

Game warden

Assistant to primary care physician

Wildlife preservationist
Forestry worker

Environmental scientist
Ecologist/urban planner

Biochemistry
The biochemist is well educated for careers with such federal agencies as the Environmental Protection Agency, the National Institutes of Health, the Food and Drug Administration, the Department of Agriculture, and the Veterans Administration. Typical jobs would include research assistant or clinical chemist. A wide selection of opportunities is available in research with medical institutions as well as with private and state analytical laboratories. Industrial jobs available with such industries as the pharmaceutical, cosmetic, food, and agricultural involve research, quality control, sales, and management. In many areas, advanced degrees are necessary.

Outlook   The employment outlook for biochemists is positive because graduates are uniquely qualified to handle the increasing number of environmental problems that face society. Increased demands are occurring in the areas of environmental protection, clinical chemistry, biochemical pharmacology, and foods and nutrition.

Chemistry
Chemical physics
Nuclear chemistry
Industrial chemistry
Biochemistry
Chemical analysis
Chemical control work
Science librarianship
Pollution control
Recycling and reclamation
Chemistry of pollutants
Ecological chemistry
Chemical consulting

Pesticide development
Plastics
Chemical engineering
Chemistry of medicinals
Medical research
Analytical chemistry
Inorganic chemistry
Physical chemistry
Chemical research
College teaching of chemistry (graduate training necessary)
Scientific jobs in government

Type of work B.A. degree recipients enter
Chemical sales worker
Drug sales worker
Chemical patent lawyer
   (with training in law)
Personal chemical manufacturer
Chemist
Technical library assistant

Medicine and dentistry student
Technical writer
High school chemistry teacher
Scientific instrumentation worker
Chemical marketing, sales, or production worker
Research assistant

Medical technician or analyst
Technical tester
Technical representative
Pharmaceutical representative

Oceanographer
Pollution control officer or specialist
Physician's assistant

See also Biochemistry under Biology description.

Education
Typical career opportunities for degree holders specializing in education include:

Public school teacher (N–12)
Independent school teacher (N–12)
Junior or community college teacher
Four-year college and university teacher
ACTION or Peace Corps–Vista worker
Bureau of Indian Affairs teacher
Teacher in federal correctional institution
Overseas teacher
Education specialist with federal
    government
Curriculum materials specialist with
    publishing house
Educational research specialist with
    publishing house
Communications specialist with
    publishing house
Regional educational laboratories
    researcher
Teacher Corps intern
Job Corps worker
Community action program worker
Advertising worker
Banker
Illustrator
Advertising designer
Community service worker
Educational consultant
Public relations worker
Audio-visual and media education
    specialist
Supervision and administration specialist

Writer
Editor
Promoter
Counselor
Personnel worker
Education and training unit specialist
    in business
Librarian
Public health educator
Social science analyst
Manpower analyst
Social science/work program specialist
State department of education worker
Supervisor
Foundation worker
Materials developer
Lobbyist for professional associations
Computer programmer or specialist
Youth center worker
Adult education worker
Translator
Statistician
Test designer
Evaluator
Special education teacher
Reading specialist
Learning disabilities specialist
Student personnel worker

Outlook   Although the field of teaching is presently *not* undersupplied with teaching candidates, opportunities do exist for those committed to an extensive job search. Geographical flexibility and a willingness to teach in a rural setting are two musts for graduates desiring to teach. Also, part-time experiences during college in activities related to teaching (tutoring, volunteer youth work, etc.) can also make the difference in hireability.

Nontraditional schools, private schools, juvenile homes, day care centers, and adult education centers as well as recreational and youth service-related organizations are potential employment settings for the qualified teacher.

English, speech, and theater
English

Teaching	Secretarial work
Editing	Radio, television, theater, or films
Newspaper reporting	Sales
Personnel management	Advertising
Foundations	Bookstore sales and management
Broadcasting	Public relations
Programming	Television or radio sales

Outlook   The employment area for English majors is becoming increasingly diversified. A recent detailed study shows twenty-three types of big industry that have a need for the services of English majors. The highest percentage of these can be found in personnel relations, followed by sales and marketing, public relations, management, and advertising. Editing and writing, of course, are always in demand. This broadening of occupational horizons for the English major more than offsets the recent tightening of job opportunities in that most familiar job area of all, the teaching of English.

Communications
Such a program prepares the student for both academic and nonacademic professions. Teaching, business, law, the ministry, journalism, and telecommunications are just some of the fields requiring the skills and background of the communications major.

Academic career opportunities exist in elementary and secondary schools as teachers and speech correctionists and in colleges and universities as media specialists and teachers of communications.

The nonacademic world offers career opportunities in business and industry. Representatives of various businesses agree that communications majors make excellent candidates for positions as service representatives, in public relations, in personnel work, and in management training programs. Positions in mass communications — specifically written communications and telecommunications — are available. Journalists, editors, announcers, and technical directors are among the positions that, although they require much on-the-job training, call for the special talents of the communications major.

Outlook   According to Darrell T. Pierson, Director of Personnel and Administration, IBM Information Records Division and Chairman of the Speech Communication Association ad hoc committee to study nonacademic careers for speech communication majors, college graduates with an emphasis in communications must be prepared for a diversity of jobs. His studies indicate that many individuals have been successful in the personnel field and compete favorably for entry-level jobs in public relations. Although positions in personnel, public relations, marketing, management, and administration usually require on-the-job training, the communications background is a valuable tool and asset.

Positions in radio and television are available, but they also require on-the-job training; the communications major has a head start in this field.

In speech science and correction, jobs have always been available; but with new state and federal laws that focus on health and safety standards, new careers in industrial audiology (setting up hearing tests) will be available.

According to Pierson, many health-oriented organizations are forming speaker bureaus to present their viewpoints adequately to the public. Service industries will be another source of jobs for communications graduates. Interesting career openings in social work, community service agencies, the Red Cross, and so forth, should be forthcoming. There will also be more demand for people who can work in recreational facilities with both children and adults.

Theater arts

Consistent with the liberal arts tradition, a significant number of students elect the theater arts major as an enrichment experience. They are, as such, less concerned with the direct and indirect career potentials of their training.

For the majority, however, preliminary occupational training is paramount. Such students are encouraged to investigate two major classifications of employment: jobs that are directly theatrical in nature, and jobs for which undergraduate theater training is desirable, helpful, or possible. In both instances advanced training beyond or coinciding with the undergraduate study is usually required.

Occupational areas that are directly theatrical

Professional acting	Professional stage managing
Professional directing	Theater management
Professional design	Theater education
Professional technical work	Playwriting

Indirect occupational areas

Public recreation

Elementary education

Advertising

Film industry

Professional library work

Museum management

Student personnel work

Interior design and display

Fashion and/or textile design

Commercial art

Commercial photography

Journalism and photojournalism

Publishing

Government media services

Audio-visual work in various industries

Arts management

Sales

Public relations

Personality management

Arts consulting

Speech and speech therapy

Graphic arts and printing

Government art programs

Private art foundations

Outlook   The employment outlook for theater arts graduates continues to improve rapidly. While higher and secondary education remain the chief employment outlets, the rapid expansion of regional theaters, the development and upgrading of dinner theater operations, and the increasing trend toward professional staff positions within community and civic theaters are making valuable contributions. The promised expansion of public recreation operations may further enhance the employment scene. In all instances, the prospective theater arts major should realize that employability is based on more than competent training. Talent remains the critical element, and both talent and training must be matched by an equal portion of good fortune and circumstance.

Foreign languages

Passenger agent, flight attendant,
     or reservations clerk for airlines

Radio announcer

Sales or clerical worker for
     export-import firm

Intelligence agent

Foreign correspondent

Foreign service staff member

Interpreter

United Nations guide

Foreign area specialist in federal
     government

Escort-interpreter, state department

Translator in federal government,
     United Nations, or literary agency

Trainee in foreign department of a bank

Library worker

Public relations writer or representative

Social worker

Court interpreter

Advertising copywriter for overseas
     markets

Travel agent or tour guide

Port receptionist (in port cities)

International motel organizations

Outlook At present there is an oversupply of Ph.D.s in the general area of the humanities, including the field of foreign languages. The demand for well-trained high school and community college teachers, preferably with a master's degree, remains fairly stable. The growth of international business, travel, and government relations is creating increased opportunities in nonacademic fields for the foreign language major. Many foreign language majors go on for master's degrees in business and become very employable in internationally based organizations. Also, at the undergraduate degree area, foreign language majors with strong supporting areas in business and communications are hireable in business and industry with international affiliations.

History

Many history graduates go into the traditional careers: teaching, research, archival work, and government service. Others use a history major as a base for prelaw or premedical preparations. Surprisingly, a major employment trend today is the tendency of large industries to hire history majors for public relations departments. Numerous companies have come to the conclusion that history majors are best prepared to understand and handle programs relating to persons of diverse character.

Owing to the wide variety of job offerings available to history majors, it is not possible to estimate salary ranges. Stipends will continue to depend on both the type of job and the quality of the individual applicant.

Outlook At the moment, the teaching profession has an excess of available and trained personnel. Only the best applicants can expect to obtain suitable employment. In contrast, the field of law needs more persons than it currently has, and industry has displayed no move to abolish the current trend of hiring history majors for public relations work and associated jobs. While many of the areas traditionally employing history graduates are short on job opportunities, a number of new vistas have opened that promise novel and exciting challenges.

It can be helpful to combine a concentration in history with strong supporting course work in business, psychology, and English to increase employment opportunities following graduation.

Mathematics

Mathematics

Computer-related positions (sales for computer-related industry, data processing for industry and government, and systems analysis) and teaching are traditional career opportunities. Mathematics teaching positions appear more prevalent than most other disciplines.

Outlook   At present the employment market is selective, meaning that employers can hire only the most outstanding students. The students choosing nine to fifteen hours each of computer sciences, statistics, and business courses to supplement their mathematics courses are in the stronger positions when seeking employment. Other directions include:

Actuarial trainee   Market research analyst
Computer programmer   Statistician
Mathematician   Surveyor's assistant
Navigator   Cartographer
Meteorologist trainee   Cryptographer
Engineering trainee   Accounting clerk
Engineering scheduler   Operations research analyst
Fiscal analyst   Systems analyst
Insurance underwriter

Statistics

The most frequent employer of graduates with a B.A. has been the federal government. Many of its branches — the Census Bureau; the Department of Health, Education and Welfare, Social and Economic Statistics Administration; the Bureau of Labor Statistics; and others — all employ people with widely varied training and experience. Some departments of the United States government have training programs for beginning employees. These programs supplement their undergraduate studies with specialized training for the job at hand. Other employers include manufacturing and utility companies. Some traditional positions or areas of work are as follows:

Actuarial statistics — insurance companies
Biostatistics — public health department of government
Economic statistics — Departments of Commerce and Labor
Quality control — manufacturing plants
Research and development — many industries especially those producing fuels, foods, and pharmaceuticals
Survey planning and analysis — market research, opinion polls

Outlook   Unlike highly trained personnel in some scientific fields, statisticians are still in demand and receive higher than average salaries. Both the opportunities and the salaries are, of course, much greater for those with graduate degrees than those with only a B.A.

With the growing interest in pollution control and environmental impact studies, there is increasing demand for statisticians with training in biology and sanitary engineering.

Also see Computer Specialists under *Business Administration*.

Music

Although the B.A. in music is not a terminal degree, there are many opportunities in music-related fields for persons holding the degree. The following is an outline of some of these fields:

A. Professional positions
    1. Composer
    2. Performer
       a. Available areas for the above:
          1. Studio recording — film, television, radio
          2. Theater orchestras
          3. Popular bands
          4. Orchestras — symphony, ballet, opera, studio
B. Academic positions
    1. Teaching — elementary, secondary, college, supervision, coordination
    2. Performance — solo, band, choral, chamber, symphonic, conducting
    3. Research — musicology, acoustics, design, social
C. Commercial positions
    1. Sales — instruments, recordings, compositions, publications
    2. Publications — individual, company
    3. Consultants — historian, programmer, mass media, advertising acoustician
D. Civic Directors
    1. Religious
    2. Secular
    3. Educational
    4. Community development

Outlook   The employment outlook for music graduates remains positive. Degree recipients in music from schools throughout the nation have either continued with graduate studies, accepted positions, or gone into private practice.

Physics

Physics

Physicists have traditionally found employment throughout industry, but particularly with those industries in the forefront of new development relying heavily on electronics and related instrumentation, especially computers. Career directions are extremely varied.

Physics	Medicine
Biophysics	Environmental sciences
Chemical physics	Engineering
Mathematics	Law
High school teaching	Politics

Astronomy	Space technology
Computer science	Oceanography
Engineering physics	Radiology
Instrumentation	Radiation safety
Nuclear science	Industrial research

With an undergraduate degree in physics, supported by courses in mathematics, communications, and computer application, an individual has a wide range of opportunities available. Education, sales, assisting in research, environmental areas, city planning, and journalism are just a few ideas.

For the undergraduate major, the ability to apply part-time work experience and classroom or private research to an industrial operation can increase chances for finding employment. Researching employers thoroughly and identifying employment areas where undergraduate skills and learnings are applicable can make the critical difference in attaining a job.

Outlook   Until the late 1960s the appetite of employers for physicists at all levels and in all specialties appeared nearly insatiable. Reduction in government support for research and curtailment of much aerospace work brought about a sharp decline in the number of students in physics and in most fields of engineering. Demand now seems to be catching up with supply, and it is anticipated that within the next two or three years, there will, once again, be many more jobs for degree recipients in physics than persons trained to fill them. This should be followed by an improvement in the job prospects for persons holding graduate degrees.

Graduate school in physics

Approximately three-fourths of the students in physics who can qualify for graduate or other professional training do so. In the recent past, physics undergraduates were strongly encouraged to go on to graduate school in physics. In the present job market, only the best and most enthusiastic students receive this encouragement officially, although they are subject to heavy recruiting pressure from graduate programs. An increasing fraction of physics undergraduates are going to graduate school in applied science fields and in professional fields such as law, business, and medicine.

Physical education

Health and physical education — directors, administrators, teachers, and coaches in public and private elementary and secondary schools, colleges, and universities. See descriptions under Teacher Education.

Government — organizer or administrator of physical activities programs for the Armed Forces.

Public recreation and park departments — supervisors, center directors, specialists, and other in federal, state, and local governments.

Youth service agencies — executives, assistants, and specialists in such organizations as the Boy Scouts, Girl Scouts, Camp Fire Girls, YMCA, YWCA.

Industrial and commercial recreation — recreation directors in resorts, airlines, and industrial enterprises.

Ill, handicapped, and aged: — directors, supervisors, and leaders in various hospitals, penal institutions, and schools in related areas of health, physical education, and recreation.

Outlook   Physical education is becoming a more prevalent force in our schools and in society as a whole. Skilled and experienced personnel are needed in community, educational, and governmental organizations to develop, administer, and teach physical education programs. One's skill and competency in the health sciences, leadership, and business administration can be an asset to these positions. (Also see "Outlook" under Teacher Education).

Philosophy and religion

A student majoring in philosphy receives a strong liberal arts education, with courses in other fields reinforcing his or her major. With liberal arts education as a primary objective, the student will be prepared to adapt himself or herself for a number of careers. He or she should not regard his or her academic background as a limiting factor, but should consult his or her own interests and aptitudes in considering a particular direction. Under-graduate philosophy majors can consider graduate work in law, the ministry, and other fields of employment in the wide variety of occupations open to liberal arts majors. As in other liberal arts areas, strong supporting course areas in business, psychology, English, and/or education can increase employment opportunities following graduation. Also, part-time work or experiential learning as well as a sound knowledge of his or her skills can result in increased hireability for the candidate.

Outlook   Graduates have gone into teaching, nursing, the ministry, law, business, the professional military, public service, and industry. Philosophy can enrich the student's background in other liberal arts and sciences. Philosophers seek to clarify basic concepts and principles and to explore interrelationships between fields of study. Since there is no final, fixed subject matter called philosophy, and since the examination of philosophical issues (like other liberal studies) is intended to open the mind, not to close it, philosophy students should be adaptable to a variety of roles.

Political science

Political science

The political science curriculum is not specifically job- or career-oriented. It is intended to complement a general education in the liberal arts or in fields that train one for a specific occupation. Students interested in career development may request individual advice on ways to use elective credit hours in pursuit of a particular career or credential. The range, scope, and variety of career objectives that a student may pursue as an undergraduate are limited only by the student's imagination and the courses the college has to offer.

Political science majors have chosen traditionally to use their degrees as bases for careers in secondary and college teaching, law, government service, journalism, public relations, political consulting, survey research, business, and politics.

Outlook   The employment outlook for people with a bachelor's degree in political science changes constantly. At this writing, careers in state and local government are particularly promising for students with elective hours in business, economics, accounting, and urban affairs. Law school is also a typical direction for political science majors. On the other hand, careers in education, particularly high school teaching, seem less bright than five years ago. Positions in higher education seem also to be more restricted than previously.

International studies

There is no typical job for individuals studying an "international discipline." Civilians working for governmental agencies abroad perform specific tasks in given categories. Missionaries do a variety of jobs besides teaching and preaching. Multinational corporations have various employment needs. Airline and travel industry functions are also varied.

Outlook   The employment outlook in international study-related occupations is cautiously positive. Some majors choose to go on to graduate school, but such students are usually interested in further academic study and probably will teach in the field. Overseas job openings should continue to hold strong for the foreseeable future; the multinational corporation is here to stay. It should be noted that the process of obtaining a job overseas either with an international company in the states or an organization abroad is a difficult and complex one. The graduate should be committed to lots of hard work to secure such a position.

Psychology

With this undergraduate background, students are prepared to enter occupations for which a liberal arts education is sufficient. Graduates typically accept positions with prisons, courts, school systems, rehabilitation centers, schools, industry, and governmental agencies. Some representative duties include those of personnel officer, research technician, probation officer, social work trainee, and behavior technician.

Outlook   It is important to note that a career as a professional psychologist requires graduate training, usually at the master's or doctoral level. About 25 percent of undergraduate psychology majors enter graduate school each year in order to become professional psychologists in subspecialties such as clinical psychology, counseling psychology, developmental psychology, educational psychology, engineering psychology, experimental psychology, industrial psychology, physiological psychology, school psychology, and social psychology.

Sociology

Sociology

An undergraduate degree in sociology does not prepare anyone for a particular job. It is, however, a degree that can be used as a steppingstone toward a variety of career objectives, including medicine, law, education, and social service. Relative to social service activities, a sociology degree combined with part-time and extracurricular activities can produce skills necessary for careers in youth services, recreation, and community agencies as well as government organizations. Examples include:

Councils of social agencies
Social service exchanges
Church Social service departments
Charities
Public opinion research
Human relations studies
Departments of public recreation
Foster home placement
Aid to families with dependent children
Hospital social services

Juvenile courts
Peace Corps and related overseas
 service
Workman's Compensation Bureau
American Red Cross
Pension bureaus
Youth groups
Detention homes
Penal institutions

Outlook   If you plan to terminate your formal education with a B.S. in sociology and have chosen one of the narrow specialties outlined in this report, you should not expect many recruiters to visit campus looking for you during your senior year. Rather, you will have to actively seek off-campus interviews to obtain the kind of job for which you have attempted to prepare yourself. Therefore, you must be able to develop a good résumé that emphasizes those skills, talents, experiences, and courses that are likely to qualify you for the job you seek. Also, remember that you should seek to develop a wide circle of acquaintances who can provide good letters of recommendation when you apply for a job.

Urban affairs

Students interested in such areas of concern as housing, transportation, public service delivery systems, recreation, the management of public resources, poverty and social justice programs, or in general, how the city functions (or fails to function) in response to social, economic, and political demands will find adequate opportunity to explore these issues in an urban affairs curriculum. Although this is not a formal part of a sociology curriculum, the relationship of issues allows us to discuss it in this context. Students graduating from this type of program will find a wide range of challenging careers in public service (government, social service agencies, housing and redevelopment authorities, urban planning, human resource councils, and so on); additionally, they will have an excellent background for graduate studies in urban affairs, urban and public administration, and related fields.

Liberal arts in general

Despite the complexity and diversity of the following list, the key to its effective use is student *exploration*. If you can identify job titles that strike a chord of interest and then explore resources (written or personal) that give you information about that particular career area, you can develop your interests. Once you have solidified your objectives or decided on areas of continued interest, additional exploration in terms of curricular and experiential planning can result in positive directions. *Not* that this planning commits you to a particular career field, but rather that through continued exploration you can develop a sense of direction based on interests, abilities, and aspirations. Other career options for persons with a concentration in the liberal arts include:

Community action worker
Community agency worker
Foreign service officer
City planning trainee
Anthropologist
Archeologist
Assistant to curator, museum consultant
Classification worker
Exhibit arranger
Field assistant
Library assistant
Airlines worker
International organization worker
Tourist guide
Travel agent
Intelligence agency analyst
Business librarian
Economic survey aide or interviewer
Market research aide or interviewer
Assistant to labor or agricultural
   economist

Test development assistant
Test administrator and scorer
Social science research trainee
Occupational analyst trainee
Personnel research trainee
Preschool educator
Clinical assistant
Employment interviewer or counselor
Educational counselor or assistant
Personnel administrative trainee
Social work aide
Parish worker, social worker
Philosopher
Theologian
Counselor
Clergyman (woman)
Missionary
Evangelist
Lay church worker
Researcher
Research aide (market, population,

Financial analyst
Housing administration trainee
Data processing system specialist
Industrial or labor relations trainee
Assistant to production manager
Statistical aide or clerk
Systems analyst
Urban planner
Geographer
Map librarian
Cartographer
Map worker
Weather observer
Military, diplomatic, economic, social, cultural, or geneological historian
Diplomatic or consular assistant
Historian
Archivist assistant
Reference librarian's assistant
Museum assistant
Researcher
Survey assistant
Lobbyist
Budget assistant
Administrative and budget analysis trainee
Labor organizer
Training assistant
Public opinion or market research analyst
Second lieutenant or ensign in armed forces
Teacher

public opinion, migration, or class stratification studies)
Juvenile delinquency specialist, investigator
Hospital case worker
Probation and parole officer
Recreation or camp leader
Welfare aide (housing, case work, or race relations)
Labor research trainee or assistant
Criminologist trainee
Labor relations trainee
Administrative assistant
Bank officer trainee
Business or executive trainee
Claims examiner
Credit investigator
Government service trainee
Human resources trainee
Insurance underwriter
Interviewer (community or other studies)
Laboratory assistant or aide
Management trainee
Personnel assistant
Research assistant or aide
Salesperson
Security analysis trainee
Service representative
Writer

An argument for liberal arts

Oh liberal arts please tell me true
Just why am I involved with you?
For investment or consumption
What, pray tell, is your main function?

Scholars advise, "Do what you can,
Develop yourself as a Renaissance Man;

Always search for the ultimate TRUTH
On bathroom walls or telephone booths."

So, I've taken English, History and Psych;
Studied Shakespeare, Gibbon and Reich.
Read philosophy with persistance,
And questioned the value of existence.

Graduation's here — I'm very annoyed
Joining the ranks of the unemployed.
Interviewed by everyone under the sun;
Jack of all trades, master of none.

What's the goal of education?
Years of futile preparation?
For you L.A. I hardly can clap;
'Tween you and reality — a credibility gap!*

In the above poem Mr. Jacobus gives us one example of the frustration felt by many students who do not understand the meaning of a liberal arts education. Through the following discussion, as well as the sections on identifying and demonstrating skills and the Bolles approach to the job search in Chapter 5, you will see that it is the student's outlook, not liberal arts, that put him or her in the "ranks of the unemployed."

One of the most controversial arguments facing college students, high school graduates, their related institutions, and their parents concerns the value (or lack thereof) of a liberal arts education. In other words, where can one go and what can one do with a liberal arts degree? From our point of view, many people suffer from the frustration and misunderstanding illustrated in the foregoing poem, particularly regarding the idea that liberal arts graduates are not readily employable. Our position quickly dispels such views. (Such a viewpoint is quite understandable — it is not so much nonsensical as it is ill informed.)

You have only to look at the number of individuals in high-level positions throughout business, industry, education, social and community services, and government to see that a liberal arts education can prepare a person for almost any career. Unequivocally, a vast majority of these high-level position holders have backgrounds in the liberal arts. The old idea that liberal arts graduates either teach or work for the government is ridiculous. Supporting this belief, refer to the previous section, "Typical College Majors

*From Peter H. Jacobus, "Liberal Arts: Education and Employability," Pennsylvania Department of Education, Harrisburg, 1973. Used by permission of the author and the Pennsylvania Department of Education.

and Their Typical Career Directions,'' and view the wide range of career directions resulting from liberal arts majors. There are too many to even discuss in this context.

Need more factual information? Check out *What Can I Do with a Major In?* by Lawrence Malnig and Sandra Morrow. It contains research results that demonstrate that liberal arts graduates are presently in as wide a range of career fields as imaginable. Philosophy majors are business executives, science majors are educational administrators, English majors are accountants, and the list goes on and on. The conclusions from this are numerous, but we will discuss only the following three:

1. The choice of an academic major has some influence on, but by no means completely determines, one's career. Specialized and graduate education beyond the four-year degree or part-time experience outside one's major area of study, combined with numerous other factors, can result in hireability for other career fields.

2. The kinds of skills, interests, motivations, and aspirations that come from a liberal arts education as a whole — not merely an academic major, but also extracurricular activities, part-time work experience, independent studies, hobbies, internships, etc. — help one to function effectively in a wide variety of work settings. Briefly, liberal arts develops skills that are applicable to, and needed by, employers. The key is for you to know explicitly what those skills are in your own case (''self-awareness'' sound familiar?) and how they fit explicitly with work situations. (You might look ahead to Chapter 4, ''Career Awareness,'' as well as to the description of Richard Bolles's job-search approach in Chapter 10 for supplemental information.)

3. Attaining a job is a very individualized process, and your success is determined by a lot of immeasurable factors: personal commitment, individual skills in selling yourself, access to resources that identify employment vacancies or organizations, being in the right place at the right time . . . to continue the list would just be boring and serve no purpose. To illustrate: An English major with mathematical skills, whose ambitions are goal oriented, who can sell herself or himself, and who is in the right place at the right time could get a job as an underwriter for an insurance company — a position traditionally filled by a person with a mathematics background. To restate the point — an individual who is career-directed and can market his or her skills to an employer can obtain a job regardless of the academic major. Needless to say, there are no guarantees (there never are, unfortunately) . . . just a strong optimistic statement that emphasizes skill identification, personal commitment, and plain hard work, while simultaneously deemphasizing the content of academic learning within a college major as it applies to the job-search process. This is *not* to say that one's cumulative education from a major field of study has no bearing on a career direction. In certain situations (usually where technical expertise is required) and with certain employers, especially when combined with worthwhile experiences, the right major can be important. However, if you do not have the right major, you should by no means be deterred from pursuing a position consistent with your interests, skills, and goals.

In quick summary, a liberal arts education can in itself be career preparation. For what? For just about anything you want it to be! Needless to say, this does not mean you can drift through four years of college majoring in anything, and presto, upon graduation, you'll have ten job offers waiting for you. No way!

However, if you have selected a college major that is consistent with your interest, skills, and a broad career direction; included courses that not only bolster this major but also provide a breadth of learning; involved yourself in extracurricular, practical, and experiential activities (internships, volunteer tutoring, summer or part-time jobs, independent studies, etc.); explored the work-world structure by talking to employers, determining how your skills and background fit into this work world, and finally, during your senior year, developing successful marketing techniques for these skills (résumé, interviewing confidence, letter writing, and credentials file), *you are extremely employable!*

Sound hard and complicated? Not really. It takes commitment (no more lectures on commitment, don't worry), but it honestly doesn't detract from an enjoyment of your college experience. And the benefits? Suffice it to say that the contentment and confidence of knowing where you're going and how you're going to get there are pretty worthwhile.

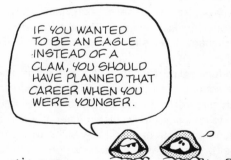

Typical community college programs of study or training and related career directions

As earlier emphasized, the best source of information about any college's program of academic studies available to students is a catalog or printed material from that particular institution. Community college programs vary considerably depending on their location and specialization. The following discussion and listing is representative of the programs of study or training typically offered at a comprehensive community college, a college offering both technical and certificate programs as well as liberal arts courses for transfer to a four-year college.

Because you must choose a program of study at a community college very early — usually as early as first-term registration — the question of which program is critical. Decisions basically involve the following considerations:

1. Select a program that you can transfer to a four-year college or one that you complete in one or two years at the community college.
2. Decide on an area of specialization consistent with your answer to consideration 1.
3. Consider length of program and whether it is a degree (Associate of Arts or Associate of Science — usually two years) or a certificate program (less than two years).
4. If you plan to transfer to a four-year college or university, decide whether you want to specialize at the community college (business administration, journalism, etc.) or just take general liberal arts.

Ideally, you should explore your own interests, abilities, and aspirations as well as the options available at the community college prior to registration — possibly during the orientation period or, better still, during the latter part of your senior year in high school. If you plan to transfer to a four-year college or university and are taking general liberal arts courses (math, English, science, history, etc.), this decision may not be so critical yet. Before registration, however, it is a good idea to study the following programs (here and in the college's catalog) and answer the ever-present questions: Where do I want to go? Which program will best take me there? Review "Self-awareness," look ahead to Chapter 5 on decision making, and talk to your counselor if it's time to answer these questions. It's probably *not* too early.

An outline of community college programs*

Agriculture

Agribusiness
Agricultural power and machinery
Agricultural resources
Agricultural supplies and services
Agronomy
Animal science — horses
Animal science — production
   management
Floriculture
Horticulture
Natural resources management and
   security

Landscape nursery and garden center
Parks and natural resources
Recreation grounds management
Turf management
Wildlife and range management

Business

Accountant specialist
Accounting (junior)
Aviation administration
Bank and finance

*Contributed especially for this book by Daniel Schaeffer, Professor of Business Education, Kirkwood Community College. Used by permission.

Data processing
    computer programmer
    key punch operator
    systems analyst
    computer operator
Fashion merchandising
Finance and credit
Food marketing
Home furnishing
Hospitality industry
    food service management
    hotel-motel management
    institutional management
Industrial marketing
Insurance
International trade
Petroleum
Public relations and advertising
Real estate
Retail management
Secretarial science
    clerk typist
    receptionist
    administrative secretary
    general secretary
    insurance secretary
    legal secretary
    medical secretary
Traffic and transportation management

Health occupations
Dental assistance
Dental laboratory technology
Dietetics
Environmental health assistance
Environmental health technology
Health care facility administration
Medical assistance
Medical emergency technology
Medical laboratory assisting

Medical laboratory technology
Nursing assistance (aide)
Nursing (A.A. degree)
Occupational therapy assistance
Operating room technology
Orthopedic physicians assistance
Practical nursing
Respiratory therapy
Surgical technology

Trade and industrial
Air conditioning
Aircraft maintenance
Architectural drafting
Automotive mechanics
Automotive collision repair
Automotive repair
Broadcast engineer
Chemical engineering
Civil engineering
Construction
    building construction
    cabinet making
    carpentry
    masonry
    plumbing
    welding
Commercial art occupations
Commercial photography
Cosmetology
Custodial services
Diesel mechanics
Drafting, mechanical
Drafting, structural
Electrician
Electronic communications
Electronic computer maintenance
Electronics engineering
Food service (cook/chef)
Graphic arts

Heavy equipment — construction
Industrial electrician
Industrial electronics
Industrial management
Lineman (woman)
Machine operations
Machine shop
Meat cutting
Mechanical engineering technology
Piano tuning
Radio/television
Tool-and-die making
Truck driving
Welding and cutting

Public and human services
Air traffic control
Community and social services
Corrections science
Educational services
    child care worker
    early childhood development assistant
    teacher/aide
Fire science
Governmental services
Institutional security

Police science
Public administration
Recreation and parks
Cosmetology
Media technician
Mental health worker
Radio broadcasting
Library technology

College transfer
Art
Art education
Fine arts
Liberal arts
Music
Theater arts
Journalism
Business administration
Education/teaching
Engineering
Science
International trade
Library science
Law enforcement

Program descriptions (nontransfer)*

The following descriptions are elaborations on selected examples of the above programs. As these are just a sampling, you are encouraged to consult your community college catalogs for additional program descriptions.

Accounting

Accountant specialist   The two-year accountant specialist program is designed to provide students with general and specialized accounting courses. Students typically spend a portion of the two years in an on-the-job business internship to gain actual work

*Contributed especially for this book by Daniel Schaeffer, Professor of Business Education, Kirkwood Community College. Used by permission.

experience. In addition to terminal training in accounting, the program is flexible and is usually readily adaptable to a transfer program.

Career opportunities
Cost accountant
Payroll clerk
Governmental accountant
Office manager
Internal accountant
General accountant
Accounting clerk

Salary range
$450–$900 per month starting

Junior accounting   Junior Accounting is usually a short-term (one year) program designed to provide a fundamental knowledge of accounting, understanding of basic concepts, familiarity with definitions and terminology, and insight into the characteristics and methods of operating accounting systems. The program usually provides some on-the-job training through which the student gains actual work experience.

Career opportunities
Accounting clerks
Accounts payable clerks
Payroll clerks
Bookkeepers
Office managers

Salary range
$350–$650 per month starting

Secretarial science
Clerical-receptionist   A clerical-receptionist program (usually nine months) prepares students for entry into clerical-receptionist positions in an office.

Career opportunities
Clerk typist
Filing clerk/receptionist in
    business offices
    professional offices
    industrial plants
    department stores
    government agencies
    institutions
    wherever correspondence,
    recording, and computations
    are involved

Salary range
$325–$450 per month starting

General secretary   A general secretary program (nine months to one year in length) prepares students for entry and advancement in secretarial positions. Length of the program usually depends on the skills of the student entering the program.

Career opportunities
Banks
Industry
Advertising
Travel agencies
Educational institutions
Government offices

Salary range
$350–$450 per month starting

Administrative or executive secretary   An executive secretary program is usually two academic years in length and is designed to prepare a student for a skilled position in the office. It also permits the student to receive a well-rounded education that makes him or her a skilled secretary and a participating member of an executive team.

Career opportunities
Government secretarial positions
    private
    supervisory
Education
Business
Industry

Salary range
$425–$575 per month starting

Legal secretary   A legal secretary program is usually a full year in length and provides instruction for students interested in working in offices that require the knowledge of legal secretarial procedures and terminology. In addition to training in basic office skills, (typing, shorthand, filing, machine transcription, accounting, communication skills, etc.) students receive specialized training in business law, income tax procedures, legal terminology, legal typing, and law office procedures.

Career opportunities
Law offices
Trust departments of banks
Insurance offices
Real estate offices
Legal departments of industrial firms
Government agency offices

Salary range
$425—$500 per month starting

Insurance secretary   An insurance secretary program is usually one year in length and is

designed to prepare students for entry into secretarial positions in an insurance office
On-the-job training is usually a part of this program.

Career opportunities   *Salary range*
Claims offices $350–$475 per month starting
Agents' offices
Home offices of insurance companies

Medical secretary   A medical secretary program is usually one year in length and is
designed to provide instruction for students interested in working in offices and hospitals
that require knowledge of medical secretarial procedures and terminology.

Career opportunities   *Salary range*
Doctors' offices $375–$500 per month starting
Insurance companies
Medical specialists
Clinics
Hospitals

Marketing and distribution

Retail management   This program is designed to prepare students for careers in the
retailing industry. The program stresses an understanding of business procedures and
knowledge of retailing principles. The program is two years in length and generally
combines classroom instruction with on-the-job training. Students who complete the
program usually receive an Associate of Applied Science degree.

Career opportunities   *Salary range*
Department stores $400–$800 per month starting
Mass merchandising (discount stores)
Specialty stores (owner/manager)
Manufacturing representative's positions
Buying positions in department stores

Food marketing   This program is designed to prepare people for careers in the retail or
wholesale food industry. Through specialized training students are provided with the
background and skills necessary to meet the requirements of this vast and expanding
field of work. The program is two years in length and usually combines on-the-job training
with classroom learning.

Career opportunities   *Salary range*
Management training programs $550–$900 per month starting
    with major food chains

Fashion merchandising   Fashion merchandising provides technical training for individuals interested in retailing fashion products. This program will vary from one to two years in length generally. The program usually provides on-the-job training that gives actual work experience in retail firms.

Career opportunities

Management trainees
Assistant retail department managers
Fashion buyers
Bridal consultants
Fashion coordinators
Department managers

Salary range

$275–$500 per month starting

Home furnishings   This program is designed to provide education and training for persons interested in middle-management and sales careers in the home furnishings industry. The home furnishings program is planned to provide training in the principles of color and design related to interiors, home decorating, and care and selection of fabrics. Students interested in this field should have a good sense of color, line, and proportion.

Career opportunities

Assistants to interior designers
Consultants in furniture, paint, wallpaper, and wall covering
Middle-management positions
Salespersons in the home-furnishings industry

Salary range

$350–$700 per month starting

Food service training (cook/chef training)   Food service training is a nine-month program that includes technical and specialized experience in quantity food preparation. There are also food preparation skill courses, general education, and related instruction including nutrition, sanitation, safety, and food composition, which prepare students to assume quantity food preparation and service responsibilities.

Career opportunities

Restaurants
Cafeterias
Drive-ins
Supper clubs
Hotels, motels
Private clubs
Schools
Hospitals, nursing homes
Private homes

Salary range

$350–$500 per month starting

Food service management   Food service management is usually two academic years (18 months) and is designed to provide technical and specialized training in both food preparation procedures and managerial skills. The first year of study concentrates on food preparation skills and related instruction in nutrition, sanitation, safety, food composition, and general studies. The second year offers managerial studies in supervision, cost control and accounting procedures, business law, general studies, and such technical studies as equipment design and layout and dining room management.

Career opportunities
Kitchen supervisors
Production supervisors
Assistant Managers (franchise units)

Salary range
$400–$700 per month starting

Positions are available in
Specialty shops
Delicatessens
Catering services
Restaurants
Hotels and motels

Floriculture   A floriculture program might vary in length from six months to one year. The program is designed to prepare people for careers in the floral industry. A one-year program would cover three phases: (1) retailing and sales promotion, (2) floral design, and (3) basic principles of growing and caring for plants and flowers. Students gain practical experience in growing and designing with flowers.

Career opportunities
Sales personnel in florist shop
Wholesalers
Greenhouse growers
Commercial flower producers
Floral designers
Garden center operators

Salary range
$400–$600 per month starting

Health

Medical assistance   This program usually consists of one year of study and concentrates on the following academic areas: (1) medical office procedures, (2) secretarial skills, and (3) routine laboratory procedures plus a period of clinical experience in physicians' offices, clinics, and industry. Employment in the field is good nationwide but depends on the applicant's competency. The medical assistant is trained to assist in a physician's office, to assist with physical examinations and treatment, to set up instrument trays, to sterilize instruments, to help with patient histories, and to handle appointments.

Career opportunities
Private physicians' offices
Hospitals
Research laboratories
Medical clinics
Nurses in industry

Salary range
$375–$500 per month starting

Respiratory therapy   The respiratory therapist is trained in oxygen administration, ventilatory support, blood gas analysis, chest-physiotherapy, and pulmonary rehabilitation. Classroom and laboratory training is provided in most programs. Two full years of study are generally required.

Career opportunities
Private hospitals
Public hospitals
Veterans Administration hospitals

Salary range
$650–$900 per month starting

Operating room technology   Usually a year of study is provided. An operating room technician is prepared to function under the supervision of an R.N. assisting surgeons and anesthesiologists in the operating room. She or he is knowledgeable in the function of surgical instruments and equipment and can identify and prepare instruments for a variety of operative procedures, is able to set up the operating room suite and sterile tables, and can prepare the patient for an operative procedure during which she or he utilizes aseptic techniques in passing instruments and assisting the surgical team as directed. Most programs would include a clinical section as well as classroom preparation.

Career opportunities
Hospitals (private and public)

Salary range
$450–$650 per month starting

Dental assistance   Usually a year of study is provided for dental assistants. The objective of a dental assistant program is to prepare the students to directly assist the dentist in the treatment of patients, to manage a smoothly functioning business office, and to perform basic laboratory procedures in a dental office. The program would generally lead to a diploma.

Career opportunities
Private dental offices
Group practices

Salary range
$280–$425 per month starting

Dental services
Clinics
Hospitals (public and private)
Public health institutions

Occupational therapy assistance   Programs usually consist of one full year of classroom instruction and clinical experiences. The work includes crafts and manual arts and other rehabilitative activities designed to assist handicapped individuals.

Career opportunities
Hospitals
Mental health clinics
Rehabilitation centers
Nursing homes
Health centers

Salary range
$425–$625 per month starting

Dental laboratory technology   This program usually is two years in duration. As part of the dental laboratory technician program students box, pour, and articulate models; set up, wax up, invest, and process full dentures; cast inlays, crowns, bridges, acrylic and porcelain jackets, and porcelain on metal; and construct many other special appliances. The program usually leads to an Associate of Applied Science degree.

Career opportunities
Commercial dental laboratories
University laboratories
Private dental offices
Veterans Administration laboratories
Self-employment

Salary range
$280–$1,000 per month starting

Orthopedic physicians assistant program   This is usually a two-year program with theory and practice integrated and offered concurrently during the program. Orthopedic physicians assistants are trained to work with the orthopedic surgeon in the emergency room, cast room, operating room, and other hospital areas as well as in clinics and private offices. Their duties, which are performed under medical direction, include preparing and maintaining the surgical equipment of the department, assisting the orthopedic surgeon, making and applying plaster limb or body casts, and setting up traction and suspension equipment on wards.

Career opportunities
Physicians' offices
Hospitals (public and private)
Clinics

Salary range
$500–$850 per month starting

Agriculture

Parks and natural resources   The parks and natural resources program may vary in length from college to college but is usually a two-year program leading to an Associate of Applied Science degree. It is designed to prepare students for entry-level employment, or employment advancement, in the area of parks and natural resource.

Career opportunities
County conservation officers
Lake officers
Park attendants
Conservation exhibit officers
Park workers
Wildlife managers

Salary range
$600–$800 per month starting

Agribusiness   The agribusiness program is designed to prepare students to enter the field of farm-supply distribution and service. Students receive preparation leading to careers in feed, seed, fertilizer, and general farm-supply work. The program may vary in duration from one to two years and usually features options in the area a student may wish to emphasize.

Career opportunities
Agricultural supply center managers
Sales representatives
Feed processing supervisors
Chemical fieldmen (women)
Feed and seed salespeople
Farm products inspectors
Elevator middle managers

Salary range
$550–$1,100 per month starting

Production agriculture   Production agriculture is designed to prepare students for entry-level employment or employment advancement in the science of food production. Students receive preparation leading to employment in careers such as farm operators, livestock technicians, buyers for agriculture product businesses, and crop technicians. Special emphasis is placed on management and decision making in most programs of this type. A program in production agriculture may vary in length from one to two years and, in some cases, may work as a transfer program with a cooperating institution.

Career opportunities
Livestock farmers
Crop farmers
Farm managers
Custom operators
Livestock herders

Salary range
$450–$1,000 per month starting

Trade and industrial occupations

Automotive mechanics   An automotive mechanics program is usually designed to provide the post-high-school-age student with basic auto mechanics. Most automotive programs allot 25 to 30 percent of their time to the classroom and laboratory shop and the balance of their time to the automotive shop.

Career opportunities   *Salary range*
Automotive dealerships $300–$575 per month starting
Franchised automotive centers
Fleet maintenance operations
Independent garages
Service stations

Automotive collision repair   Students enrolled in a program of this type will learn how to use hydraulic jacks, rams, air and electric grinders, sanders, buffers, drills, panel cutters, welders, torches, paint guns, damage dozers, alignment tools, and specialized hand tools. Most programs of this type would entail nine months of full-time study.

Career opportunities   *Salary range*
Body and fender shops $325–$650 per month starting
Garages with repair service
Automotive manufacturers
Automotive dealerships
Trucking, taxicab, and bus companies

Graphic arts   Graphic arts programs introduce the student to basic printing fundamentals, processes, functional typography, letterpress operations, lithography, layout and design, mathematics, and bindery operations. Advancing through a program of this type the student would learn more about lithography including camera and darkroom, photo composition, theory of color, stripping and platemaking, advanced letterpress and offset problems, estimating, production control, plant operations and layout, industrial relations, and related technical data. This program would usually be a full year in length.

Career opportunities   *Salary range*
Printshops $300–$650 per month starting
Newspapers

Architectural drafting   This program is designed to prepare a student for entry employment in an architect's office. It includes the drawing or redrawing of plans, elevations, details, and plumbing, electrical, and mechanical layouts. Attention is given to accuracy, neatness, and proper drawing procedure. A program of this type is generally one year in length.

Career opportunities
Civil engineer's office
Mechanical engineer's office
Local government
Architect's office
Construction company
Lumber company

Salary range
$400–$700 per month starting

Mechanical engineering technology Mechanical engineering technology is usually a two-year program leading to an associate's degree. The curriculum includes practical experience in the drafting room, shop, and laboratory, but it is more heavily weighted toward technical studies in the classroom. The graduate will have a high degree of ability in analytical problem solving as well as the ability to translate his own and others' thoughts into graphical representations. A thorough knowledge of the machine and manufacturing processes will allow him to follow a design to its conclusion in the actual manufacture and ultimate production of a special tool or product.

Career opportunities
Civil engineer's office
Mechanical engineer's office
Engineer technician's office
Small manufacturers
Engineering firms
County, state, and city governments
Large manufacturing companies
  (technicians)

Salary range
$700–$850 per month starting

Welding Welding programs will vary in length from school to school depending upon the degree of proficiency needed. Generally nine months of training is suggested. Generally the curriculum for a welding program would be divided into the "how" of welding and instructional methods related to the "why" of welding. The award the student would receive would depend on the time spent in the program. Welding is generally available on a part-time as well as a full-time basis.

Career opportunities
Metal manufacturing companies
General welding repair shops
Maintenance in industrial plants
Construction work

Salary range
$500–$850 per month starting

Machinist programs Machinist programs are designed for the person who is generally mechanically inclined, likes to work with machines and tools, and is interested in learning a trade that can be rewarding in terms of both job satisfaction and remuneration. The major objectives of the machinist trade are: (1) to provide a solid foundation in the basic principles of the machinist trade, and (2) to allow students to advance as far beyond the basics as time and individual interests and abilities allow. The general length of a machinist program is nine months.

Career opportunities   *Salary range*
Machine operators $450–$700 per motnh starting
General machinists
Tool-and-die apprentices
Model shop machinists
Maintenance machinists

Electronics

Electronic communications   Electronic communications is oriented toward radio and television broadcasting and radio/television servicing. Major emphasis is on maintenance and troubleshooting of existing equipment. Successful completion of a program of this type typically qualifies the students for an entry job as a radio/television serviceman (woman), broadcast engineer, two-way radio serviceman (woman), test technician, commercial sound engineer, and so forth. Generally this program takes one year and students receive diplomas.

Career opportunities   *Salary range*
Radio and television broadcasting $350–$700 per month starting
   stations
Communications sound system
   companies
Home service electronics
   television repair
   radio repair
Service of electronic devices in
    industry

Electronics engineering   This program is oriented toward research and development electronics. Major emphasis is on circuit analysis, basic design, and modification. Successful completion of this program qualifies the student for an entry job as a research and development technician, an engineering associate, or an instrumentation technician in certain industries. The program is generally two years in length and students are awarded the associate's degree.

Career opportunities
Design technicians
Industrial electronics technicians
Sales representatives
Field engineers
Electronics draftsman (woman)

Salary range
$600–$800 per month starting

Public and human services

Library technology   This is a one- to two-year certificate or diploma program at most comprehensive community colleges. Studies involve research techniques, cataloguing, organization of library and community resources, and some practical on-the-job training.

Career opportunities
Large law or medical offices
Private business
School systems
Public libraries
College career planning offices

Salary range
$5,000–$9,000 per year depending
    on experience and location

Social service aide program   Social and community agencies as well as day care centers require personnel to assist directors, social workers, and counselors in their daily responsibilities. Many community colleges offer programs of preparation for these aides with courses and training in interviewing techniques, interpersonal relationships, community resources, and organizational and personnel management.

Career opportunities
Day care centers
Preschools
Health clinics
Hospitals
State, federal, and community agencies

Salary range
$5,000–$8,000 per year

Career development model—Chapter 4

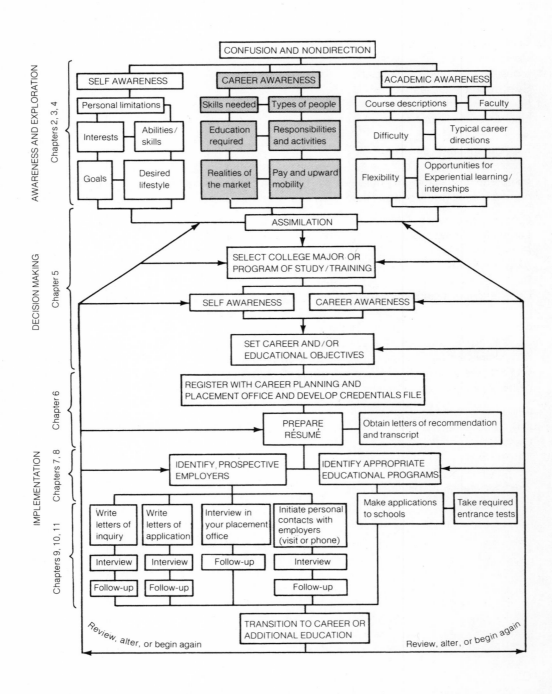

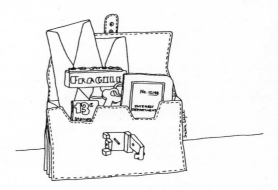

4 Career awareness

As was briefly mentioned in Chapter 3, "Academic Awareness," exploring study programs as well as career fields is essential to your career development. Unless you possess information about the various study and career fields, all the insight (self-awareness) you have about yourself (likes, dislikes, interests, skills, goals, etc.) is useless. You need to take this information about yourself and use it in viewing and exploring careers. You can then draw conclusions about how your make-up fits with what you are learning about a career. Unfortunately, this essential task in determining a direction for yourself can be the most painstaking, and, unless you can imagine yourself in the career field you're exploring, it can also be the most frustrating.

Information about careers

When we discuss career exploration, we are simply talking about your assimilation of career information — either through reading, listening, viewing, or experiencing. By its name alone, career information seems to imply material that is probably unreadable and certainly uninteresting at best. A counselor may have given you a huge book entitled *The Dictionary of Occupational Titles* and said something like, "This is all you need to help you in a career-related problem — go to it." You took one look at the confusing and lengthy listings as well as the complex classification system and decided that there was no way you were going to waste time trying to figure it out, much less read it. Because of the dominant role that reading plays in our lives (especially in academics), we all back off a bit when we consider reading about career information. Fortunately, there are new approaches to gathering this all-important type of information. The fact remains, however, that sound, successful career decisions are based on career information. Acquiring it is an essential step in our career development model. In many cases, spending time reading this type of information is the only way we can find out if the career is consistent with what we are all about and, therefore, self-discipline is, in some cases, the only way to go.

Students spend literally thousands of hours studying courses for the prized college degree. Doesn't it make sense then to spend some time, energy, and effort trying to figure out what to do following that degree? This exploration — gathering and organizing information about different careers — which may have influenced some of your answers in Chapter 1, is essential to this figuring-out process. Still, we know all too well that after spending four hours in class, working at a job for two, and then studying for three more, the last thing you want to do is sit down and read about careers. Well, let's look at some alternatives then.

Career exploration: Nonwritten resources

The big thing now in career information is the use of the audio-visual media, such as films, audio cassettes, and filmstrips. You've got to admit that getting important information about careers via this method sure beats reading some thick text. Check with your career counseling or planning and placement service and see what types of audio-visual material they have. There are many different kinds and types pertaining to the various steps of our model. In this chapter, however, we are concerned only with career awareness — becoming aware of the numerous aspects of a particular career or job. We will discuss what these specific aspects are that you should be aware of shortly.

So-called career kits or multimedia kits, media approaches to gaining career information, can be helpful as well as enjoyable. When you use these kits to explore career fields you usually complete a selection criteria exercise prior to the actual career exploration. In this way, you can explore only those careers that are based on the criteria (abilities, interests, likes, etc.) that you evidenced in the preliminary exercise. In a sense, they combine Chapters 2, 3, and 4 of this book. You must view them as a single source of information and not as the actual decision maker, however.

Different audio-visual media that can help you explore and become aware of careers are listed, discussed, and evaluated in the College Placement Council publication, *Audio Visual Media in Career Development*. See your career counselor or director of career planning and placement to see if he or she is aware of it.

Another method of career exploration is to meet and talk with people who are actually in the careers in which you're interested. Career Days, Career Colloquia, and similar opportunities bring representatives from various careers to your campus. They can be an easy place to gain important information. In these situations, either a formal presentation of information may be made or facilities to provide informal dialogue between you and a career representative may be arranged.

Initiating interviews (not employment — although they frequently do lead to future employment) with various career professionals as well as meetings and tours within career areas that are available in your college or university community is another way of getting some firsthand information. Here again, your career counselor and placement director can help facilitate these meetings and tours. Many career planning and placement offices have special programs that bring you together with people from various career fields. Check them out. Again, although you are merely seeking information from an employer, these personal contacts can lead to a career or summer employment. Look ahead to Chapter 10, "Initiating Personal Contact with Employers," if you are really interested in how this approach can work for you.

Other firsthand information about careers can be obtained through your professors, faculty, and student personnel administrators as well as through survey courses and independent studies in many major areas of study.

A final approach to collecting important information about careers, as well as about yourself, is to actually experience a career. This can be done through work-study projects, part-time jobs, off-campus programs, volunteer activities, internships, and summer employment. Take advantage of the programs offered by your college or university. We think the old adage "experience is the best teacher" is most appropriate here. There is no better way ultimately to answer the question, Is this career for me? than by actually "living" the daily activities and responsibilities, meeting people in the job, and getting a feel for the career. Not only does this experience help you decide upon the field as a career direction, but it provides valuable skill development that is marketable in numerous employment settings.

The following section speaks specifically to this point as summer job and internships are discussed relative to the entire career development process.

The summer job: An opportunity for exploring and experiencing*

Summer employment can do much more than just put necessary money in your pockets. When it is incorporated within a career and life planning program, it can be a very important and useful tool to help you make career and life decisions. Also, it gives you practice in everything discussed in *Directions:* gaining self-awareness and career awareness, setting objectives, writing résumés and letters, interviewing, identifying

---

*This section combines an untitled, unpublished pamphlet on summer jobs by Donald Brandt (1974) and "So You Want a Summer Job" by Bonnie Cejka, an unpublished resource in the Coe College Center for Academic and Career Planning (1975). Each is used by permission of the author.

prospective employers, and job-hunting techniques. You can try out your skills before you have to do it for real in the pursuit of your initial career position. As we see it, then, summer employment can be more than just a job; it is a learning laboratory for testing out career interests and developing marketable skills.

"Okay, okay," you may be saying, "so it's important. But how do I actually obtain a meaningful and financially rewarding summer job these days?" Let's take a look at a couple of things — to begin with, let's examine a couple of decisions that you need to make.

First things first

Let's ask a question: *Why* do you want to work? Do you want to work strictly for money? (If that is your main reason for seeking employment, decide which fields are most likely to provide you with that kind of money over the summer. Be realistic in both the amount you think you must earn, and the field you choose to earn it in.) Or, do you want to work to gain experience or to help you decide on a future career direction? If you think you have already found a career that interests you, it might be a good idea to get some related experience to see what working in the field is actually like. Getting general work experience and learning to meet and get along with people is another good reason for working, and in that case too, you need to consider summer job resources from other than just a monetary standpoint. Now, if you are looking for excitement or travel, your search will have to be more widespread. But once you know what your purpose is, it will be easier for you to find a job that meets your specific needs, and it will make your summer more rewarding. Also, you need to consider where you want to work: Do you want to be near home, or do you have no geographical preference? This decision will dictate your resources and approach to finding a job.

Near or at home

1. *Early* in the spring (possibly during spring vacation), contact all factories, fast food chains, and/or construction companies in the area. Drop by, fill out applications, and *follow up.**

2. Use the Yellow Pages — see the index in back of the telephone directory for employers to visit.

3. Pore over want ads in the newspaper; call or write about jobs that sound promising.

4. Investigate openings and register at your state employment service.

5. Call or drop into city and county personnel offices to check on openings for playground directors or park and road construction crews. Complete an application.

6. Visit your career planning and placement office to see the latest local job vacancies; note the numerous booklets and pamphlets described a few pages ahead.

Follow up means just that. After visiting an office or individual for an information-seeking appointment, and leaving your résumé, be sure to stop back again to see what's happening there. See if anything has opened up.

7. Ask parents and relatives in the business community for suggestions. Let them know you're looking and need their help!

8. If the idea of being a self-made entrepreneur is appealing, be innovative. Dream up your own job! Caring for or walking dogs, tending houseplants, washing windows, planting gardens, helping harried mothers with small children, painting houses, and doing odd jobs — or how about weeding gardens, organizing or pricing for garage sales, making and selling box lunches to construction crews and beach and lake visitors, waxing floors and cleaning rugs, guiding city tours.

9. Vacationing families sometimes hire housesitters to protect the premises, water the plants, and take care of the family pet — all at once. Go door-to-door in your neighborhood to get business.

10. Don't forget hotel and motel jobs in any location: bellhops, switchboard operators, kitchen workers, desk clerks, and custodians.

No geographical preference (or seeking an experience-related position at home)

1. Write a résumé (see examples in Chapter 6).

2. *Write letters of application and inquiry* (see examples in Chapter 9).

3. Use the following resources in your career planning and placement office to identify summer job employers and/or vacancies:

a. want ads from large city newspapers — beginning mid-April

b. summer job resources in your career planning and placement office

c. *College Placement Annual*

d. summer job vacancy binders

e. Yellow Pages

f. state and federal government summer intern programs

4. If working abroad interests you, be sure to read through the *Directory of Overseas Summer Jobs*. There are numerous opportunities.

5. There are several businesses that typically offer summer jobs for students: Pioneer Seed Company of Des Moines for one (crew leaders for corn detasseling), Southwestern Company of Nashville, Tennessee, for another. Southwestern publishes and markets educational and religious books and offers a sales training program plus a very fine cash incentive. The latter job is for the more adventurous soul, however, since salespersons are both trained and assigned to work all over the country. Check the *College Placement Annual* and other resources in your career planning and placement office.

6. Contact temporary help firms, such as Manpower and Kelly Services, for assignments. Manpower, in many cities, sponsors a free summer-job clearing-house called Youth Power. Check locally to see if there is such an office near you and when it will open.

Selling yourself

After deciding on the geographical location and type of summer job (money or experience) you want, the next task to take on is the responsibility of selling yourself — your skills, interests, abilities, and experiences — to a prospective employer. There is one main point — it's what you can do for the employer that counts, not what the employer can do for you. (Ever heard that one before?) Someone will hire you for a job because she or he thinks you can perform a service for the business or organization. Since competition for summer jobs will be stiff, you must find some way to convince this prospective employer that *you* are the one. And that takes knowing yourself, basically. Just think about it for a minute. What can you comfortably do? What kinds of things do you *like* to do? What do others think you do well? What kinds of things do you do naturally in your spare time? What makes you *different* from the next person? In his book *A Strategy for Daily Living* (1973), Dr. Ari Kiev points out that "the real trick is not in acquiring a greater fortune, more prestige or more power, but in finding out your gift and putting it to good use — and you won't find this gift outside of yourself, but in your own activities." If the answers to these questions seem to be coming slowly, you might consider reviewing "Self-awareness" or scheduling an appointment with a counselor in your career planning and placement office.

Seeking information and communicating skills

As previously mentioned, summer employment can do much more than just put necessary money in your pocket; it can also be an important and useful tool in helping you make career and life decisions. It allows you to practice job-hunting techniques and offers a learning lab for testing out career interests and developing marketable skills. Again, you may be saying that you understand the value of a good summer job but to actually obtain a meaningful summer job these days is impossible! Before putting all your faith behind that belief, let's look at a real-life example. One student described how he got employment for the 1975 summer like this:

> When I was home during the winter break in December 1974, I began to think seriously about my plans for the summer. I began to narrow down a specific field of employment. I chose media sales as my preferred area of employment with the full knowledge that the chances of getting into media sales for the summer were slim — simply because television and radio stations *"never"* hire students to work in the sales department. In fact, most managers informed me that I was the only person to their knowledge to apply for a summer job in that area. So my problem of getting a job wasn't so much the competition, but rather to get one of these stations to create an opening for me.
>
> My next step was to obtain from a close personal acquaintance, a person knowledgeable about the local media sales scene, a list of names of persons who were in the position to hire me in each of the different stations in the area. So that I could get some interviews, this was important for me because it allowed me to easily get in touch with most of these persons. In the interview, I particularly tried to impress upon my interviewer how much I was interested in the field of media sales, what my skills were, and that I was willing to work for a relatively low salary.

> Most of the interviews ended with the interviewer telling me how much he would like to hire me, but there were no openings for summer help. However, a few interviewers told me that they were interested in hiring me and "would see what could be done." They told me to keep in touch.
>
> In March, I returned to New Orleans to personally follow up my interviews. I told them that I was still very interested in working in their organization in media sales and that I would like to be notified at their earliest convenience. I also contacted the chemical warehouse where I worked last summer to let them know that I would like to work for them again. As a result, I felt fairly secure with the knowledge that I would have some source of income for the summer, though not necessarily my chosen one.
>
> When I returned to school, I sent follow-up letters to three of my most promising prospects. I simply thanked them for their consideration and cooperation in my search for a summer job.
>
> Eventually one of these stations contacted me and offered me a job for the summer in their sales department. That's where I am now. And the job is fantastic!!

This example described a freshman who was trying to decide if he would like to become involved in some way with either radio or television as a career. Through his growing self-awareness, he found that he possessed some skills that could be used in radio and television. In order to be able to try on this career, he created his own work experience. He wanted to get into the sales department so that he could get a good overview of the total station's operation. So, take heart, and read on!

Seeking advice

Let's look at a second approach. Another related method for finding summer employment is for you not to ask for a job! Why? Most employers really do not like to be asked if they have a job opening, for they don't like to say no. Likewise, you don't like to be told no. Therefore, you need to create a relaxed and comfortable atmosphere so that the employer does not have to reject you and you do not have to feel rejected.

If you don't ask for a job, then how do you find employment? Utilizing a very well developed résumé (look ahead to the section on résumés in Chapter 6) you can seek out employers to ask them for advice concerning your résumé, your job-hunting techniques, and where your particular skills can be utilized within any organization in your community. Once again, you are not asking for a job, you are merely seeking advice and information. Almost anyone is willing to take the time to give you some advice — even the busiest executive in an organization.

When you ask for advice about your résumé and summer job search, the potential employer will get to know you better and he or she will further question you about your skills. If you feel that the person with whom you are talking does not have a serious interest in hiring you, you should ask to be referred to another person who can provide you with additional advice. It will be the information that you provide about yourself that will allow a referral to take place. No one is going to do a very good job of referring you if they know little about you. Talk about yourself! Many times, the person you're talking with will provide referrals to you — before you ever get the chance to ask!

When seeking advice from the person to whom you were referred, simply state that Mr. or Mrs. _____referred you. Once again, you are not asking for a job at this time. You are merely seeking advice about your résumé and the best methods for finding summer employment. Within this system, you will eventually find someone who can use your skills and who begins to discuss job opportunities.

Researching your community

The following is a slightly different approach to the summer job search. Suppose you are interested in social work as a career, but you are unaware of summer employment opportunities. You desire this kind of experience because it will help you decide whether or not social work is a potential career field for you. To set up some interviews, consult the Yellow Pages for the name of an organization and an address and, through a phone conversation, initiate an information-seeking meeting. During your "interview" ask if your interviewer knows of any summer jobs that could give you experience in or exposure to social work. Make sure that you give the person a copy of your résumé so that you can ask his or her advice concerning it and methods for finding summer employment. Many times, this type of informal discussion can result in employment leads.

Don't forget that a lot of research can be done in your current community (where you're going to school) that is applicable to another community. Can you still expect to be referred? Sure, you can! As mobile as people are within our society, you never know whom the person you are talking with knows in another community. Implicit in all the previous discussion is the need to begin this process early — the first day of summer vacation is not going to make it.

As Eli Djeddah describes in his book *Moving Up* (1971), there are only twelve ways for anyone to find employment. The unpublished employment market contains about 80 percent of all employment. The published market accounts for about 20 percent of all employment. The published market includes such listings as are found in newspapers, employment agencies, and professional organizations. It has been estimated that 90 percent of all people utilize the published listing to find their employment experience. It is to your advantage to begin *now* to learn how you can control the job market to your advantage, rather than allowing it to control you. The referral process described previously is a good way to gain control over your destiny in the summer employment world — and to polish your skills for similar "control" regarding your initial life and career position.

Using your summer job

You must decide what type of employment you want and go out and find it. Realistically, we know that circumstances will prevent you from doing this from time to time. In short, you may get stuck doing something that is totally unexciting during the summer. Don't let this employment situation get you down, however, for you can turn it into a more meaningful and more exciting job. How? Practice your skill in collecting career and life information. Collect this information even though you are with people that you do not necessarily wish to emulate. For example, even if you are working on an assembly line in a factory, ask the people you meet during the breaks such questions as: How did you get your job with this company? How did you advance to your current position within the company? What do you like or dislike about your company? What do you like or dislike about the work you are doing? Begin to define for yourself such things as the type of people you want to work with, the type of lifestyle you desire, the type of living and working conditions that are important to you.

Another idea! If you are working in a factory and are seriously interested in business as a career, why not make an appointment with one of the company executives before or after work, during the lunch hour, whenever. As we stated earlier, almost anyone is willing to give you advice if you are seriously interested. If you are shy, take a friend who shares your interest. There are no reasons why two people cannot see a company executive to seek out career information. We want you to incorporate this concept of discovering career and life information as part of your daily routine — not only for today, but for each day of your life.

Don't forget to consider volunteer work as a summer work experience. Many students shy away from volunteer work because there is no salary, but we would like to point out that many times this is an incorrect assumption. Though the positions are not numerous, we have seen several volunteer organizations provide salaries between $600 to $1,000. Many situations provide at least room and board.

In his book *Go Hire Yourself an Employer* (1973), Richard K. Irish answers the question, "Does it make any sense to volunteer for no pay to work in the field you want where you have no qualifications?" We like the way he answers: "You bet it does. Half the political hotshots in the country started off as unpaid canvassers in some obscure campaign. And advertising geniuses often begin licking stamps for free in the mail room. Volunteer work — especially in glamor jobs such as the theater, communications and political action — is useful training and make the volunteer, especially if he becomes rapidly indispensable, highly visible to decision-makers who are quick to recognize and promote competence."

As you build up your level of consciousness of various career areas through volunteer experiences, you also build up a tremendous amount of experience that can prove very useful in selling your skills to a future graduate school or employer. For example, in an interview or on your résumé, you could describe your organizational and planning skills thus:

Organized, planned, and helped execute Democratic party activities on a countywide basis for six weeks prior to the November 1974 elections. Involvements included con-

> ducting canvasses, assembling computer data, working on fund-raising projects, and informing the campus community about the candidates and the issues.

Or you could demonstrate your leadership skills by pointing out:

> Very instrumental through the Health Services Committee in establishing gynecological services for college women based upon surveys of needs and attitudes.

If you enjoyed working with children, your teaching skills could be demonstrated by:

> Organizing and conducting a story hour for first graders twice weekly. Tutoring three sixth-grade boys in reading. Working with kindergarten teacher with reading and reading readiness groups. Leading group of special education Campfire Girls. Co-leading group of third-grade Bluebirds. Nursery school teacher at Unitarian Church for three years.

Though they may state it in many different ways, employers or graduate schools are really asking only one question: "What can you do for me that is so important that I want to know about it — that makes you so different from the next person I will be talking with?" Through a statement of your skills, you can answer this question in your interviews, letters, and résumé. Though the subject of skills will be discussed in another chapter of this book, we bring it to your attention here because of its critical importance. Knowledge of your skills is as important to your working self as your heart is to your biological self. *Know your skills and watch yourself gain in confidence!*

Six important points in conclusion

1. Before going after a summer job, first decide what your major reasons for getting a summer job are and whether or not you are geographically mobile. Answers to these questions will make your search more efficient.

2. The previous approaches require confidence, practice, and skills that many of us have not yet developed. Be sure to seek out assistance from your career planning and placement office in these areas. Their support and advice can be valuable.

3. For summer jobs or any job, other sections of this resource can be valuable. Look ahead especially to Chapter 6, "Developing a Credentials File" (especially the section on résumés); Chapter 8, "Identifying Prospective Employers"; Chapter 9, "Letters of Inquiry, Application, and Follow-up"; and Chapter 11, "The Employment Interview Process." But, in closing, no matter where you decide to apply for work, please remember the following little items:

4. Include positive references. Ask the professors and former employers who think you're good to put in a word for you. Don't select someone you're not sure of.

5. Give an employer a glimpse into your background experiences, noting extracurricular activities and travel; and even if you only have some babysitting as previous work experience, it will give someone an idea of your dependability, at least.

6. Look neat and clean when appearing for any interview: hair combed, gleaming bright teeth, sincere smile, firm handshake (no cold fishes), and pressed clothes.

Sources of information on summer jobs

We have listed some sources of information that can be very helpful to you as you research and develop your own summer employment laboratory experience. Your college or university library and/or career planning and placement office will probably have most of them.

Summer Employment Directory of the U.S.

Mynena A. Leith, National Director Service, Inc.

252 Ludlow Avenue, Cincinnati, Ohio 45220

Ms. Leith is one of the nation's leading authorities concerning summer employment. Her directory lists over 90,000 positions: Boy Scouts of America, Camp Fire Girls, Girl Scouts of America, YMCA, YWCA, summer theaters, national parks, ranches, resorts, hotels, restaurants, and business and industry.

The Directory of Overseas Summer Jobs, 1976

Charles J. James, National Directory Service, Inc.

252 Ludlow Avenue, Cincinnati, Ohio 45220

Over 50,000 vacancies listed. Information concerning visa, residence, and work permit regulations. Presents opportunities for volunteer work.

Seasonal Employment

This government publication is designed to answer questions concerning seasonal employment with the United States Park Service and nongovernmental park concessionaires.

Invest Yourself

Commission on Voluntary Service and Action

475 Riverside Drive, Room 635, New York, New York 10027

Discusses volunteer experiences with community service organizations, work camps, work-study programs and seminars, and community development.

Mort's Guide to 100,000 Vacation Jobs

CMG Publishing Company, Inc.

Princeton, New Jersey 08540
Information is provided on finding employment in business, camps, the circus, domestic service, dude ranches, farms and ranches, resorts, restaurants, parks, ski resorts, summer theaters, travel, and yachts.

College Placement Annual
This directory includes 1,400 corporate and government employers with a special section on summer employment.

The Directory of Summer Jobs in Britain
Sally E. Hunt, Vacation-Work
9 Park End Street, Oxford, England
Information provided on visa and work permit regulations. Includes vacancies for business and industry, teaching, farms, resorts, hotels, and volunteer work.

Jobs in Social Change
Social and Education Research Foundation (SERF)
3416 Sansom Street, Philadelphia, Pennsylvania 19104
Provides an in-depth description of 175 major Washington, D.C., public interest groups. Areas presented include Nader network, environment, urban affairs, consumerism, prison reform, education, population, media, women, health, social planning, children's rights, civil liberties, political reform, and public interest law. Discusses internships and summer jobs with social change groups.

Summer Jobs in Federal Agencies
Announcement N. 414.
Discusses all federal jobs, except with the United States Postal Service.

National Directory of Summer Internships for Undergraduate College Students
Prepared by the Career Planning Offices of Bryn Mawr and Haverford Colleges. Inquiries can be addressed to Summer Internship Research Project, Career Planning Office, Bryn Mawr College, Bryn Mawr, Pennsylvania 19019. As described by the authors, the internships "should give qualified students professional experience in positions similar in degree of responsibility and initiative to those held by college graduates beginning a career." Listings include social service, government, communications, health professions, conservation and environmental sciences, scientific research, business and finance, education, engineering and architecture, and museums.

Summer Studies Abroad
Edited by Gail Caben, published by the Institute of International Education, 809 United Nations Plaza, New York, New York 10017. It lists opportunities for summer study abroad and the universities or colleges that offer off-campus study abroad.

The Directory of Overseas Summer Jobs (1976 edition)
National Directory Service

252 Ludlow Ave.
Cincinnati, Ohio 45220
This book lists as wide a variety of job openings as possible in as many countries as possible —
information on employment prospects and details of work available with individual employers.

Summer Jobs
Pamphlet published by United States Civil Service Commission, November 1975. Majority of jobs are
in large metropolitan areas, limited opportunities. Deadlines and procedures for applying are given.

Summer Employment Guide 1975
University Publications, Denver, Colorado
United States and Canadian job listings, study programs abroad, scholarships, farm jobs, and
government employment.

Back to the written word

Unfortunately, because media in most cases are quite expensive, meetings and tours difficult to coordinate, and work experience not always easy to obtain, the old printed word, in many instances, is still your best source of *beginning* information. The following are good resources that contain important career information essential to your career awareness and ultimately your career choice. Check with your career planning and placement office or library and begin exploring them.

1. *Occupational Outlook Handbook:* This is a very comprehensive resource published by the Department of Labor. It discusses just about every career imaginable. Careers are discussed in depth according to many of the criteria listed on the chart on pp. 82–124.
Beware of the overly optimistic approach to the number-of-jobs-available information.
2. *Dictionary of Occupational Titles (DOT):* Perhaps the most thorough, yet complex, system of career classification, this resource discusses all careers in regard to all-important criteria — including aptitudes, interests, and skills — needed for the career. Not enough counselors and students use this resource.
3. Company literature: Businesses and industries publish literature describing their career opportunities; usually not recommended for beginning exploration, but rather for gathering detailed, specific career information.
4. Professional organizations' material: Just about every career field has a professional organization or union to which it belongs and which makes available related career information. Information is usually excellent, useful, up to date, free of charge, and available in your career planning and placement office.
5. Career descriptions file: Almost every career planning and placement office has a file of career descriptions, usually made up of easy-to-read brochures and similar information. This type of material can be read quickly, and you can decide (without wasting much time) whether or not you're interested in the field and wish to pursue it further. This type of information also serves as a good point of departure for your exploration. If you can see yourself doing the things discussed in the brochure, then you should probably do some

further reading and try talking to people as well as actually experiencing some aspects of the field.

6. *Encyclopedia of Careers:* This resource is very similar to the *Occupational Outlook Handbook,* with a little more emphasis on the activities and daily involvements of career fields. Many times, actual examples of a typical day are discussed.

7. *Matching Technicians to Jobs* (World Trade Academy Press): This is an excellent informational resource providing a breakdown of all technical fields by specialty, nature of the work, working conditions, and supply and demand figures for personnel.

Occupational Outlook Handbook in brief

The following compilation is an example of a comprehensive and easy-to-use source of career information. It is essentially a selection of some 275 occupations from the *Occupational Outlook Handbook.* It summarizes employment outlook to 1985 for these occupations. The jobs are grouped into thirteen clusters of related jobs. The clusters can relate the outlook materials to school curriculums and occupational training programs, career ladders, and fields of interest for those engaged in career exploration and planning.

Occupational outlook handbook in brief (1976–1977 edition)

Occupation	Estimated employment 1974	Average annual openings[1] 1974–1985	Employment trends and prospects
Industrial production and related occupations			
Foundry occupations			
Coremakers	24,500	550	Employment expected to change little as more cores are made by machine instead of by hand. Nevertheless, replacement needs will create several hundred openings annually.
Molders	60,000	1,300	Employment expected to change little due to laborsaving innovations. However, replacement needs will create hundreds of openings annually.
Patternmakers	20,500	500	Employment expected to change little due to increased use of metal patterns and other technical improvements. Most of relatively small number of openings created by replacement needs will be for metal patternmakers.

Occupation	Estimated employment 1974	Average annual openings[1] 1974–1985	Employment trends and prospects
Machining occupations			
All-round machinists	335,000	14,500	Employment expected to increase about as fast as average for all occupations due to expansion of metalworking activities and rising demand for machined goods.
Instrument makers (mechanical)	5,500	150	Employment expected to increase at slower rate than average for all occupations due to laborsaving technological innovations. Very few job opportunities.
Machine tool operators	600,000	18,000	Despite slower than average employment growth, many job opportunities should result from large replacement needs.
Setup workers (machine tools)	50,000	1,350	Despite growth in consumer and industrial demand for machined goods, increasing use of numerically controlled machine tools will result in slower than average employment growth. Most opportunities will arise from replacement needs.
Tool-and-die makers	170,000	6,600	Employment expected to grow about as fast as average for all occupations as result of expansion in metalworking industries.
Printing occupations			
Bookbinders and related workers	35,000	1,900	Employment expected to increase about as fast as average for all occupations due to expansion of metalworking activities and rising demand for machined goods.
Composing room workers	165,000	3,900	Employment expected to decline due to use of high-speed phototypesetting and typesetting computers that require few operators. Few thousand openings annually resulting from replacement needs. Best prospects for those who have completed posthigh school programs in printing technology.
Electrotypers	4,000	20	Employment expected to decline as result of

Occupation	Estimated employment 1974	Average annual openings[1] 1974–1985	Employment trends and prospects
and stereotypers			offset printing and other laborsaving developments. Opportunities will be very limited.
Lithographic workers	85,000	4,300	Employment expected to grow faster than average for all occupations as offset presses are increasingly used in place of letter presses. Best prospects for those who have completed posthigh school programs in printing technology.
Photoengravers	17,000	250	Employment expected to decline as result of offset printing, which requires no photoengraving, and other technological advances. Limited opportunities.
Printing press operators and assistants	140,000	5,600	Despite increased use of faster, more efficient presses, employment expected to increase about as fast as average for all occupations due to growth in volume of printed materials. Particularly good outlook for webpress operators.

Other industrial production and related occupations

Occupation	Estimated employment 1974	Average annual openings 1974–1985	Employment trends and prospects
Assemblers	1,140,000	63,000	Employment expected to increase about as fast as average for all occupations due to growing demand for consumer products and industrial machinery and equipment. However, applicants may find opportunities limited during some years since employment is concentrated in durable goods industries which are highly sensitive to changes in business conditions and national defense needs.
Automobile painters	25,000	900	Employment expected to increase about as fast as average for all occupations due to growing number of vehicles damaged in traffic accidents. Best opportunities in metropolitan areas.
Blacksmiths	9,000	50	Employment expected to decline, as blacksmiths are replaced by welders and

Occupation	Estimated employment 1974	Average annual openings[1] 1974–1985	Employment trends and prospects
			machines in forge shops. Some openings due to replacement needs.
Blue-collar worker supervisors	1,460,000	61,000	Employment expected to grow about as fast as average for all occupations. Most of increase in employment due to expansion of nonmanufacturing industries. Competition for supervisory jobs usually is keen. Best prospects for workers who have leadership ability plus some college.
Boilermaking workers	45,000	2,700	Employment expected to increase faster than average for all occupations due to construction of many new electric powerplants and expansion of chemical, petroleum, steel, and shipbuilding industries.
Boiler tenders	90,000	2,100	Employment expected to decline as more new boilers are equipped with automatic controls. However, hundreds of openings will arise annually due to replacement needs.
Electroplaters	34,000	1,250	Employment expected to grow about as fast as average for all occupations due to expansion of metalworking industries and increased use of electroplating on metals and plastics.
Forge shop workers	65,000	1,750	Employment expected to grow more slowly than average for all occupations because of improved forging techniques and equipment, despite expansion in automobile and energy-related industries. Most job openings due to replacement needs.
Furniture upholsterers	34,000	1,200	Employment expected to grow at a slower rate than average for all occupations because furniture is being constructed with less upholstery and because of trend toward buying new furniture instead of reupholstering the old. Most job openings due to replacement needs.
Inspectors (manufacturing)	790,000	51,000	Employment expected to increase faster than average for all occupations because of indus-

Occupation	Estimated employment 1974	Average annual openings[1] 1974–1985	Employment trends and prospects
			trial expansion and growing complexity of manufactured products.
Millwrights	95,000	3,800	Employment expected to increase about as fast as average for all occupations as result of construction of new plants, improvements in existing plants, and building and maintenance of increasingly complex machinery.
Motion picture projectionists	18,000	1,000	Employment expected to grow more slowly than average for all occupations because of laborsaving innovations in equipment and theater design. Applicants are likely to face keen competition.
Ophthalmic laboratory technicians	22,000	2,100	Employment expected to increase much faster than average for all occupations due to rising demand for eyeglasses.
Photographic laboratory workers	50,000	3,300	Employment expected to increase faster than average for all occupations due to increasing use of photography in business, government, research and development activities, and growth of amateur photography.
Power truck operators	347,000	9,100	Employment expected to increase about as fast as average for all occupations as more firms use power trucks in place of hand labor.
Production painters	125,000	5,000	Employment expected to grow about as fast as average for all occupations, but will not keep pace with manufacturing output because of increased use of automatic sprayers and other laborsaving innovations.
Stationary engineers	193,000	5,000	Employment expected to change little because of increased use of more powerful and centralized equipment. However, several thousand openings will arise annually due to replacement needs.
Waste water treatment plant operators	62,000	6,100	Employment expected to increase much faster than average for all occupations as result of construction of new plants to process growing

Occupation	Estimated employment 1974	Average annual openings[1] 1974–1985	Employment trends and prospects
			amount of domestic and industrial waste water.
Welders	645,000	27,000	Employment expected to increase faster than average for all occupations due to favorable outlook for metalworking industries and greater use of welding. Very good opportunities, particularly for skilled welders in nuclear power plant, pipeline, and ship construction jobs.

Office occupations

Clerical occupations

Bookkeeping workers	1,700,000	121,000	Employment expected to increase at slower rate than average for all occupations because of increasing automation in recordkeeping. Most job openings will result from replacement needs.
Cashiers	1,111,000	97,000	Because of very high turnover and average employment growth in response to increased retail sales, thousands of job openings for cashiers expected annually. However, future growth could slow with widespread adoption of automated checkout systems.
Collection workers	63,000	4,500	Employment expected to grow faster than average for all occupations as continued expanded use of credit results in increasing numbers of delinquent accounts. Best opportunities in collection agencies and retail trade firms.
File clerks	275,000	25,000	Increased demand for recordkeeping should result in some job openings. However, employment is not expected to grow as fast as in past years due to increasing use of computers to arrange, store, and transmit information. Most job openings will be created by replacement needs.

Occupation	Estimated employment 1974	Average annual openings[1] 1974–1985	Employment trends and prospects
Hotel front office clerks	54,000	4,250	Employment expected to grow about as fast as average for all occupations as new hotels and motels are built. Most openings, however, will result from replacement needs.
Office machine operators	170,000	12,800	Employment expected to grow more slowly than average for all occupations as result of more centralized and computerized recordkeeping and processing systems. Most job openings due to replacement needs.
Postal clerks	293,000	9,700	Employment expected to change little due to modernization of post offices and installation of new equipment which will increase efficiency of clerks. Thousands of openings annually due to replacement needs.
Receptionists	460,000	57,500	Employment expected to grow faster than average for all occupations due to expansion of firms providing business, personal, and professional services. Work is of personal nature and prospects should not be affected by automation.
Secretaries and stenographers	3,300,000	439,000	The increasing use of dictating machines will limit opportunities for office stenographers. Very good prospects for skilled shorthand reporters and secretaries.
Shipping and receiving clerks	465,000	20,500	Employment expected to grow about as fast as average for all occupations as business expansion results in increased distribution of goods.
Statistical clerks	325,000	23,000	Employment expected to grow about as fast as average for all occupations as numerical data increasingly are used to analyze and control activities in business and government. Increased use of computers may eliminate some routine positions.
Stock clerks	490,000	26,000	Employment expected to grow about as fast as average for all occupations as business

Occupation	Estimated employment 1974	Average annual openings[1] 1974–1985	Employment trends and prospects
			firms continue to expand. Competition anticipated as many young people seek this work as a first job.
Typists	1,000,000	125,000	Employment expected to grow faster than average for all occupations as business expansion results in increased paperwork. Very good opportunities for typists, particularly those familiar with automatic typewriters and new kinds of word processing equipment.

Computer and related occupations

Computer operating personnel	500,000	27,500	Employment of keypunch operators expected to decline because of advances in other data entry techniques and equipment. Employment of console and auxiliary equipment operators should grow faster than average for all occupations in response to the expanding use of computer hardware, especially terminals.
Programmers	200,000	13,000	Employment expected to grow faster than average for all occupations as computer use expands, particularly in medical, educational, and data processing services. Best opportunities for programmers with some training in systems analysis.
Systems analysts	115,000	9,100	Employment expected to grow faster than average for all occupations in response to advances in hardware and computer programs resulting in expanded computer applications. Also, as users become more familiar with computer capabilities, they will expect greater efficiency and performance from their systems.

Banking occupations

Bank clerks	517,000	54,000	Excellent employment opportunities due to large replacement needs and faster than average growth as banking services expand.

Occupation	Estimated employment 1974	Average annual openings[1] 1974–1985	Employment trends and prospects
			Best prospects for those trained in computer techniques.
Bank officers	240,000	16,000	Employment expected to grow faster than average for all occupations as increasing use of computers and expansion of banking services require more officers to provide sound management. Good opportunities for college graduates as management trainees.
Bank tellers	270,000	30,000	Good employment opportunities due to large replacement needs and faster than average employment growth as banking services expand. Many openings will arise for part-time tellers to work during peak business hours.

Insurance occupations

Occupation	Estimated employment 1974	Average annual openings 1974–1985	Employment trends and prospects
Actuaries	10,700	700	Best opportunities for college graduates who passed at least one actuarial examination while in school and have strong mathematical and statistical backgrounds. However, competition may be keen because of large number of qualified applicants.
Claim representatives	125,000	6,600	Employment expected to grow about as fast as average for all occupations in response to expanding insurance sales and claims. Limited opportunities for adjusters specializing in automobile claims in States with no-fault insurance plans; favorable prospects for other types of adjusters. Less favorable prospects for claim examiners due to increased computer processing.
Insurance agents, brokers, and underwriters	470,000	19,400	Employment expected to increase about as fast as average for all occupations as insurance sales continue to expand. Selling expected to remain competitive, but ambitious people who enjoy sales work will find favorable opportunities as agents and brokers. Good prospects for underwriters.

Occupation	Estimated employment 1974	Average annual openings[1] 1974–1985	Employment trends and prospects
Administrative and related occupations			
Accountants	805,000	45,500	Very good opportunities. Because of growing complexity of business accounting requirements, college graduates, particularly those who worked part time for an accounting firm while in school, will be in greater demand than nongraduates. Employers also prefer applicants trained in computer techniques.
Advertising workers	170,000	7,100	Employment expected to increase about as fast as average for all occupations as the growing number of consumer goods and expanding competition in many product and service markets cause advertising expenditures to rise. Favorable opportunities for highly qualified applicants; keen competition for others.
Buyers	110,000	9,000	Employment expected to grow faster than average for all occupations as retailers place greater emphasis on the selection of goods they have for sale. However, keen competition anticipated as merchandising attracts large numbers of college graduates.
City managers	2,900	150	Employment expected to grow faster than average for all occupations. However, persons without at least a master's degree in public administration or related management experience likely to face keen competition.
College student personnel workers	50,000	[2]	Tightening budgets in both public and private colleges and universities will limit employment growth, resulting in competition for available positions. Over short run, most openings will result from replacement needs.
Credit managers	66,000	4,500	Employment expected to increase faster than average for all occupations due to expanded use of credit by both businesses and consumers. Best opportunities in large metropolitan areas.

Occupation	Estimated employment 1974	Average annual openings[1] 1974–1985	Employment trends and prospects
Hotel managers and assistants	120,000	6,500	Employment expected to grow about as fast as average for all occupations as additional hotels and motels are built and chain and franchise operations spread. Best opportunities for those with degrees in hotel administration.
Industrial traffic managers	20,500	[2]	Employment expected to grow more slowly than average for all occupations. Best opportunities for college graduates with majors in traffic management or transportation.
Lawyers	342,000	26,400	Continued increase in number of law school graduates is expected to create keen competition for salaried positions. Prospects for establishing new practice probably best in small towns and expanding suburban areas.
Marketing research workers	25,000	3,000	Employment expected to grow much faster than average for all occupations as marketing activities are stimulated by demand for new products and services. Best opportunities for those with graduate training in marketing research or statistics.
Personnel and labor relations workers	320,000	23,000	Employment expected to increase faster than average for all occupations as employers implement new employee relations programs in areas of occupational safety and health, equal employment opportunity, and pensions. Although growing public employee unionism will spur demand for labor relations workers, keen competition is anticipated. Best opportunities for applicants with advanced degrees.
Public relations workers	100,000	6,500	Employment expected to increase about as fast as average for all occupations as organizations expand their public relations efforts. However, keen competition for beginning jobs as glamorous nature of the occupation attracts many applicants.

Occupation	Estimated employment 1974	Average annual openings[1] 1974–1985	Employment trends and prospects
Purchasing agents	189,000	11,700	Employment expected to increase faster than average for all occupations. Strongest demand for those with graduate degrees in purchasing management. Firms manufacturing technical products will need engineering and science graduates.
Urban planners	13,000	700	Employment expected to grow faster than average for all occupations in response to need for quality housing, transportation systems, health care, and other social services. Best opportunities for graduates with advanced degrees.

Service occupations

Cleaning and related occupations

Occupation	Estimated employment 1974	Average annual openings 1974–1985	Employment trends and prospects
Building custodians	1,900,000	146,000	Employment expected to grow about as fast as average for all occupations as construction of office buildings, schools, and hospitals increases demand for maintenance services. Many opportunities for part-time and evening work.
Hotel house-keepers and assistants	18,000	1,450	Employment expected to grow about as fast as average for all occupations, but competition is likely to be keen. Best opportunities in newly built hotels and motels.
Pest controllers	27,000	2,100	Employment expected to grow faster than average for all occupations. Because pests reproduce rapidly and tend to develop resistance to pesticides, control of them is never-ending problem.

Food service occupations

Occupation	Estimated employment 1974	Average annual openings 1974–1985	Employment trends and prospects
Bartenders	233,000	15,200	Employment expected to increase faster than average for all occupations as new restaurants, hotels, and bars open.

Occupation	Estimated employment 1974	Average annual openings[1] 1974–1985	Employment trends and prospects
Cooks and chefs	955,000	78,600	Employment expected to increase faster than average for all occupations. Most starting jobs in small restaurants serving simple food.
Dining room attendants and dishwashers	370,000	17,200	Favorable opportunities due to average employment growth and high replacement needs, particularly for part-time workers.
Food counter workers	350,000	29,200	Favorable opportunities due to average employment growth and high replacement needs, particularly for part-time workers.
Meatcutters	202,000	5,000	Employment expected to change little but thousands of openings annually will be created by replacement needs.
Waiters and waitresses	1,180,000	105,000	Favorable opportunites due to average employment growth and very high replacement needs, particularly for part-time workers. Keen competition for jobs in swank restaurants.

Personal service occupations

Barbers	130,000	5,550	Employment expected to change little with most openings resulting from replacement needs. Better opportunities for hairstylists than for conventional barbers.
Bellhops and bell captains	17,000	600	Employment expected to grow more slowly than average for all occupations due to growing popularity of economy motels. Best opportunities in motels, small hotels, and resort areas open only part of year.
Cosmetologists	500,000	50,800	Employment expected to grow about as fast as average for all occupations in response to rise in demand for beauty shop services. Good opportunities for both newcomers and experienced cosmetologists, including those seeking part-time work.
Funeral directors and embalmers	45,000	1,400	Employment expected to change little. Nevertheless, prospects are good for mortuary school graduates due to openings created by replacement needs.

Occupation	Estimated employment 1974	Average annual openings[1] 1974–1985	Employment trends and prospects
Private household service occupations			
Private household workers	1,200,000	52,000	Despite expected decline in employment, good opportunities as demand is likely to continue to exceed supply. Low wages, tedious nature of work, and lack of advancement opportunities discourage many prospective employees.
Protective and related service occupations			
Construction inspectors (government)	22,000	1,700	Employment expected to increase faster than average for all occupations. Best opportunities for those with some college education and knowledge of specialized type of construction.
FBI special agents	8,600	[2]	Rising employment as FBI responsibilities grow. Traditionally low turnover rate.
Firefighters	220,000	7,300	Employment expected to increase about as fast as average for all occupations in response to growing need for fire protection and replacement of volunteer fire companies by professional fire departments. Keen competition for jobs in urban areas; better opportunities in smaller communities.
Guards	475,000	26,000	Employment expected to grow more slowly than average for all occupations due to increased use of remote cameras, alarm systems, and other electronic surveillance equipment. Replacement needs will create most openings. Best opportunities for those seeking night work.
Health and regulatory inspectors (government)	110,000	7,900	Employment expected to increase faster than average for all occupations in response to public concern for improved quality and safety of consumer products. Employment of health inspectors expected to grow more rapidly than that of regulatory inspectors.

Occupation	Estimated employment 1974	Average annual openings[1] 1974–1985	Employment trends and prospects
Occupational safety and health workers	25,000	1,100	Employment expected to increase faster than average for all occupations as growing concern for occupational safety and health and consumer safety continues to generate programs and jobs. Best prospects for graduates of occupational safety or health curriculums.
Police officers	480,000	22,000	Good prospects for those with college training in law enforcement. Women and minority applicants sought to make police departments more representative of the populations they serve.
State police officers	45,500	3,600	Employment expected to increase much faster than average for all occupations primarily due to growing demand for officers to work in highway patrols.

Other service occupations

Mail carriers	267,000	5,600	Employment expected to change little due to more efficient mail delivery, but several thousand openings annually will result from replacement needs. Openings concentrated in metropolitan areas.
Telephone operators	390,000	28,000	Employment expected to change little due to increased direct dialing, but thousands of openings will arise annually as result of replacement needs.

Education and related occupations

Teaching occupations

College and university teachers	527,000[3]	14,000	Applicants expected to face keen competition. Number of new master's and Ph.D. degree recipients expected to more than meet the demand for college and university teachers. Best prospects in junior and community colleges.

Occupation	Estimated employment 1974	Average annual openings[1] 1974–1985	Employment trends and prospects
Kindergarten and elementary school teachers	1,276,000	94,000	If past trends continue, number of persons qualified to teach in elementary schools will exceed number of openings. Therefore, applicants are likely to face competition. Re-entrants also will face increasing competition from new graduates.
Secondary school teachers	1,086,000	37,500	Supply of secondary school teachers expected to exceed greatly anticipated demand, and applicants are likely to face keen competition. However, a recent survey found that teacher supply was least adequate in mathematics, natural and physical sciences, industrial arts, special education, and some vocational-technical subjects.

Library occupations

Occupation	Estimated employment 1974	Average annual openings[1] 1974–1985	Employment trends and prospects
Librarians	125,000	10,400	Applicants are likely to face competition for choice positions. Best opportunities for new graduates in public and special libraries.
Library technicians and assistants	135,000	14,100	Employment expected to grow faster than average for all occupations. Best opportunities in large public and college and university libraries, particularly for graduates of academic programs.

Sales occupations

Occupation	Estimated employment 1974	Average annual openings[1] 1974–1985	Employment trends and prospects
Automobile parts counter workers	75,000	3,500	Employment expected to increase faster than average for all occupations as more parts will be needed to repair growing number of motor vehicles.
Automobile salesworkers	130,000	5,500	Employment expected to grow as demand for automobiles increases. However, employment may fluctuate from year to year because car sales are highly sensitive to economic conditions and consumer preferences.
Automobile service advisers	20,000	800	Employment expected to increase about as fast as average for all occupations as au-

Occupation	Estimated employment 1974	Average annual openings[1] 1974–1985	Employment trends and prospects
			tomobiles increase in number and complexity. Most openings in large dealerships located in metropolitan areas.
Gasoline service station attendants	450,000	12,700	Employment expected to grow over next few years, although trends toward cars with improved gas mileage and self-service gas stations might limit growth over long run. Nevertheless, replacement needs will create thousands of openings annually.
Manufacturers' salesworkers	380,000	9,500	Employment expected to increase more slowly than average for all occupations. Some growth will occur in response to rising demand for technical products. Good opportunities for those with sales ability. Most job openings due to replacement needs.
Models	9,000	800	Employment expected to grow faster than average for all occupations, but applicants are likely to face keen competition. Glamour of modeling attracts many more persons than needed.
Real estate salesworkers and brokers	400,000	28,500	Employment expected to increase about as fast as average for all occupations in response to growing demand for housing and other properties. However, highly competitive nature of occupation will result in many beginners having to transfer to other fields of work after short period of time.
Retail trade salesworkers	2,800,000	190,000	Employment expected to grow about as fast as average for all occupations as volume of sales rises and stores continue to remain open longer. Good opportunities for full-time, part-time, and temporary employment due to growth and high replacement needs.
Route drivers	190,000	3,700	Employment expected to change little, but several thousand openings annually will result from replacement needs.

Occupation	Estimated employment 1974	Average annual openings[1] 1974–1985	Employment trends and prospects
Securities salesworkers	100,000	6,100	Employment expected to grow faster than average for all occupations as funds available for investment increase. Due to competitive nature of occupation, replacement needs are relatively large. Those seeking part-time work will be limited to selling shares in mutual funds.
Wholesale trade salesperson	770,000	30,000	Employment expected to grow about as fast as average for all occupations as wholesalers sell wider variety of products and improve services to their customers. Good opportunities for persons suited to competitive nature of selling.

Construction occupations

Occupation	Estimated employment 1974	Average annual openings 1974–1985	Employment trends and prospects
Asbestos and insulation workers	30,000	2,300	Employment expected to grow much faster than average for all occupations in response to increased construction activity and need for energy-saving insulation. Best opportunities in metropolitan areas, where most insulation contractors are located.
Bricklayers and stonemasons	165,000	6,500	Employment expected to grow about as fast as average for all occupations in response to increased construction activity and expanding use of brick for decorative work. Little change expected in employment of stonemasons due to cost of stone relative to other materials.
Carpenters	1,060,000	49,100	Plentiful opportunities over long run resulting from high replacement needs and average employment growth due to increased construction activity.
Cement masons (cement and concrete finishers)	90,000	4,300	Favorable opportunities due to faster than average employment growth in response to increased construction activity and greater use of concrete.
Construction workers	865,000	28,400	Employment expected to grow more slowly than average for all occupations because of greater use of laborsaving equipment such as

Occupation	Estimated employment 1974	Average annual openings[1] 1974–1985	Employment trends and prospects
			trenching machines and forklifts. However, replacement needs will create many openings.
Drywall installers and finishers	60,000	1,900	Employment expected to grow faster than average for all occupations due to increases in construction activity. Best opportunities in metropolitan areas.
Electricians (construction)	245,000	11,700	Employment expected to increase faster than average for all occupations as more electrical fixtures and wiring will be needed in homes, offices, and other buildings.
Elevator constructors	19,000	1,050	Employment expected to increase faster than average for all occupations due to growth in number of high rise apartment and commercial buildings.
Floor covering installers	85,000	2,400	Employment expected to increase about as fast as average for all occupations due to more widespread use of resilient floor coverings and carpeting. Best opportunities for those who can install both carpeting and resilient flooring.
Glaziers	9,000	500	Employment expected to increase faster than average for all occupations as more glass is used in building design. Best opportunities in metropolitan areas where most glazing contractors are located.
Lathers	25,000	200	Employment expected to change little as drywall materials are increasingly used in place of lath and plaster. Some openings annually due to replacement needs.
Marble setters, tile setters, and terrazzo workers	40,000	[2]	Employment expected to grow more slowly than average for all occupations due to increasing use of competing materials such as carpeting, paving brick, and plastic coated wallboard usually installed by other skilled workers.
Operating engineers	400,000	27,000	Employment expected to grow much faster than average for all occupations due to in-

Occupation	Estimated employment 1974	Average annual openings[1] 1974–1985	Employment trends and prospects
(construction machinery operators)			creased activity in construction, highway maintenance, and movement of materials in factories and mines.
Painters and paperhangers	470,000	18,100	Employment of painters expected to grow more slowly than average for all occupations, but many openings annually will result from high replacement needs. Despite average employment growth for paperhangers, stimulated by rising popularity of wallpaper and vinyl wallcovering, there will be fewer job opportunities than for painters because of small number in occupation.
Painters	450,000	16,700	
Paperhangers	20,000	1,400	
Plasterers	26,000	450	Employment expected to change little as drywall materials are increasingly used in place of plaster. Replacement needs will create several hundred openings annually.
Plumbers and pipefitters	375,000	23,500	Employment expected to grow faster than average for all occupations due to increased construction activity and growth in areas which use extensive pipework, such as chemical and petroleum refineries and coal gasification and nuclear power plants. Also, trend toward more air-conditioning, appliances, and disposal equipment will create additional demand for these workers.
Roofers	90,000	5,000	Employment expected to increase faster than average for all occupations due to increases in construction activity, roof repairs, and waterproofing.
Sheet-metal workers	65,000	2,000	Employment expected to increase about as fast as average for all occupations due to need for air-conditioning and heating ducts and other sheet-metal products in homes, stores, offices, and other buildings.
Structural-, ornamental-, and reinforcing-ironworkers,	85,000	3,900	Employment in all ironworking occupations expected to increase faster than average for all occupations. Growing use of structural steel, ornamental panels, metal framing, and

Occupation	Estimated employment 1974	Average annual openings[1] 1974–1985	Employment trends and prospects
riggers, and machine movers			prestressed concrete should create additional jobs for structural-, ornamental-, and reinforcing-ironworkers; need to handle increasing amount of heavy construction machinery will result in additional jobs for riggers and machine movers.

Occupations in transportation activities

Air transportation occupations

Occupation	Estimated employment 1974	Average annual openings 1974–1985	Employment trends and prospects
Air traffic controllers	22,000	750	Employment expected to grow about as fast as average for all occupations as number of aircraft increases, but applicants may face keen competition. Best opportunities for college graduates with experience as controllers, pilots, or navigators.
Airplane mechanics	130,000	3,200	Employment expected to increase about as fast as average for all occupations, but opportunities in various areas of aviation will differ. Good opportunities in general aviation; keen competition for airline jobs; opportunities in Federal Government dependent upon defense spending.
Airplane pilots	79,000	2,800	Employment expected to grow faster than average for all occupations, but applicants likely to face keen competition. Best opportunities for recent college graduates with flying experience.
Flight attendants	41,000	6,400	Employment expected to grow faster than average for all occupations as number of airline passengers increases. However, keen competition for available positions.
Reservation, ticket, and passenger agents	56,000	4,250	Employment expected to grow faster than average for all occupations due to anticipated increase in airline passengers. Nevertheless, applicants likely to face keen competition because of popularity of airline jobs.

Occupation	Estimated employment 1974	Average annual openings[1] 1974–1985	Employment trends and prospects
Merchant marine occupations			
Merchant marine officers	7,500	150	Employment expected to change little as number of ships in merchant fleet not expected to increase significantly. Best opportunities for graduates of maritime academies to fill openings created by replacement needs.
Merchant marine sailors	20,000	50	Employment expected to decline as more ships become equipped with laborsaving features. Keen competition for positions created by replacement needs.
Railroad occupations			
Brake operators	73,000	700	Employment expected to decline due to technological innovations which increase efficiency of freight movement, but some openings will result from replacement needs.
Conductors	39,500	1,250	Employment expected to grow more slowly than average for all occupations as a result of technological innovations which increase efficiency of freight movement. Most openings due to replacement needs.
Locomotive engineers	37,000	1,350	Employment expected to grow more slowly than average for all occupations due to technological innovations which increase efficiency of freight movement. Most openings due to replacement needs.
Shop trades	75,000	[4]	Employment expected to decline as shop efficiency increases and as newer, more durable railroad cars replace older models.
Signal department workers	11,500	250	Employment expected to change little due to installation of new signal systems requiring less maintenance. However, some openings annually will result from replacement needs.
Station agents	7,600	[4]	Employment expected to decline as more customer orders and billings are handled by cen-

Occupation	Estimated employment 1974	Average annual openings[1] 1974–1985	Employment trends and prospects
			trally located stations and as smaller stations are serviced by mobile agents.
Telegraphers, telephoners, and tower operators	11,000		Employment expected to decline due to wider use of automatic signaling and train control systems.
Track workers	57,000	1,050	Employment expected to change little due to increased productivity of track workers and installation of improved train control systems requiring less track. However, some openings annually due to replacement needs.

Driving occupations

Occupation	Estimated employment 1974	Average annual openings 1974–1985	Employment trends and prospects
Intercity busdrivers	25,000	850	Employment expected to change little. Applicants are likely to face keen competition for openings created by replacement needs.
Local transit busdrivers	71,000	2,900	Employment expected to increase more slowly than average for all occupations, but many openings will result from replacement needs. Keen competition for available positions.
Local truck-drivers	1,600,000	38,500	Employment expected to increase more slowly than average for all occupations, but applicants are likely to find favorable opportunities. Thousands of openings annually due to replacement needs in this very large occupation.
Long distance truckdrivers	540,000	12,000	Employment expected to grow more slowly than average for all occupations as result of increased efficiency of freight movement. Keen competition for available openings.
Parking attendants	42,000	1,800	Employment expected to grow more slowly than average for all occupations as trend to self-parking systems continues. Most job opportunites will be in large commercial parking lots in urban areas.
Taxicab	92,000	2,450	Employment expected to change little, but

Occupation	Estimated employment 1974	Average annual openings[1] 1974–1985	Employment trends and prospects
drivers			applicants should find good opportunities due to high replacement needs.

Scientific and technical occupations

Conservation occupations

Occupation	Estimated employment 1974	Average annual openings[1] 1974–1985	Employment trends and prospects
Foresters	24,000	950	Employment expected to grow about as fast as average for all occupations. However, number of forestry graduates each year expected to exceed number of annual openings, creating competition for jobs.
Forestry technicians	10,500	500	Employment expected to increase faster than average for all occupations. However, due to anticipated large number of qualified applicants, even those with specialized posthigh school training may face competition.
Range managers	2,500	150	Good employment opportunities expected. Demand stimulated by need to increase output of rangelands while protecting their ecological balance.
Engineering occupations	1,100,000[5]	52,500[5]	Employment expected to grow faster than average for all occupations. Very good opportunities for engineering school graduates as supply is likely to fall short of demand. Many openings also will be filled by upgraded technicians and graduates in related fields.
Aerospace engineers	52,000	1,100	Employment, largely dependent upon Federal expenditures on defense and space programs, expected to grow about as fast as average for all occupations. Expenditures expected to increase by mid-1980's but remain below their peak levels of 1960's.
Agricultural engineers	12,000	500	Employment expected to grow faster than average for all occupations in response to increasing demand for agricultural products, modernization of farm operations, and increasing emphasis on conservation of resources.

Occupation	Estimated employment 1974	Average annual openings[1] 1974–1985	Employment trends and prospects
Biomedical engineers	3,000	150	Employment expected to grow faster than average for all occupations, but actual number of openings not likely to be very large. Strong demand for master's and Ph.D. degree holders in teaching and medical research.
Ceramic engineers	12,000	550	Employment expected to grow faster than average for all occupations as result of need to develop and improve ceramic materials for nuclear energy, electronics, defense, and medical science.
Chemical engineers	50,000	1,850	Employment expected to grow faster than average for all occupations in response to industrial expansion, particularly in chemicals industry.
Civil engineers	170,000	9,300	Employment expected to increase faster than average for all occupations as result of growing needs for housing, industrial buildings, electric power generating plants, and transportation systems. Work on environmental pollution and energy self-sufficiency also will result in openings.
Electrical engineers	290,000	12,200	Employment expected to increase faster than average for all occupations. Growing demand for computers, communications and electric power generating equipment, military and consumer electronics goods, and increased research and development in nuclear power generation will spur demand.
Industrial engineers	180,000	7,200	Employment expected to grow faster than average for all occupations due to industry growth, increasing complexity of industrial operations, expansion of automated processes, and greater emphasis on scientific management and safety.
Mechanical engineers	185,000	7,900	Employment expected to increase faster than average for all occupations resulting from growing demand for industrial machinery and

Occupation	Estimated employment 1974	Average annual openings[1] 1974–1985	Employment trends and prospects
			machine tools and increasing complexity of industrial machinery and processes.
Metallurgical engineers	17,000	550	Employment expected to grow about as fast as average for all occupations to develop new metals and alloys, adapt current ones to new needs, solve problems associated with efficient use of nuclear energy, and develop new ways of recycling solid waste materials.
Mining engineers	5,000	350	Employment will grow, spurred by efforts to attain energy self-sufficiency and resulting increase in demand for coal, development of more advanced mining systems, and further enforcement of mine health and safety regulations.
Petroleum engineers	12,000	750	Employment expected to increase faster than average for all occupations. Efforts to attain energy self-sufficiency will result in growing demand for petroleum and natural gas and will require increasingly sophisticated recovery methods.

Environmental science occupations

Occupation	Estimated employment 1974	Average annual openings[1] 1974–1985	Employment trends and prospects
Geologists	23,000	1,300	Employment expected to increase faster than average for all occupations because of demand for petroleum and minerals. Good employment opportunities for bachelor's degree holders; very good opportunities for those with advanced degrees.
Geophysicists	8,200	450	Employment expected to grow faster than average for all occupations as petroleum and mining companies need additional geophysicists for increased exploration activities. Excellent opportunities for graduates at all degree levels.
Meteorologists	5,600	200	Favorable opportunities in industry, weather consulting firms, radio and television, government, and colleges and universities.

Occupation	Estimated employment 1974	Average annual openings[1] 1974–1985	Employment trends and prospects
Oceanographers	2,500	100	Applicants are likely to face competition. Those with Ph.D. degrees should have favorable opportunities, but those with less education may be limited to routine analytical work as research assistants or technicians.

Life science occupations

Occupation	Estimated employment 1974	Average annual openings 1974–1985	Employment trends and prospects
Biochemists	12,400	800	Employment expected to grow faster than average for all occupations. Favorable opportunities for those with advanced degrees due to increased activities in medical research and environmental protection.
Life scientists	190,000	10,700	Good opportunities for those with advanced degrees due to increased activities in medical research and environmental protection. Although those with lesser degrees may face competition, they may become research assistants or laboratory technologists or enter health care field.

Mathematics occupations

Occupation	Estimated employment 1974	Average annual openings 1974–1985	Employment trends and prospects
Mathematicians	40,000	1,550	Keen competition expected, particularly for those seeking teaching positions in colleges and universities. Holders of advanced degrees in applied mathematics should have least difficulty in finding satisfactory employment.
Statisticians	24,000	1,250	Employment expected to grow faster than average for all occupations due to increasing use of statistical techniques in business and government. Favorable opportunities for those who combine training in statistics with knowledge of field of application such as engineering.

Occupation	Estimated employment 1974	Average annual openings[1] 1974–1985	Employment trends and prospects
Physical science occupations			
Astronomers	2,000	30	Employment expected to grow more slowly than average for all occupations because funds available for basic research in astronomy not expected to increase enough to create many new positions. Keen competition as number of degrees granted in astronomy probably will exceed number of job openings.
Chemists	135,000	6,400	Good opportunities for graduates at all degree levels. Increased demand for plastics, man-made fibers, drugs, and fertilizers in addition to activities in health care, pollution control, and energy will contribute to need for additional chemists.
Food scientists	7,200	350	Employment expected to grow faster than average for all occupations. Favorable opportunities, particularly for those with advanced degrees, in research and product development. Increased demand for food scientists in quality control and production.
Physicists	48,000	1,700	Employment expected to grow faster than average for all occupations. Good employment opportunities overall, but keen competition for teaching positions in colleges and universities.
Other scientific and technical occupations			
Broadcast technicians	22,000	1,350	Employment expected to increase about as fast as average for all occupations as new radio and television stations go on air and cable television stations broadcast more of their own programs.
Drafters	313,000	17,300	Employment expected to increase faster than average for all occupations as more drafters

Occupation	Estimated employment 1974	Average annual openings[1] 1974–1985	Employment trends and prospects
			will be needed to support growing number of scientists and engineers. Also, increasingly complex design problems require additional drafters. Best opportunities for holders of associate degrees in drafting.
Engineering and science technicians	560,000	32,000	Employment expected to grow faster than average for all occupations as result of industrial expansion and increasingly important role of technicians in research and development. Favorable employment opportunities, particularly for graduates of postsecondary school technician training programs.
Surveyors	55,000	3,600	Employment expected to increase much faster than average for all occupations in response to rapid development of urban areas. Best opportunities for those with postsecondary school training in surveying.

Mechanic and repairer occupations

Telephone craft occupations

Occupation	Estimated employment 1974	Average annual openings 1974–1985	Employment trends and prospects
Central office craft occupations	110,000	2,900	Employment of frame wirers, trouble locators, and central office repairers expected to increase about as fast as average for all occupations in response to growing demand for telephone services.
Central office equipment installers	30,000	800	Employment expected to increase about as fast as average for all occupations because of need to install equipment in thousands of new telephone central offices and to replace obsolete equipment.
Line installers and cable splicers	55,000	150	Employment expected to change little due to laborsaving technological developments. Some openings will arise annually as result of replacement needs.
Telephone and PBX	115,000	2,400	Growing demand for telephones and private branch exchange (PBX) and central exchange

Occupation	Estimated employment 1974	Average annual openings[1] 1974–1985	Employment trends and prospects
installers and repairers			(CENTREX) systems will result in employment growth slower than average for all occupations.

Other mechanic and repairer occupations

Occupation	Estimated employment 1974	Average annual openings[1] 1974–1985	Employment trends and prospects
Air-condition- ing, refrigeration, and heating mechanics	200,000	10,900	Employment expected to increase faster than average for all occupations. Most openings for air-conditioning and refrigeration mechanics. Employment of furnace installers and gas burner mechanics should follow growth trends in new construction, while employment of oil burner mechanics should grow as heating systems are serviced more frequently to conserve oil.
Appliance repairers	135,000	5,600	Employment expected to grow about as fast as average for all occupations in response to increases in population and income, in addition to introduction of new appliances and improvements in existing ones.
Automobile body repairers	145,000	4,700	Employment expected to increase about as fast as average for all occupations as result of rising number of vehicles damaged in traffic accidents.
Automobile mechanics	735,000	24,400	Employment expected to grow about as fast as average for all occupations as more automobiles will be equipped with pollution control devices, air-conditioning, and other features that increase maintenance requirements. Good opportunities because of these factors and high replacement needs.
Boat-motor mechanics	11,000	550	Employment expected to increase faster than average for all occupations due to growth in number of boats and related vehicles such as minibikes and snowmobiles. Particularly favorable opportunities for those with knowledge of electricity and electronics.
Bowling-pin-	5,000	150	Employment expected to grow more slowly

Occupation	Estimated employment 1974	Average annual openings[1] 1974–1985	Employment trends and prospects
machine mechanics			than average for all occupations due to improvements in pinsetting machines. Limited number of openings will become available because of replacement needs.
Business machine repairers	65,000	3,100	Employment expected to grow faster than average for all occupations. Opportunities particularly favorable for those with training in electronics.
Computer service technicians	50,000	4,300	Employment expected to grow much faster than average for all occupations due to increased use of computers.
Diesel mechanics	95,000	3,400	Employment expected to grow faster than average for all occupations due to expansion of industries which are major users of diesel engines and continued replacement of gasoline engines by diesel engines.
Electric sign repairers	9,000	450	Employment expected to grow faster than average for all occupations in response to rapid increase in number of signs.
Farm equipment mechanics	60,000	2,700	Employment expected to grow about as fast as average for all occupations as increase in size and complexity of farm equipment will lead to more maintenance requirements.
Industrial machinery repairers	500,000	42,500	Employment expected to increase much faster than average for all occupations because of the growing amount of complex factory machinery requiring maintenance and repair.
Instrument repairers	110,000	6,600	Employment expected to increase faster than average for all occupations because of anticipated increased use of instruments for energy conservation and exploration, air and water pollution monitoring, and medical diagnosis.
Jewelers	18,000	750	Employment expected to change little. While demand for jewelry grows, improved production methods will limit need for new workers. For openings created by replacement needs, priority will be given to applicants who have

Occupation	Estimated employment 1974	Average annual openings[1] 1974–1985	Employment trends and prospects
			completed technical school courses in jewelry design, construction, and repair.
Locksmiths	9,000	400	Employment expected to grow faster than average for all occupations as result of more security conscious public. Particularly favorable opportunities for those who can install and service electronic security systems.
Maintenance electricians	280,000	13,800	Employment expected to grow faster than average for all occupations due to increased use of electrical and electronic equipment by industry.
Motorcycle mechanics	11,000	[2]	Employment expected to increase much faster than average for all occupations in response to growing number of motorcycles, minibikes, and snowmobiles. Most full-time jobs in large dealerships located in suburban metropolitan areas.
Piano and organ tuners and repairers	8,000	350	Employment expected to change little as number of pianos and organs will be limited by competition from other forms of entertainment. However, some openings annually due to replacement needs.
Shoe repairers	30,000	1,300	Employment expected to decline, largely because number of people entering trade has been insufficient to meet replacement needs. Good opportunities for experienced repairers who wish to open their own shops.
Television and radio service technicians	135,000	6,600	Employment expected to increase faster than average for all occupations in response to growing number of radios, television sets, phonographs, tape recorders, and other home entertainment products.
Truck mechanics and bus mechanics	135,000	5,600	Employment of truck mechanics expected to grow faster than average for all occupations due to significant increases in transportation of freight by trucks. Employment of bus mechanics, however, expected to grow more slowly than average.

Occupation	Estimated employment 1974	Average annual openings[1] 1974–1985	Employment trends and prospects
Vending machine mechanics	24,000	600	Slower than average employment increase. Some growth as additional machines are installed to meet demands of increasing population. However, most openings will result from replacement needs.
Watch repairers	17,000	800	Employment expected to grow at slower rate than average for all occupations, because many watches now made cost little more to replace than to repair. Nevertheless, good opportunities for graduates of watch repair schools.

Health occupations

Dental occupations

Dental assistants	120,000	14,500	Employment expected to grow faster than average for all occupations in response to increasing use of assistants by dentists. Excellent opportunities, especially for graduates of approved programs. Favorable outlook for part-time work.
Dental hygienists	23,000	6,300	Employment expected to grow much faster than average for all occupations in response to increasing use of hygienists by dentists. Very good prospects for graduates of approved programs.
Dental laboratory technicians	32,000	2,600	Employment expected to grow faster than average for all occupations in response to increasing demand for dentures. Very good opportunities for graduates of approved programs.
Dentists	105,000	6,200	Employment expected to grow faster than average for all occupations as dental services increase in response to expansion of prepayment arrangements. Excellent opportunities for qualified dentists.

Occupation	Estimated employment 1974	Average annual openings[1] 1974–1985	Employment trends and prospects
Medical practitioners			
Chiropractors	18,000	1,200	Employment expected to increase faster than average for all occupations in response to broader public acceptance of profession. Best opportunities in areas with comparatively few established practitioners.
Optometrists	19,000	900	Favorable employment opportunities. Employment expected to grow about as fast as average for all occupations.
Physicians and osteopathic physicians	350,000	23,000	Very good employment outlook. Particular demand in primary care areas such as general practice, pediatrics, and internal medicine, especially in rural areas.
Podiatrists	7,500	400	Favorable opportunities for graduates to establish their own practices as well as to enter salaried positions.
Veterinarians	29,000	1,450	Favorable employment opportunities as result of growth in pet population and number of livestock and poultry and increase in veterinary research.
Medical technologist, technician, and assistant occupations			
Electrocardiographic technicians	11,000	1,000	Employment expected to increase faster than average for all occupations because of growing reliance on electrocardiograms in diagnosis and physical examinations.
Electroencephalographic technicians	3,800	350	Employment expected to grow faster than average for all occupations in response to increased use of electroencephalographs in surgery, in diagnosis, and in monitoring patients with brain diseases.
Medical assistants	220,000	27,200	Employment expected to increase faster than average for all occupations in response to growth of number of physicians. Excellent opportunities, particularly for graduates of accredited junior college programs.

Occupation	Estimated employment 1974	Average annual openings[1] 1974–1985	Employment trends and prospects
Medical laboratory workers	175,000	18,000	Employment expected to increase faster than average for all occupations as physicians make wider use of laboratory facilities. However, applicants may face competition for choice positions.
Medical record technicans and clerks	53,000	11,500	Very good outlook for clerks due to anticipated expansion in medical facilities and record-keeping. Favorable prospects for technicians with at least associate degree; those with less education may face strong competition.
Operating room technicians	28,000	2,700	Employment expected to grow faster tnan average for all occupations as operating room technicians increasingly assume more of routine nursing tasks in operating room. Good opportunities, particularly for graduates of 2-year junior college programs.
Optometric assistants	11,500	1,800	Employment expected to grow much faster than average for all occupations in response to greater demand for eye care services. Excellent opportunities for those who have completed formal training programs.
Radiologic (X-ray) technologists	82,000	8,600	Despite faster than average employment growth as X-ray equipment is increasingly used to diagnose and treat diseases, even graduates of AMA-approved programs may face competition for choice positions. Part-time workers will find best opportunities in physicians' offices and clinics.
Respiratory therapy workers	38,000	6,800	Employment expected to grow much faster than average for all occupations due to many new uses for respiratory therapy. Favorable employment opportunities.

Nursing occupations

Licensed practical	495,000	93,000	Very good opportunities as public and private health insurance plans expand and as LPN's

Occupation	Estimated employment 1974	Average annual openings[1] 1974–1985	Employment trends and prospects
nurses			assume duties previously performed by registered nurses.
Nursing aides, orderlies, and attendants	970,000	123,000	Employment expected to increase much faster than average for all occupations. Although most openings will arise from replacement needs, many new openings will be in nursing homes, convalescent homes, and other long term care facilities.
Registered nurses	860,000	71,000	Favorable opportunities, especially for nurses with graduate education seeking positions as teachers and administrators. Strong demand in some southern States and many inner-city locations.

Therapy and rehabilitation occupations

Occupational therapists	9,400	1,000	Employment expected to grow faster than average for all occupations due to public interest in rehabilitation of disabled persons and success of established occupational therapy programs. Favorable opportunities for graduates of approved programs.
Occupational therapy assistants	7,900	1,150	Employment expected to grow faster than average for all occupations due to public interest in rehabilitation of disabled people. Very good opportunities, particularly for graduates of approved programs.
Physical therapists	20,000	2,400	Employment expected to grow much faster than average for all occupations due to expansion of rehabilitation programs and facilities. Favorable opportunities for new graduates, particularly in suburban and rural areas.
Physical therapist assistants and aides	10,500	1,400	Employment expected to grow much faster than average for all occupations, resulting in excellent opportunities for both assistants and aides.

Occupation	Estimated employment 1974	Average annual openings[1] 1974–1985	Employment trends and prospects
Speech pathologists and audiologists	31,000	3,700	Employment expected to increase much faster than average for all occupations. Favorable opportunities for master's degree holders; limited opportunities for bachelor's degree holders. Very keen competition for teaching positions in colleges and universities.

Other health occupations

Occupation	Estimated employment 1974	Average annual openings 1974–1985	Employment trends and prospects
Dietitians	33,000	3,200	Employment expected to grow faster than average for all occupations due to increasing demand for expertise in fields of nutrition and food management. Good opportunities for those with at least bachelor's degree in foods and nutrition or institution management.
Dispensing opticians	17,000	1,550	Employment expected to increase much faster than average for all occupations in response to growing demand for prescription lenses. Best opportunities for those with associate degrees.
Health services administrators	150,000	17,400	Employment expected to grow much faster than average for all occupations as quality and quantity of patient services increase and hospital management becomes more complex. Best opportunities for those with graduate degrees.
Medical record administrators	12,000	1,100	Employment expected to grow faster than average for all occupations as increased use of health facilities will add to volume and importance of medical record systems. Very good opportunities for graduates of approved programs.
Pharmacists	117,000	6,500	Employment expected to grow about as fast as average for all occupations due to establishment of new pharmacies and more extensive use of pharmacists in hospitals and clinics. Very good outlook as number of job openings expected to exceed number of pharmacy school graduates.

Occupation	Estimated employment 1974	Average annual openings[1] 1974–1985	Employment trends and prospects
Social science occupations			
Anthropologists	3,800	250	Ph.D.'s may face keen competition for choice professional positions. Master's degree holders are expected to face very keen competition but may find positions as college instructors or in other areas such as urban planning or mental and public health.
Economists	71,000	4,700	Economists with master's and Ph.D. degrees may face keen competition for positions in colleges and universities but may find good opportunities in private industry and government. Bachelor's degree holders are expected to face keen competition in all areas.
Geographers	9,000	650	Favorable employment opportunities for Ph.D.'s in teaching and research. Master's and bachelor's degree holders are likely to face competition for jobs. In addition to positions as instructors or teaching assistants, opportunities may be available in regional planning and development, environmental quality control, and cartography.
Historians	26,000	1,300	Ph.D.'s are expected to face keen competition for choice academic positions. Master's degree holders may encounter very keen competition, but some positions may be available in small colleges and some high schools. Limited opportunities for bachelor's degree holders.
Political scientists	11,500	600	Ph.D.'s may face keen competition for choice academic positions. Master's degree holders may face very keen competition for teaching positions, but those with specialized training may find jobs in government and industry. Limited opportunities for bachelor's degree holders.
Psychologists	75,000	5,200	Very good opportunities for Ph.D. and some master's degree holders, particularly in clini-

Occupation	Estimated employment 1974	Average annual openings[1] 1974–1985	Employment trends and prospects
			cal and counseling psychology. However, those wishing to teach or do research in large colleges and universities may face keen competition.
Sociologists	14,000	750	Ph.D.'s may face competition for choice academic positions. Master's degree holders are likely to face keen competition for academic positions but may find jobs in government and private research organizations. Sociologists well trained in research methods, advanced statistics, and use of computers are expected to have widest choice of jobs.

Social service occupations

Counseling occupations

Occupation	Estimated employment 1974	Average annual openings 1974–1985	Employment trends and prospects
College career planning and placement counselors	4,100	250	Favorable prospects for well-qualified workers, particularly those with specialized training in junior and community college career counseling. However, financial problems in colleges and universities may limit growth, resulting in competition for available positions.
Employment counselors	7,000	650	Applicants with master's degrees or experience in related fields expected to face competition in both public and community employment agencies. Employment growth largely dependent on Federal Government funding and State allocation of money to employment service.
Rehabilitation counselors	19,000	2,100	Favorable prospects, particularly for those with graduate work in rehabilitation counseling or related fields. Employment growth largely dependent on government funding for vocational rehabilitation.
School counselors	44,000	2,050	Employment expected to increase more slowly than average for all occupations due to expected continuing decline in school enroll-

Occupation	Estimated employment 1974	Average annual openings[1] 1974–1985	Employment trends and prospects
			ments during late 1970's. However, some positions will be available in elementary schools. Opportunities largely dependent upon Federal Government's Career Education Program.
Clergy	245,000	[2]	
Protestant ministers	183,000	[2]	Keen competition in most denominations and geographic areas. Many ministers will find employment in social work and education and as chaplains in Armed Forces, hospitals, and institutions.
Rabbis	4,000	[2]	As some established congregations have closed and fewer new ones are being built, many newly ordained rabbis will take positions in smaller communities and in related fields such as social work and education.
Roman Catholic priests	58,000	[2]	Growing number needed. Number of priests ordained insufficient to meet needs of increasing Catholic population.
Other social service occupations			
Home economists	128,000	9,000	Although employment is expected to grow more slowly than average for all occupations, many jobs will become available due to replacement needs. Those wishing to teach in high schools may face keen competition, while those with graduate degrees may find good prospects in college and university teaching.
Recreation workers	65,000	5,900	Employment expected to grow faster than average for all occupations in response to increased demand for recreation programs. Favorable outlook for those with at least bachelor's degree in recreation. Good opportunities for part-time and summer employment.

Occupation	Estimated employment 1974	Average annual openings[1] 1974–1985	Employment trends and prospects
Social service aides	70,000	8,400	Employment expected to grow much faster than average for all occupations as social welfare programs expand and aides perform tasks formerly handled by professional personnel. Good opportunities for part-time work.
Social workers	300,000	30,500	Employment expected to increase faster than average for all occupations. Best opportunities for those with professional social work training at all degree levels.

Art, design, and communications-related occupations

Performing artists

Actors and actresses	10,000	900	Overcrowding in field expected to persist resulting in keen competition. Moreover, many are employed for only part of year.
Dancers	7,000	950	Those seeking professional careers in dance likely to face keen competition, despite expected faster than average rate of employment growth. Teaching offers best opportunities.
Musicians	85,000	5,200	All but highest caliber symphonic players likely to face keen competition. Better prospects for those qualified as teachers as well as musicians than for those qualified as performers only.
Singers	36,000	2,400	Keenly competitive field, despite expected faster than average rate of employment growth. Some opportunities will arise from expanded use of television satellites, cable television, and wider use of video cassettes, but best prospects are in teaching.

Design occupations

Architects	40,000	3,000	Employment expected to increase much faster than average for all occupations as result of growth of nonresidential construction. Most openings will be in architectural firms. Favorable opportunities.

Occupation	Estimated employment 1974	Average annual openings[1] 1974–1985	Employment trends and prospects
Commercial artists	64,000	4,000	Talented and well-trained commercial artists may face competition for employment and advancement in most kinds of work. Those with only average ability and little specialized training will encounter keen competition and have limited advancement opportunities.
Display workers	34,000	2,200	Employment expected to grow about as fast as average for all occupations due to construction of additional stores and increased emphasis on window and interior displays.
Floral designers	33,000	3,300	Employment expected to increase faster than average for all occupations in response to growing demand for floral arrangements. Good prospects.
Industrial designers	10,000	450	Employment expected to grow about as fast as average for all occupations. Best prospects for those with college degrees in industrial design.
Interior designers	34,000	1,550	Competition for beginning jobs. Best opportunities for talented college graduates who majored in interior design and graduates of professional schools of interior design. Those with less talent or without formal training are likely to face increasingly keen competition.
Landscape architects	12,000	900	Employment expected to grow much faster than average for all occupations as result of increased interest in city and regional environmental planning.
Photographers	80,000	3,400	Employment expected to grow about as fast as average for all occupations. Good opportunities in technical fields such as scientific and industrial photography. Portrait and commercial photographers are likely to face keen competition.

Communications-related occupations

Interpreters	600	[2]	Competition expected for limited number of openings. Only highly qualified applicants may find favorable opportunities.

Occupation	Estimated employment 1974	Average annual openings[1] 1974–1985	Employment trends and prospects
Newspaper reporters	40,000	2,200	Favorable opportunites for those with exceptional writing talent and ability to handle highly specialized scientific and technical subjects. Best prospects on weekly or daily newspapers in small towns and suburban areas.
Radio and television announcers	19,000	600	Despite average employment growth as new radio and television stations are licensed and as more cable television stations begin their own programming, applicants likely to face keen competition. Better opportunities in radio than in television.
Technical writers	20,000	1,150	Employment expected to grow about as fast as average for all occupations. Best opportunities for those with good writing ability and appropriate technical background.

Footnotes

[1]Due to growth, deaths and retirements, and other causes of separation from labor force. Does not include transfers out of occupations.

[2]Estimate not available.

[3]Excludes part-time junior staff.

[4]For the Nation as whole, projected decrease in employment expected to be greater than number of openings resulting from deaths and retirements. However, in some localities decline in employment may be less than national average. In such cases, job openings resulting from deaths and retirements may be greater than decline in employment. In some areas, employment growth may occur.

[5]Totals do not equal sum of individual estimates because all branches of engineering are not covered separately in *Handbook*.

SOURCE: *Occupational Outlook Quarterly*, 20, no. 1 (Spring 1976), United States Government Printing Office, Washington, D.C.

Toward matching personal and job characteristics

The information on careers in the *Occupational Outlook Handbook in Brief* consists of a general overview of the job market and some specific information on hiring potential for the future. In most cases, this information provides you with only limited assistance in determining which career fields interest you. Although it has its place in the overall process of gathering information about careers, we believe that there are other important kinds of information for you to consider and explore the types of activities in which workers engage, the skills and level of education necessary to enter the field, and the satisfaction to be derived from the work, to name just a few. The following table uses the same job titles as the *Occupational Outlook Handbook in Brief* and can provide you with this new and important information. Read the list of twenty-five common job characteristics and requirements carefully and then get involved in the table, identifying careers and job fields that are consistent with your own interests, abilities, and aspirations. Before you begin, you may want to check back to some of your conclusions from Chapter 2, "Self-awareness." Then, once you've identified five to ten careers, compare them with the careers that you identified earlier.

As with all the information and exercises in this book, this information is not meant to and isn't capable of deciding for you which career field you will eventually enter. It can, however, supply you with important information about yourself and about career options that, along with other information, will help you in the career development process. Be patient. Don't jump to conclusions. Soon we will be discussing setting goals and making decisions.

Twenty-five common job characteristics and requirements

1. High school degree — high school diploma generally required.

2. Technical school of apprenticeship — some form of nondegree posthigh school training required.

3. Junior college — requires Associate in Arts degree.

4. College degree — requires at least a bachelor's degree.

("C" = BA degree; "G" = graduate work or first professional degree.)

5. Jobs widely scattered — jobs are located in most areas of the United States.

6. Jobs concentrated in localities — jobs are highly concentrated in one or a few geographical locations.

7. Works with things — job generally requires manual skills.

8. Works with ideas — uses one's intellect to solve problems.

9. Helps people — assists people in a helping relationship.

10. Works with people — job generally requires pleasing personality and ability to get along with others.

11. Able to see physical results of work — work produces a tangible product.

12. Opportunity for self-expression — freedom to use one's own ideas.

13. Works as part of a team — interacts with fellow employees in performing work.

14. Works independently — requires initiative, self-discipline, and the ability to organize.

15. Work is closely supervised — job performance and work standards controlled by supervisor.

16. Directs activities of others — work entails supervisory responsibilities.

17. Generally confined to work area — physically located at one work setting.

18. Overtime or shift work required — works hours other than normal daytime shifts.

19. Exposed to weather conditions — works outside or is subjected to temperature extremes.

20. High level of responsibility — requires making key decisions involving property, finances, or human safety and welfare.

21. Requires physical stamina — must be in physical condition for continued lifting, standing, and walking.

22. Works with details — works with technical data, numbers, or written materials on a continuous basis.

23. Repetitious work — performs the same task on a continuing basis.

24. Motivates others — must be able to influence others.

25. Competititve — competes with other people on the job for recognition and advancement.

INDUSTRIAL PRODUCTION AND RELATED OCCUPATIONS

Column key:
1. High school diploma
2. Technical school or apprenticeship
3. Junior college
4. College degree
5. Jobs widely scattered
6. Jobs concentrated in localities
7. Working with things
8. Working with ideas
9. Helping people
10. Working with people
11. Able to see physical results of work
12. Opportunity for self-expression
13. Works as part of a team
14. Works independently
15. Directs activities of others
16. Work is closely supervised
17. Generally confined to work area
18. Overtime or shift work required
19. Exposed to weather conditions
20. High level of responsibility
21. Requires physical stamina
22. Works with detail
23. Repetitious work
24. Motivates others
25. Competitive

Occupation	1	2	3	4	5	6	7	8	9	10	11	12	13	14	15	16	17	18	19	20	21	22	23	24	25
Foundry occupations																									
Patternmakers	X	X		X		X					X		X		X		X					X			
Molders		X		X		X					X		X		X		X					X			
Coremakers		X		X		X					X		X		X		X					X			
Machining occupations																									
All-round machinists		X		X		X					X			X			X				X	X	X		
Instrument makers (mechanical)	X	X			X	X					X		X		X							X			
Machine tool operators		X		X		X					X			X			X				X	X	X		
Set-up workers (machine tools)	X	X			X	X					X			X			X				X	X			
Tool-and-die makers		X			X	X					X			X	X		X	X				X	X		
Printing occupations																									
Bookbinders	X	X		X		X					X		X		X							X			
Composing room workers	X	X			X	X						X		X		X	X					X	X		
Electrotypers and stereotypers	X	X			X	X				X		X		X		X	X					X	X		
Lithographic workers	X	X			X	X							X		X		X	X				X	X		
Photoengravers	X	X			X	X				X		X					X	X				X	X		
Printing press operators and assistants	X	X			X	X							X				X			X					
Other industrial and related occupations																									
Assemblers					X	X					X		X		X							X			
Automobile painters		X		X		X				X		X	X	X								X			
Automobile trimmers and installers				X		X				X		X		X								X			
Blacksmiths		X		X		X				X		X		X					X			X			
Blue-collar-worker supervisors	X			X					X				X		X	X		X							

	1	2	3	4	5	6	7	8	9	10	11	12	13	14	15	16	17	18	19	20	21	22	23	24	25
Other industrial and related occupations																									
Boilermakers		X			X		X				X		X					X			X	X			
Electroplaters		X			X		X				X			X			X					X			
Forge shop workers					X		X				X		X		X		X				X		X		
Furnace tenders					X		X							X				X							
Furniture upholsterers		X			X		X				X			X			X					X			
Inspectors (manufacturing)						X	X						X	X	X		X	X			X	X			
Millwrights		X			X		X				X		X		X						X	X			
Motion picture projectionists		X			X		X							X			X	X				X			
Photographic laboratory workers					X		X				X			X			X				X	X			
Power truck operators					X		X						X		X							X			
Production painters					X		X						X		X		X					X			
Stationary engineers	X	X			X		X							X			X				X				
Waste water treatment plant operators					X		X							X			X	X	X		X	X			
Welders and oxygen arc cutters					X			X			X			X			X				X				
OFFICE OCCUPATIONS																									
Clerical occupations																									
Bookkeeping workers	X				X								X		X		X					X	X		
Cashiers					X					X			X	X			X					X	X		
File clerks	X				X			X					X		X							X	X		
Hotel front office clerks	X				X				X	X				X			X	X				X			
Office machine operators	X				X	X							X		X		X					X	X		
Postal clerks					X		X							X			X	X			X		X		
Receptionists	X				X				X	X				X			X								
Shipping and receiving clerks					X		X						X		X		X				X		X		

Occupation	1	2	3	4	5	6	7	8	9	10	11	12	13	14	15	16	17	18	19	20	21	22	23	24	25
Clerical occupations																									
Statistical clerks	X			X			X					X		X		X						X	X		
Stock clerks				X		X						X		X						X					
Stenographers	X			X		X			X				X	X		X						X	X		
Typists	X			X		X			X				X	X		X						X	X		
Computer and related occupations																									
Electronic computer operating personnel	X			X		X						X		X		X	X					X	X		
Programmers	1*	1		X				X				X				X	X					X			
Systems analysts			C	X				X				X										X			
Banking occupations																									
Bank clerks	X			X								X		X		X						X	X		
Bank officers			C	X					X	X			X		X					X		X			
Bank tellers	X			X					X	X			X	X		X						X			
Insurance occupations																									
Actuaries			C			X		X			X		X			X						X	X		
Claim adjusters	X			X					X	X			X					X				X			
Claim examiners	X			X				X					X		X				X			X	X		
Underwriters			C			X		X					X									X			
Administrative and related occupations																									
Accountants			C	X				X					X			X						X	X		
Advertising workers			C			X		X			X	X				X								X	X
City managers			C	X					X	X			X			X				X		X			
College student personnel workers			C	X					X	X			X			X				X				X	
Credit officials	X			X				X					X		X	X				X		X	X		
Hotel managers and assistants			C	X					X	X			X			X		X		X		X			

* See footnotes at end of table.

Column key:
1. High school diploma
2. Technical school or apprenticeship
3. Junior college
4. College degree
5. Jobs widely scattered
6. Jobs concentrated in localities
7. Working with things
8. Working with ideas
9. Helping people
10. Working with people
11. Able to see physical results of work
12. Opportunity for self-expression
13. Works as part of a team
14. Work is closely supervised
15. Works independently
16. Directs activities of others
17. Generally confined to work area
18. Overtime or shift work required
19. Exposed to weather conditions
20. High level of responsibility
21. Requires physical stamina
22. Works with detail
23. Repetitious work
24. Motivates others
25. Competitive

Occupation	1	2	3	4	5	6	7	8	9	10	11	12	13	14	15	16	17	18	19	20	21	22	23	24	25
Administrative and related occupations																									
Industrial traffic managers			C	X				X						X		X				X		X			
Lawyers			G	X				X	X			X		X			X		X	X		X		X	X
Marketing research workers			C			X		X					X									X			X
Personnel workers			C	X					X	X			X			X				X		X			
Public relations workers			C			X		X			X	X					X					X		X	X
Purchasing agents			C	X				X						X		X				X		X		X	X
SERVICE OCCUPATIONS																									
Cleaning and related occupations																									
Building custodians				X		X								X	X					X					
Hotel housekeepers and assistants				X					X					X		X						X			
Pest controllers	X			X		X								X				X		X					
Food service occupations																									
Bartenders				X					X	X				X				X	X						
Cooks and chefs		X		X		X		X				X				X		X							
Meatcutters		X		X		X								X		X				X		X			
Waiters and waitresses				X					X	X			X					X		X					
Personal service occupations																									
Barbers		X		X					X	X	X					X							X		
Bellhops and bell captains				X					X	X				X				X		X					
Cosmetologists		X		X					X	X	X						X								
Funeral directors		X		X					X	X				X		X		X							
Private household service occupations																									
Private household workers				X		X		X						X	X					X					

	1	2	3	4	5	6	7	8	9	10	11	12	13	14	15	16	17	18	19	20	21	22	23	24	25
Protective and related service occupations																									
FBI special agents				G		X			X	X			X					X		X	X	X			
Firefighters	X			X		X			X				X					X	X		X				
Guards				X										X				X		X	X				
Police officers	X			X					X	X			X	X				X	X	X	X	X			
State police officers	X			X					X	X			X	X				X	X	X	X	X			
Health and regulatory inspectors (Government)			C	X			X						X					X			X		X		
Construction inspectors (Government)	X	X		X			X						X					X	X	X	X				
Other service occupations																									
Mail carriers				X		X	X						X					X		X					
Telephone operators	X			X		X	X						X			X	X								
EDUCATION AND RELATED OCCUPATIONS																									
Teaching occupations																									
Kindergarten and elementary school teachers			C	X				X	X	X		X		X		X		X		X			X	X	
Secondary school teachers			C	X				X	X	X		X		X		X		X		X				X	
College and university teachers			G	X				X	X	X		X		X		X								X	
Library occupations																									
Librarians			G	X					X					X				X				X			
Library technicians		X		X					X				X					X				X			
SALES OCCUPATIONS																									
Automobile parts counter workers				X		X			X	X				X											
Automobile salesworkers	X			X					X	X				X				X					X	X	X
Automobile service advisers	X			X					X	X		X													
Gasoline service station attendants				X		X			X					X				X			X				
Insurance agents and brokers	X			X					X	X				X				X				X		X	X

	1	2	3	4	5	6	7	8	9	10	11	12	13	14	15	16	17	18	19	20	21	22	23	24	25
Manufacturers' salesworkers			C	X					X	X			X					X		X		X		X	X
Models	X				X				X		X							X		X					X
Real estate salesworkers and brokers	X			X					X	X			X					X		X		X		X	X
Retail trade salesworkers				X					X	X			X					X						X	X
Route workers				X					X	X			X					X	X		X		X		
Securities salesworkers			C	X				X	X	X			X					X		X				X	X
Wholesale trade salesworkers	X			X					X	X			X					X				X		X	X

CONSTRUCTION OCCUPATIONS

	1	2	3	4	5	6	7	8	9	10	11	12	13	14	15	16	17	18	19	20	21	22	23	24	25
Asbestos and insulating workers		X		X		X				X			X			X			X		X				
Bricklayers		X		X		X				X	X								X		X				
Carpenters		X		X		X				X	X								X		X				
Cement masons (cement and concrete finishers)		X		X		X				X	X				X			X	X		X				
Construction laborers and carpenter's helpers				X		X				X		X						X	X		X		X		
Electricians (construction)		X		X		X				X	X								X		X				
Elevator constructors				X		X				X	X										X				
Floor covering installers		X		X		X				X			X								X				
Glaziers	X	X		X		X				X			X						X		X				
Lathers		X		X		X					X										X				
Marble setters, tile setters, and terrazzo workers				X		X				X			X			X					X				
Operating engineers (construction machinery operators)	X	X		X		X				X			X						X	X	X				
Painters and paperhangers		X		X		X				X			X								X				
Plasterers		X		X		X				X	X										X				
Plumbers and pipefitters		X		X		X				X			X								X				
Roofers		X		X		X				X			X						X		X				

Occupation	High school diploma	Technical school or apprenticeship	Junior college	College degree	Jobs widely scattered in localities	Jobs concentrated in localities	Working with things	Working with ideas	Helping people	Working with people	Able to see physical results of work	Opportunity for self-expression	Works as part of a team	Works independently	Work is closely supervised	Directs activities of others	Generally confined to work area	Overtime or shift work required	Exposed to weather conditions	High level of responsibility	Requires physical stamina	Works with detail	Repetitious work	Motivates others	Competitive
	1	2	3	4	5	6	7	8	9	10	11	12	13	14	15	16	17	18	19	20	21	22	23	24	25
Sheet-metal workers	X	X			X		X				X		X				X			X					
Stonemasons		X			X		X				X			X					X		X				
Structural-, ornamental-, and reinforcing-iron workers, riggers, and machine movers		X			X		X				X		X						X		X				

OCCUPATIONS IN TRANSPORTATION ACTIVITIES

Air transportation occupations

Occupation	1	2	3	4	5	6	7	8	9	10	11	12	13	14	15	16	17	18	19	20	21	22	23	24	25
Air traffic controllers	X				X		X				X					X	X	X		X		X			
Aircraft mechanics	X	X			X	X					X								X	X		X			
Flight attendants	X				X				X	X	X							X			X				
Airline dispatchers				C	X		X				X					X		X		X		X			
Flight engineers	X				X	X					X					X		X		X		X			
Ground radio operators and teletypists	X				X				X	X	X					X				X		X			
Pilots and copilots	X				X	X					X					X	X	X		X	X	X			
Traffic agents and clerks	X				X				X	X			X			X	X								

Merchant marine occupations

Occupation	1	2	3	4	5	6	7	8	9	10	11	12	13	14	15	16	17	18	19	20	21	22	23	24	25
Merchant marine officers				C	X		X				X					X		X		X	X				
Merchant marine sailors					X	X					X			X		X	X			X					

Railroad occupations

Occupation	1	2	3	4	5	6	7	8	9	10	11	12	13	14	15	16	17	18	19	20	21	22	23	24	25
Brake operators and couplers					X		X				X					X	X			X	X	X			
Bridge and building workers					X		X			X	X		X					X		X					
Clerks	X				X						X		X	X								X	X		
Conductors					X				X	X			X			X		X		X		X			
Locomotive engineers	X				X		X							X		X	X	X	X	X	X	X			
Locomotive firemen (helpers)	X				X		X				X			X		X	X			X			X		

	1	2	3	4	5	6	7	8	9	10	11	12	13	14	15	16	17	18	19	20	21	22	23	24	25
	High school diploma	Technical school or apprenticeship	Junior college	College degree	Jobs widely scattered	Jobs concentrated in localities	Working with things	Working with ideas	Helping people	Working with people	Able to see physical results of work	Opportunity for self-expression	Works as part of a team	Works independently	Work is closely supervised	Directs activities of others	Generally confined to work area	Overtime or shift work required	Exposed to weather conditions	High level of responsibility	Requires physical stamina	Works with detail	Repetitious work	Motivates others	Competitive
Railroad occupations																									
Shop trades workers	X			X		X							X		X				X						
Signal department workers				X		X							X						X		X				
Station agents				X					X	X			X				X	X					X		
Telegraphers, telephoners, and tower workers				X		X							X		X		X	X							
Track workers				X		X					X		X		X				X		X				
Driving occupations																									
Intercity busdrivers				X		X		X					X				X	X	X						
Local transit busdrivers				X		X		X					X				X	X	X						
Local truckdrivers				X		X							X				X	X	X		X				
Long-distance truckdrivers				X		X							X				X	X	X		X				
Parking attendants				X		X		X					X				X	X	X		X				
Taxi drivers					X	X		X					X				X	X	X						X
SCIENTIFIC AND TECHNICAL OCCUPATIONS																									
Conservation occupations																									
Foresters			C	X		X							X		X		X	X	X	X					
Forestry aides and technicians		X		X		X						X					X	X	X						
Range managers			C	X			X						X				X		X						
Soil conservationists			C	X			X			X			X				X		X	X					
Engineers																									
Aerospace			C		X		X			X	X	X		X			X		X						
Agricultural			C		X		X			X	X	X		X					X						
Biomedical			C		X		X			X	X	X		X					X						
Ceramic			C		X		X			X	X	X		X					X						
Chemical			C		X		X			X	X	X		X					X						
Civil			C	X			X			X	X	X		X			X		X						

	1	2	3	4	5	6	7	8	9	10	11	12	13	14	15	16	17	18	19	20	21	22	23	24	25
	High school diploma	Technical school or apprenticeship	Junior college	College degree	Jobs widely scattered	Jobs concentrated in localities	Working with things	Working with ideas	Helping people	Working with people	Able to see physical results of work	Opportunity for self-expression	Works as part of a team	Works independently	Work is closely supervised	Directs activities of others	Generally supervised	Overtime or shift work required	Exposed to weather conditions	High level of responsibility	Requires physical stamina	Works with detail	Repetitious work	Motivates others	Competitive
Engineers																									
Electrical				C	X			X			X	X	X			X						X			
Industrial				C	X			X				X	X			X				X		X	X		
Mechanical				C	X			X			X	X	X			X						X			
Metallurgical				C		X		X			X	X	X			X						X			
Mining				C		X		X			X	X	X			X			X	X		X			
Environmental scientists																									
Geologists				G		X		X				X		X								X			
Geophysicists				C		X		X				X		X								X			
Meteorologists				C		X		X				X		X				X				X			
Oceanographers				C		X		X				X	X			X		X				X			
Life scientists																									
Biochemists				C	X			X				X										X			
Life scientists				G	X			X				X		X								X			
Soil scientists				C	X			X				X		X								X			
Mathematics occupations																									
Mathematicians				C	X			X				X		X			X					X			
Statisticians				C	X			X				X	X				X					X			
Physical scientists																									
Astronomers				C		X		X				X		X											
Chemists				C	X			X				X		X											
Food scientists				C	X			X				X		X											
Physicists				C	X			X				X		X											
Technicians																									
Broadcast technicians	X			X		X						X			X		X		X			X			

	1	2	3	4	5	6	7	8	9	10	11	12	13	14	15	16	17	18	19	20	21	22	23	24	25
Technicians																									
Drafters (draftsmen)			X		X			X					X		X		X					X			
Engineering and science technicians			X		X	X							X		X							X			
Food processing technicians			X		X	X							X		X							X			
Surveyors	X	2¹	2		X			X					X			X			X			X			
MECHANICS AND REPAIRERS																									
Telephone craft occupations					X		X							X											
Central office craft occupations	X				X		X				X			X			X	X					X	X	
Line installers and cable splicers	X				X		X						X		X			X	X			X	X		
Telephone installers and repairers	X				X		X							X				X	X			X	X		
Other mechanics and repairers																									
Air-conditioning, refrigeration, and heating mechanics					X		X				X			X				X							
Appliance repairers					X		X							X						X					
Automobile body repairers		X			X		X				X			X			X					X			
Automobile mechanics		X			X		X				X			X			X					X			
Boat-motor mechanics					X		X				X			X				X							
Bowling-pin-machine mechanics					X		X							X				X			X		X		
Business machine repairers	X	X			X		X							X								X			
Computer service technicians					X		X							X											
Diesel mechanics		X			X		X				X			X			X					X			
Dispensing opticians and optical technicians	X	X			X		X	X	X		X			X								X			
Electric sign repairers					X		X				X			X				X	X			X	X		
Farm equipment mechanics		X			X		X				X			X				X	X		X				
Industrial machinery repairers	X	X			X		X							X				X			X	X			
Instrument repairers	X	X			X		X							X			X					X			

* See footnotes at end of table.

	1	2	3	4	5	6	7	8	9	10	11	12	13	14	15	16	17	18	19	20	21	22	23	24	25
Other mechanics and repairers																									
Jewelers and jewelry repairers		X		X		X							X			X						X			
Locksmiths				X		X							X									X			
Maintenance electricians		X		X		X							X												
Motorcycle mechanics				X		X					X		X												
Piano and organ tuners and repairers	X					X	X						X												
Shoe repairers				X		X					X		X			X						X	X		
Television and radio service technicians		X		X		X	X				X		X									X			
Truck and bus mechanics		X		X		X							X								X				
Vending machine mechanics					X	X					X		X	X				X			X	X			
Watch repairers		X		X		X					X		X	X		X						X			
HEALTH OCCUPATIONS																									
Dental occupations																									
Dentists				G	X				X	X	X	X		X					X			X			
Dental assistants			X		X				X	X				X		X	X						X		
Dental hygienists			X		X				X	X				X			X						X		
Dental laboratory technicians	X	X				X					X			X		X	X					X	X		
Medical practitioners																									
Chiropractors				C	X				X	X	X	X		X						X		X			
Optometrists				G	X				X	X	X	X		X					X	X		X			
Osteopathic physicians				G	X				X	X	X	X		X					X	X		X			
Physicians				G	X				X	X	X	X		X					X	X		X			
Podiatrists				G	X						X	X		X						X		X			
Veterinarians				G	X						X	X		X				X	X	X		X			

	1	2	3	4	5	6	7	8	9	10	11	12	13	14	15	16	17	18	19	20	21	22	23	24	25
Medical technicians, technologists, and assistants occupations																									
Electrocardiograph technicians			X		X				X	X			X		X							X	X		
Electroencephalograph technicians			X		X				X	X			X		X							X	X		
Medical assistants			X		X				X	X			X		X			X				X			
Medical laboratory workers	X	3*	3	3	X	X	X						X		X			X		X		X			
Medical record technicians and clerks			C	X		X								X								X	X		
Operating room technicians	X			X				X	X				X		X							X			
Optometric assistants	X			X					X	X			X		X							X			
Radiologic (X-ray) technologists			C	X		X			X				X		X			X		X		X			
Respiratory therapists	X			X					X	X			X		X			X				X			
Nursing occupations																									
Registered nurses	X	4*	4	4	X				X	X			X		X	X		X		X		X			
Licensed practical nurses		5*	5		X				X	X			X		X			X				X			
Nursing aides, orderlies, and attendants					X				X	X			X		X			X							
Therapy and rehabilitation occupations																									
Occupational therapists			C	X					X	X	X	X		X		X						X			
Occupational therapy assistants	X			X					X	X	X		X	X											
Physical therapists			G	X					X	X	X	X		X		X				X		X			
Physical therapy assistants		5*	5	X					X	X	X		X	X											
Speech pathologists and audiologists			G	X					X	X	X	X		X		X				X		X			
Other health occupations																									
Dietitians			C	X			X	X					X		X							X			
Hospital administrators			G	X						X			X		X		X		X	X		X		X	
Medical record administrators			C	X		X							X									X	X		

* See footnotes at end of table.

	1 High school diploma	2 Technical school or apprenticeship	3 Junior college	4 College degree	5 Jobs widely scattered	6 Jobs concentrated in localities	7 Working with things	8 Working with ideas	9 Helping people	10 Working with people	11 Able to see physical results of work	12 Opportunity for self-expression	13 Works as part of a team	14 Works independently	15 Work is closely supervised	16 Directs activities of others	17 Generally confined to work area	18 Overtime or shift work required	19 Exposed to weather conditions	20 High level of responsibility	21 Requires physical stamina	22 Works with detail	23 Repetitious work	24 Motivates others	25 Competitive
Other health occupations																									
Pharmacists				G	X		X		X					X				X		X		X			
Sanitarians				C	X		X							X								X			
SOCIAL SCIENTISTS																									
Anthropologists				G	X			X				X		X								X			
Economists				C	X			X				X		X								X			
Geographers				C	X			X				X		X								X			
Historians				G	X			X				X		X								X			
Political scientists				C	X			X				X		X								X			
Sociologists				G	X			X				X		X								X			
SOCIAL SERVICE OCCUPATIONS																									
Counselors																									
School counselors				C	X				X	X			X			X				X					
Employment counselors				C	X				X	X	X			X		X	X							X	
Rehabilitation counselors				C	X				X	X				X		X				X				X	
College career planning and placement counselors				C	X				X	X				X		X								X	
Clergy																									
Protestant ministers				G	X				X	X				X		X								X	
Rabbis				G	X				X	X				X		X								X	
Roman Catholic priests				G	X				X	X				X		X								X	
Other social service occupations																									
Cooperative extension service workers				C	X				X	X						X								X	
Home economists				C	X				X	X		X		X		X								X	
Psychologists				G	X			X	X			X		X						X		X		X	
Recreation workers				C	X				X	X				X		X		X			X			X	

140

Column key:
1. High school diploma
2. Technical school or apprenticeship
3. Junior college
4. College degree
5. Jobs widely scattered
6. Jobs concentrated in localities
7. Working with things
8. Working with ideas
9. Helping people
10. Working with people
11. Able to see physical results of work
12. Opportunity for self expression
13. Works as part of a team
14. Works independently
15. Work is closely supervised
16. Directs activities of others
17. Generally confined to work area
18. Overtime or shift work required
19. Exposed to weather conditions
20. High level of responsibility
21. Requires physical stamina
22. Works with detail
23. Repetitious work
24. Motivates others
25. Competitive

Occupation	1	2	3	4	5	6	7	8	9	10	11	12	13	14	15	16	17	18	19	20	21	22	23	24	25
Other social service occupations																									
Social service aides						X			X	X			X		X			X							
Social workers			C	X					X	X			X		X			X				X			
ART, DESIGN, AND COMMUNICATIONS–RELATED OCCUPATIONS																									
Performing arts																									
Actors and actresses			X			X		X				X	X			X									X
Dancers			X			X		X				X	X			X									X
Musicians				C	6†	X		X	6			X	X			X									X
Singers				C	6†	X		X	6			X	X												X
Design occupations																									
Architects		X		C	X			X	X		X	X		X		X				X	X				X
Commercial artists		X				X		X			X	X	X		X			X			X	X			
Display workers	X				X			X			X	X		X											
Floral designers					X		X				X	X		X			X								
Industrial designers				C		X		X			X	X	X												
Interior designers		X			X			X	X		X	X		X		X						X			X
Landscape architects				C	X			X	X		X	X		X		X						X			X
Photographers	X	X			X			X			X	X		X								X			X
Urban planners				G		X		X	X			X	X			X				X		X		X	
Communications–related occupations																									
Interpreters				C		X		X		X			X				X								
Newspaper reporters				C	X			X	X		X	X	X					X		X	X	X			X
Radio and television announcers	X				X			X					X				X	X						X	X
Technical writers				C	X			X			X		X							X		X			

1. Requirements vary according to type of industry.
2. Postsecondary schooling required, usually in junior college, technical school, or vocational school.
3. Educational requirements vary according to area of work. See *Occupational Outlook Handbook* for details.
4. Type of training program depends on individual preference.
5. Training programs are available from vocational schools or junior college.
6. Teachers only.

Job outlook

As you make education and career decisions and plans, it becomes increasingly important that you have as much information as possible. An important factor to consider is *where the jobs will be* during the next decade and how many people will be applying for these positions.

The two tables "Graduate and Professional Study" and "Annual Average Supply-Demand in Selected Occupations . . . in the 1970s" represent the general supply-demand situation that exists today and projections for the 1970s.*

Graduate and professional study

	Number of applicants	Number of openings
Law School	70,000	35,000
Medical School	35,000	13,000

Annual average supply-demand in selected occupations generally requiring a bachelor's or advanced degree for entry in 1970s

	Supply	Demand
Engineers	37,000	38,000
Chemists	13,800	17,000
Physicists	3,000	3,600
Life scientists	21,000	15,000
Geologists and geophysicists	900	1,000
Mathematicians	40,000	22,000
Physicians	10,000	20,000
Dentists	1,800	4,900
Dietitians	1,500	1,800
Pharmacists	6,000	4,400
Optometrists	500	800
Elementary and secondary teachers	350,000	200,000
College and university teachers	23,000	17,000
Police officers	7,865	15,000

*Statistics compiled from United States Department of Labor sources.

Annual average supply-demand in selected occupations generally requiring a bachelor's or advanced degree for entry in 1970s (continued)

	Supply	Demand
Social workers (M.S.W.)	5,037	16,000
Lawyers	21,000	20,000
Architects	4,200	4,200
Counselors (all types)	4,500	5,500
Accountants	26,100	33,000
Sales workers		69,800
Psychologists (clinical)	5,562	3,100
Nurses	55,000	65,000
Hospital administrators	442	900
Social scientists (all)	64,000	4,800
Anthropologists	2,990	200
Economists	16,867	2,200
Historians	40,939	800
Geographers	3,338	200

Career values and activities*

The following comments on values and activities inherent in various career fields attempt to supply yet another perspective for your career awareness. Again, they will help you answer some of your questions about a career direction — one of which is: Are these values and activities consistent with what I'm all about? (Review Chapter 2, "Self-Awareness.") The career fields listed are just a sampling — be sure to consult comprehensive resources like the *Occupational Outlook Handbook* and the *Dictionary of Occupational Titles* for activities and values related to other career fields.

Accountant   Large number of vacancies exist; not limited to just business — education, government, and community services are also applicable; works with detail and figures; applies principles of accounting to install and maintain operation of general accounting systems; designs new systems or modifies existing system to provide records of assets, liabilities, and financial transactions of establishment; audits contracts, orders, and vouchers; prepares reports substantiating individual transactions before their settlement.

*Adapted from *Path: A Career Workbook for Liberal Arts Students,* by Howard E. Figler, copyright © 1975, by permission of the publisher, The Carroll Press, Cranston, R.I.

Actuary   Competitive field; computer-oriented; plans and solves mathematical problems; applies numerical analysis to insurance problems, applies knowledge of mathematics, probability, statistics, principles of finance and business to problems of life, health, social and casualty insurance, annuities, and pensions; determines mortality, accident, sickness, disability, and retirement rates.

Advertising worker   Communication skills; business minded; analyzes public needs; includes executives responsible for planning and overall supervision of advertisements, copywriters who write the text, artists who prepare the illustrations, and layout specialists who put copy and illustrations into the most attractive arrangement possible.

Anthropologist   Makes comparative studies of origin, evolution, and races of man, cultures they have created, and man's distribution and physical characteristics.

Architect   B.A. in liberal arts can enroll in some M.A. programs in architecture; closely allied to city planning; plans and designs private residences, office buildings, theaters, public buildings, factories, and other structures; organizes services necessary for construction. Landscape architects plan and design development land areas for such projects as parks and other recreational facilities, airports, highways, parkways, hospitals, schools, land subdivisions, and commercial, industrial, and residential sites.

Astronomer   Observes and interprets celestial phenomena and relates research to basic scientific knowledge or to practical problems, such as navigation.

Biologist   Studies origin, relationship, development, anatomy, functions, and other basic principles of plant and animal life; may specialize in research centering around a particular plant, animal, or aspect of biology.

Chemist   Limited positions at B.S. level; scholarly research; works alone or in small teams; performs chemical tests, performs qualitative and quantitative chemical analyses, or conducts chemical experiements in laboratories for quality of process control or to develop new products or new knowledge.

Chiropractor   Alternative to medical schools; muscle and bone specialty; knowledge of body as a whole also necessary.

City manager   Business administration oriented; interdisciplinary preparation, supervisory skills, ability to communicate to public are necessary; ability to work under conflicting people's views as well as to plan ahead is also significant.

Commercial artist   Competitive field, opportunities in public relations departments of industry and business; draws and paints illustrations for advertisements, books, magazines, posters, billboards, and catalogs.

Dentist   Expensive to begin practice; commitment to dentistry; dental schools competitive; ability to work under pressure; concern with detail and steady hands necessary.

Dietitian   Specialized undergraduate or graduate education; science interest and understanding; wide open field; administers and plans diets and meals; plans and directs food service programs in hospitals, schools, restaurants, and other public or private institutions; plans menus and diets providing required food nutrients to feed individuals and groups.
    Home economist — develops, interprets, and applies principles of homemaking to promote health and welfare of individuals and families; advises homemakers in selection and utilization of household equipment, food, and clothing; interprets homemakers' needs to manufacturers of household products.

Economist   Ph.D a necessity; math oriented; scholarly approach and communications skills needed; analyzes economic problems on the national and/or corporate level; conducts research; prepares reports; formulates plans to aid in solution of economic problems arising from production and distribution of goods and services.

Educational specialists   Speech pathologist — diagnoses, treats, and performs research related to speech and language problems; diagnoses speech and language disorders by evaluating etiology; treats language and speech impairments such as aphasia, stuttering, and articulatory problems or organic and nonorganic etiology.
    Guidance counselor — is concerned with educational, vocational, and social development of students in schools and colleges; works with students, both individually and in groups, as well as with teachers, other school personnel, parents, and community agencies; includes reading specialist or clinician, college administrator, student personnel worker, media and audio-visual specialist.

Employment counselor   Works closely with people searching for jobs; knowledge of psychology, job market, and job-hunting techniques needed; frustrating in today's market.

Financial officer   Employment in education as a business manager or financial aid officer.
    A security trader performs securities, investments, and counseling services for banks

and their customers; studies financial background and future trends in stocks and bonds; advises bank officials and customers regarding investments.

A financial analyst conducts statistical analyses of information affecting investment programs of public, industrial, and financial institutions, such as banks, insurance companies, and brokerage and investment houses.

A credit analyst analyzes credit data to estimate degree of risk involved in extending credit or lending money to firms or individuals and prepares reports of findings; contacts banks, trade and credit associations, salespeople, and others to obtain credit information.

Flight attendant Possibly not as glamorous as it appears; waitress duties, tight and hectic schedules; travel benefits; steadiness, poise; field opening up for males; puts up with rude passengers.

Forester Interdisciplinary preparation or special program; science based; varied administrative, recreational, and people-oriented activities; manages and develops forest lands and their resources for economic and recreational purposes; plans and directs projects in forestation and reforestation; maps forest areas; estimates standing timber and future growth and manages timber sales.

Soil conservationist plans and develops coordinated practices for soil-erosion control, moisture conservation, and sound land use; conducts surveys and investigations of erosion and of preventative measures needed; plans soil management practices such as crop rotation, strip cropping, contour plowing, and reforestation as related to soil and water conservation.

Range manager conducts research in range problems to provide sustained production of foliage, livestock, and wildlife; studies range lands to determine best grazing seasons and number and kind of livestock that can most profitably be grazed.

Geographer Interest in travel, world locations; concerned with detail; entails more than just land and water — economy, sociology, environment also important; studies nature and use of areas of earth's surface, relating and interpreting interactions of physical and cultural phenomena; conducts research on physical and climatic aspect of area.

Geologist Studies composition, structure, and history of earth's crust; examines rock, minerals, and fossil remains to identify and determine sequence of processes affecting development of earth.

Health technician Concern for patients' health; possesses technological skill; interest in health, anatomy, and science.

Historian   Job market extremely tough; research, writing, and teaching; prepares in narrative, brief, or outline form chronological account or record of past or current events dealing with some phase of human activity, either in terms of individuals or social, ethnic, political, or geographic groupings.

Museum curator administers affairs of museum and conducts scientific research programs; directs activities concerned with instructional, research, and public service objectives of institutions; interprets and assists in formulating museum directions; administers exchange of loan collections; obtains, develops, and organizes new collections to build up and improve educational and research facilities.

Hospital administrator   Administrative skills; business management oriented; works with doctors and surgeons; administers and coordinates activities of hospital personnel to promote care of sick and injured, furtherance of scientific knowledge, development of preventative medicine, advancement of medical and vocational rehabilitation, and participation in and promotion of community health and welfare.

Hotel manager   Ability to relate well with public; recreation oriented; business minded; involved with entertainment; administers and delegates responsibilities in a diversity of work areas; faces stiff competition.

Industrial designer   An industrial designer designs forms of new products and associated packaging and trademarks; sketches design of products such as furniture, lamps, motor vehicles, radio cabinets, and household appliances, taking into consideration appearance for sales appeal, serviceability in adapting design to function, price, cost, methods of production, and specifications stipulated by clients.

Insurance agent   Good communications skills, salesmanship, knowledge of math and figures; competitive; works mainly for commissions. Insurance underwriters decide the acceptability of various types of risks by analyzing information contained in insurance applications, reports of safety engineers, and actuarial studies (reports describing the probability of insured loss). Life insurance underwriters solicit and sell all types of life insurance, based on client's present insurance and government benefits, to establish plans for financial security; advises clients concerning life insurance, pensions, taxation, and family finance.

Interior designer   Practical application of art, varied media; plans and designs artistic interiors for homes, hotels, ships, commercial and institutional structures, and other establishments; analyzes functional requirements, moods, and purpose of finished interior based on client's needs and preferences.

Jeweler   Skilled trade requiring training, steady hand; apprenticeship required.

Journalist or editor News reporter collects and analyzes facts about newsworthy events by interview, investigation, or observation; writes newspaper stories conforming to prescribed editorial techniques and format; reports to scene, beat, or special assignment, as directed; interviews people and observes events to obtain and verify story facts and to develop leads for news items.

Copywriter consults with account executives and media and marketing representatives to obtain information about product or service and to discuss style and length of advertising copy, considering budget and media limitations; writes original copy for newspapers, magazines, billboards, and transportation advertising; writes scripts for radio and television advertising.

Book editor interviews authors, suggests changes in book manuscripts, and negotiates with authors regarding details of publication, such as royalties to be paid, publication date, and number of copies to be printed, according to knowledge of production requirements and estimate of public demand for the book.

Technical writer organizes, writes, and edits material about science and technology so that it is in a form most useful to the person who needs it, be it a technician or repairer, a scientist or engineer, an executive or a housewife.

Lawyer Law schools are very selective and competitive; hiring is decreasing, but a law degree is valuable for numerous fields; good memory for details; intense pressure; desire to serve the public; conducts criminal and civil lawsuits, draws up legal documents, advises clients as to legal rights, and practices other phases of law; gathers evidence in divorce, civil, criminal, and other cases to formulate defense or to initiate legal action.

Librarian Hiring is down; organizational skills, planning, creativity, and research; interest in student learning; maintains library collection of books, periodicals, documents, films, recordings, and other materials; assists groups and individuals to locate and obtain materials.

Library technician Mainly works by himself or herself; enjoys books and working with them; pays attention to detail and organization; activities include cataloging, working with numerical systems, and some contact with people.

Licensed practical nurse Patience and dedication with patients; desire to serve and help; knowledge of medicine; ability to act in an emergency; concerned about detail; long, tiring work hours. The term *professional nurse* is applied to persons meeting educational, legal, and training requirements to practice as professional nurses, as required by a state board of nursing; performs acts requiring substantial specialized judgment and skill in observation; in the care and counsel of ill, injured, or infirm persons; and in promotion of health and prevention of illness.

Management   Leadership, supervision over people and/or a process; business, education, social service, government at all levels; communication skills, problem solving, mediator.

Marketing research worker   Economic analysis of problems, needs assessment concerning public, selling a product or service.

Market research analyst researches market conditions in local, regional, or national area to determine potential sales of a product or a service; examines and analyzes statistical data on past sales and wholesale or retail trade trends to forecast future sales trends.

A buyer purchases merchandise for resale; selects and orders merchandise from showings of manufacturing representatives, basing selection on nature of clientele, demand for specific merchandise, and experience as buyer.

Mathematician   Federal government is a major employer; needs computer and experiential learning; conducts research in fundamental mathematics and in application of mathematical techniques to science, management, and other fields; solves or directs solutions to problems in various fields by mathematical methods.

Meteorologist   Studies and interprets atmospheric conditions and related meteorological data to forecast immediate and long-range changes in weather.

Occupational therapist   Stiff graduate school entrance requirements; rehabilitation work; patience and dedication; knowledge of anatomy. Physical therapist treats patients with disabilities, disorders, and injuries to relieve pain, develop or restore function, and maintain maximum performance, using physical means, such as exercise, massage, heat, water, light, and electricity as prescribed by physician. The occupational therapist also plans, organizes, and participates in medically oriented occupational programs in a hospital or similar institution to rehabilitate patients who are physically or mentally ill; utilizes creative and manual arts, recreational, educational, and social activities, prevocational evaluations, and training in everyday activities, such as personal care and homemaking.

Osteopathic physician   Alternate to medical school; dedication and ability in the sciences; emphasis on the structure of the body rather than organs and systems; equivalent to and in many areas equal status to M.D.'s.

Personnel worker   Involved in the hiring and firing process; employee relations; may need experience in business prior to personnel work; interpersonal relationship skills necessary.

Labor relations specialist serves as specialist on labor management relations, representing either management or labor union; studies and interprets collective bargaining agreements and current labor market conditions to assist in establishing policies and operating procedures; represents management or labor in contract negotiations and conciliation and arbitration procedures.

Personnel managers plan and carry out policies relating to all phases of personnel activities; organizes recruitment, selection, and training procedures and directs activities of subordinates directly concerned; confers with company and union officials to establish pension and insurance plans, workmen's compensation policies, and similar functions.

Pharmacist Compounds and dispenses medications, following prescriptions issued by physicians, dentists, or other authorized medical practitioners; weighs, measures, and mixes drugs and other medicinal compounds.

Pharmacologist Studies effects of drugs, gases, dusts, and other minerals on tissues and physiological processes of animals and human beings; experiments with animals, such as rats, guinea pigs, and mice to determine actions of drugs and other substances on the functioning of organs and tissues, noting effects on circulation, respiration, digestion, or other vital processes; alternative to medical school.

Photographer Photographs persons, motion-picture sets, merchandise, exteriors and interiors, machinery, and fashions to be used in advertising and selling.

Physicist Needs Ph.D.; applies physics to solving problems; conducts research on physical phenomena, develops theories and laws on basis of observation and experiments, and devises methods to apply laws and theories of physics to industry, medicine, and other fields.

Physiologist Conducts research on cellular structure and organ-system functions of plants and animals; studies growth, respiration, circulation, excretion, movement, reproduction, and other functions of plants and animals under normal and abnormal conditions.

Pilot and copilot High perception skills, excellent vision, and good nerves; ability to deal with crisis; high sense of responsibility; meticulous inspection of instruments; concern with detail.

Police officer Commitment to service and helping; long and odd working hours, including weekends; knowledge of the law; ability to handle weapons and deal with criminals.

Political scientist   Conducts research into origin, development, operation, and interrelationships of political institutions; studies phenomena of political behavior and develops political theory.

Printer   Mechanical skills; careful and concerned with perfection; neat; knowledge of grammar, spelling, and usage.

Programmer   Math skills; ability to conceptualize problems; detailed work; converts symbolic statement of business problems to detailed, logical flow charts for coding into computer language and solution by means of automatic data-processing equipment.

Psychologist   Individual and group work with people's emotional and personal problems; therapy; dedication to study for master's or Ph.D.; diagnoses mental and emotional disorders of individuals and administers treatment programs; interviews patients in clinics, hospitals, prisons, and other institutions; studies medical and social case histories.

Public relations worker   Plans and conducts public relations programs designed to procure publicity for groups, organizations, or institutions through such media as magazines, newspapers, radio, and television; selects and assembles publicity material that accords with organizational policy; writes news releases and submits photographs to newspapers.

Purchasing agent   Business and interpersonal skills; purchases machinery, equipment, tools, raw materials, parts, services, and supplies necessary for operation of an organization such as an industrial establishment, public utility, or government unit.

Radio and television announcer   Excellent communication skills; relaxed speaking in front of groups; enjoyment of entertaining; clear speaking voice; works odd hours; introduces radio or television programs, interviews guests, and acts as master of ceremonies; reads news flashes, identifies station by giving call letters; gives necessary network cues to control room so that selected stations connected by telephone lines may receive intended programs.

Recreation workers   Administration and creative skills; interdisciplinary preparation; plans and organizes activities; conducts recreation activities with assigned groups in public department or voluntary agency; organizes, promotes, and develops interest in activities such as arts and crafts, sports, games, music, dramatics, social recreation, camping, and hobbies.

Rehabilitation counselor   Dedication to helping combined with knowledge of how the body functions; works with individuals and groups; rehabilitates clients to work effectively in society; works with physical, mental, and emotional problems.

Sales worker   One of few careers where hiring is increasing; much more administrative and problem-analysis involvement than most people realize; communication skills needed.

A manufacturer's representative sells single, allied, diversified, or multiline products to wholesalers or other customers for one or more manufacturers on commission basis.

Real estate salesperson rents, buys, and sells property for clients on commission basis; studies property listings to become familiar with properties for sale; reviews trade journals to keep informed of marketing conditions and property values; interviews prospective clients to solicit listings.

Social worker   Works with poverty-stricken and underprivileged people; patience, communication, desire to help people, long hours.

A caseworker counsels and aids individuals and families requiring assistance of social service agency; interviews clients with problems in such areas as personal and family adjustments, finances, employment, and physical and mental impairments to determine nature and degree of problem.

A parole officer engages in activities related to conditional release of juvenile or adult offenders from correctional institutions; establishes relationship with offenders and familiarizes himself with offenders' social history prior to and during institutionalization.

Sociologist   Research; teaching at a college level; conducts research into origin and development of groups of human beings and patterns of culture and social organization that have arisen out of group life in society.

Statistician   Heavy on math and computer skills; solves numerical problems; plans surveys and collects, organizes, interprets, summarizes, and analyzes statistical theory and methods to provide usable information in scientific and other fields.

Stenographer or secretary   High clerical skills; good listening skills; ability to interpret and accurately record; greets clients and converses with incoming people.

Surgical technician   Steady hands and sound knowledge of medicine, medical equipment and tools; good memory; cooperative, "helping" attitude. Physician is a person with degree of doctor of medicine who diagnoses and treats disease and disorders of the human body; examines patients, utilizing all types of medical equipment, instruments, and tests, following standard medical procedures.

Systems analyst   Application of math and computer knowledge to solving business problems; analyzes business problems such as development of integrated production, inventory control, and cost analysis system to refine its formulation and convert it to programmable form for application to electronic data-processing system.

Teacher, elementary   Teaches elementary school pupils academic, social, and manipulative skills in rural, suburban, or urban communities; prepares teaching outline for course of study.

Teacher, handicapped children   Teaches handicapped pupils in elementary and secondary grades, evaluating pupils' abilities to determine training programs that will result in maximum progress; observes pupils to determine physical limitations and plans academic and recreational programs to meet individual needs.

Teacher, mentally retarded   Teaches mentally retarded children basic academic subjects in schools, centers, and institutions; plans courses of study according to pupils' levels of learning; conducts activities in subjects such as music, art, crafts and physical education, to stimulate and develop interests, abilities, manual skills, and coordination.

Teacher, secondary   Instructs students in one or more subjects, such as English, mathematics, or social studies, in private, religious, or public secondary school (high school); instructs pupils through lectures, demonstrations, and audio-visual aids; usually has some kind of extracurricular involvement with students.

Telephone operator   Daily routine; ability to converse and relay information; patience with rude customers.

Truck driver   Ability to go long periods of time without sleep; daily routine the same; mechanically minded; map reading and scheduling skills; little contact with people.

Urban planner   Requires specialized degree or interdisciplinary studies with good internships; plans community facilities from multiple perspectives — economical, architectural, sociological, and so forth; develops comprehensive plans and programs for utilization of land and physical facilities of cities, counties, and metropolitan areas; compiles and analyzes data on economic, social, and physical factors affecting land use and prepares or requisitions graphic and narrative reports on data.

Profiles of people in their careers

The career information and career resources presented in this chapter contained information that could give you a sense of direction. They allowed you to read about activities, responsibilities, types of people, necessary skills, and related information in various career fields. If you are still interested in a particular career, you should explore additional resources as well as talk to people and experience facets of the career. Except for actually talking to people, however, this career information is somewhat limited. It doesn't usually give you people's gut level feelings about the career or job. Studs Terkel's *Working: People Talk about What They Do All Day and How They Feel about What They Do* (1972, 1974) does just that. After all, work is more than activities, responsibilities, and skills — it is feelings too and, as stated by Terkel, people are "aware of a sense of personal worth or more often a lack of it in the work they do." (p. xxx)

> It is about a search, too, for daily meaning as well as daily bread, for recognition as well as cash, for astonishment rather than torpor; in short, for a sort of life rather than a Monday through Friday sort of dying. (p. xiii)*

It is this search for whatever brings satisfaction to people's lives through their work that elicits the emotional response. This emotional response can be considered along with other criteria when exploring careers. The following profiles provide sharp insight into how people view their jobs — their anxieties, joy, comfort; the plusses and minuses that they experience. We encourage you to read the entire book, *Working.* It will increase the depth and extent of your career awareness and ultimately facilitate your choice of a career direction.

Dolores Dante†

She has been a waitress in the same restaurant for twenty-three years. Many of its patrons are credit card carriers on an expense account — conventioneers, politicians, labor leaders, agency people. Her hours are from 5:00 P.M. to 2:00 A.M. six days a week. She arrives earlier "to get things ready, the silverware, the butter. When people come in and ask for you, you would like to be in a position to handle them all, because that means more money for you.

"I became a waitress because I needed money fast and you don't get it in an office. My husband and I broke up and he left me with debts and three children. My baby was six months. The fast buck, your tips. The first ten-dollar bill that I got as a tip, a Viking guy gave to me. He was a very robust, terrific atheist. Made very good conversation for us, 'cause I am too.

"Everyone says all waitresses have broken homes. What they don't realize is when

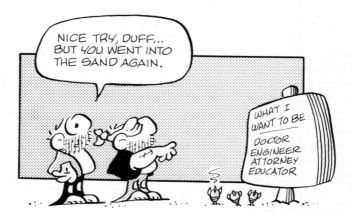

people have broken homes they need to make money fast, and do this work. They don't have broken homes because they're waitresses.''

I have to be a waitress. How else can I learn about people? How else does the world come to me? I can't go to everyone. So they have to come to me. Everyone wants to eat, everyone has hunger. And I serve them. If they've had a bad day, I nurse them, cajole them. Maybe with coffee I give them a little philosophy. They have cocktails, I give them political science.

I'll say things that bug me. If they manufacture soap, I say what I think about pollution. If it's automobiles, I say what I think about them. If I pour water I'll say, "Would you like your quota of mercury today?'' If I serve cream, I say, "Here is your substitute. I think you're drinking plastic.'' I just can't keep quiet. I have an opinion on every single subject there is. In the beginning it was theology, and my bosses didn't like it. Now I am a political and my bosses don't like it. I speak *sotto voce*. But if I get heated, then I don't give a damn. I speak like an Italian speaks. I can't be servile. I give service. There is a difference.

I'm called by my first name. I like my name. I hate to be called Miss. Even when I serve a lady, a strange woman, I will not say madam. I hate ma'am. I always say milady. In the American language there is no word to address a woman, to indicate whether she's married or unmarried. So I say milady. And sometimes I playfully say to the man milord.

It would be very tiring if I had to say, "Would you like a cocktail?'' and say that over and over. So I come out different for my own enjoyment. I would say, "What's exciting at the bar that I can offer?'' I can't say, "Do you want coffee?'' Maybe I'll say, "Are you in the mood for coffee?'' Or, "The coffee sounds exciting.'' Just rephrase it enough to make it interesting for me. That would make them take an interest. It becomes theatrical and I feel like Mata Hari and it intoxicates me.

People imagine a waitress couldn't possibly think or have any kind of aspiration other than to serve food. When somebody says to me, "You're great, how come you're *just* a waitress?'' *Just* a waitress. I'd say, "Why, don't you think you deserve to be served by me?'' It's implying that he's not worthy, not that I'm not worthy. It makes me irate. I don't feel lowly at all. I myself feel sure. I don't want to change the job. I love it.

Tips? I feel like Carmen. It's like a gypsy holding out a tambourine and they throw the coin. (Laughs.) If you like people, you're not thinking of the tips. I never count my money at night. I always wait till morning. If I thought about my tips I'd be uptight. I never look at a tip. You pick it up fast. I would do my bookkeeping in the morning. It would be very dull for me to know I was making so much and no more. I do like challenge. And it isn't demeaning, not for me.

There might be occasions when the customers might intend to make it demeaning — the man about town, the conventioneer. When the time comes to pay the check, he would do little things, ''How much should I give you?'' He might make an issue about it. I did say to one, ''Don't play God with me. Do what you want.'' Then it really didn't matter whether I got a tip or not. I would spit it out, my resentment — that he dares make me feel I'm operating only for a tip.

He'd ask for his check. Maybe he's going to sign it. He'd take a very long time and he'd make me stand there, ''Let's see now, what do you think I ought to give you?'' He would not let go of that moment. And you knew it. You know he meant to demean you. He's holding the change in his hand, or if he'd sign, he'd flourish the pen and wait. These are the times I really get angry. I'm not reticent. Something would come out. Then I really didn't care. ''Goddamn, keep your money!''

There are conventioneers, who leave their lovely wives or their bad wives. They approach you and say, ''Are there any hot spots?'' ''Where can I find girls?'' It is, of course, first directed at you. I don't mean that as a compliment, 'cause all they're looking for is females. They're not looking for companionship or conversation. I am quite adept at understanding this. I think I'm interesting enough that someone may just want to talk to me. But I would philosophize that way. After all, what is left after you talk? The hours have gone by and I could be home resting or reading or studying guitar, which I do on occasion. I would say, ''What are you going to offer me? Drinks?'' And I'd point to the bar, ''I have it all here.'' He'd look blank and then I'd say, ''A man? If I need a man, wouldn't you think I'd have one of my own? Must I wait for you?''

Life doesn't frighten me any more. There are only two things that relegate us — the bathroom and the grave. Either I'm gonna have to go to the bathroom now or I'm gonna die now. I go to the bathroom.

And I don't have a high opinion of bosses. The more popular you are, the more the boss holds it over your head. You're bringing them business, but he knows you're getting good tips and you won't leave. You have to worry not to overplay it, because the boss becomes resentful and he uses this as a club over your head.

If you become too good a waitress, there's jealousy. They don't come in and say, ''Where's the boss?'' They'll ask for Dolores. It doesn't make a hit. That makes it rough. Sometimes you say, Aw hell, why am I trying so hard? I did get an ulcer. Maybe the things I kept to myself were twisting me.

It's not the customers, never the customers. It's injustice. My dad came from Italy and I think of his broken English —*injoost.* He hated injustice. If you hate injustice for the world, you hate more than anything injustice toward you. Loyalty is never appreciated, particularly if you're the type who doesn't like small talk and are not the type who makes reports on your fellow worker. The boss wants to find out what is going on surreptitiously. In our society today you have informers everywhere. They've informed on cooks, on coworkers. "Oh, someone wasted this." They would say I'm talking to all the customers. "I saw her carry such-and-such out. See if she wrote that on her check." "The salad looked like it was a double salad." I don't give anything away. I just give myself. Informers will manufacture things in order to make their job worthwhile. They're not sure of themselves as workers. There's always someone who wants your station, who would be pretender to the crown. In life there is always someone who wants somebody's job.

I'd get intoxicated with giving service. People would ask for me and I didn't have enough tables. Some of the girls are standing and don't have customers. There is resentment. I feel self-conscious. I feel a sense of guilt. It cramps my style. I would like to say to the customer, "Go to so-and-so." But you can't do that, because you feel a sense of loyalty. So you would rush, get to your customers quickly. Some don't care to drink and still they wait for you. That's a compliment.

There is plenty of tension. If the cook isn't good, you fight to see that the customers get what you know they like. You have to use diplomacy with cooks, who are always dangerous. (Laughs.) They're madmen. (Laughs.) You have to be their friend. They better like you. And your bartender better like you too, because he may do something to the drink. If your bartender doesn't like you, your cook doesn't like you, your boss doesn't like you, the other girls don't like you, you're in trouble.

And there will be customers who are hypochondriacs, who feel they can't eat, and I coax them. Then I hope I can get it just the right way from the cook. I may mix the salad myself just the way they want it.

Maybe there's a party of ten. Big shots, and they'd say, "Dolores, I have special clients, do your best tonight." You just hope you have the right cook behind the broiler. You really want to pleasure your guests. He's selling something, he wants things right, too. You're giving your all. How does the steak look? If you cut his steak, you look at it surreptitiously. How's it going?"

Carrying dishes is a problem. We do have accidents. I spilled a tray once with steaks for seven on it. It was a big, gigantic T-bone, all sliced. But when that tray fell, I went with it, and never made a sound, dish and all (softly) never made a sound. It took about an hour and a half to cook that steak. How would I explain this thing? That steak was salvaged. (Laughs.)

Some don't care. When the plate is down you can hear the sound. I try not to have that sound. I want my hands to be right when I serve. I pick up a glass, I want it to be just right. I get to be almost Oriental in the serving. I like it to look nice all the way. To be a waitress, it's an art. I feel like a ballerina, too. I have to go between those tables, between those chairs

. . . Maybe that's the reason I always stayed slim. It is a certain way I can go through a chair no one else can do. I do it with an air. If I drop a fork, there is a certain way I pick it up. I know they can see how delicately I do it. I'm on stage.

I tell everyone I'm a waitress and I'm proud. If a nurse gives service, I say, "You're a professional." Whatever you do, be professional. I always compliment people.

I like to have my station looking nice. I like to see there's enough ash trays when they're having their coffee and cigarettes. I don't like ash trays so loaded that people are not enjoying the moment. It offends me. I don't do it because I think that's gonna make a better tip. It offends me as a person.

People say, "No one does good work any more." I don't believe it. You know who's saying that? The man at the top, who says the people beneath him are not doing a good job. He's the one who always said, "You're nothing." The housewife who has all the money, she believed housework was demeaning, 'cause she hired someone else to do it. If it weren't so demeaning, why didn't *she* do it? So anyone who did her housework was a person to be demeaned. The maid who did all the housework said, "Well, hell, if this is the way you feel about it, I won't do your housework. You tell me I'm no good, I'm nobody. Well, maybe I'll go out and be somebody." They're only mad because they can't find someone to do it now. The fault is not in the people who did the — quote — lowly work.

Just a waitress. At the end of the night I feel drained. I think a lot of waitresses become alcoholics because of that. In most cases, a waiter or a waitress doesn't eat. They handle food, they don't have time. You'll pick at something in the kitchen, maybe a piece of bread. You'll have a cracker, a little bit of soup. You go back and take a teaspoon of something. Then maybe sit down afterwards and have a drink, maybe three, four, five. And bartenders, too, most of them are alcoholics. They'd go out in a group. There are after-hour places. You've got to go release your tension. So they go out before they go to bed. Some of them stay out all night.

It's tiring, it's nerve-racking. We don't ever sit down. We're on stage and the bosses are watching. If you get the wrong shoes and you get the wrong stitch in that shoe, that does bother you. Your feet hurt, your body aches. If you come out in anger at things that were done to you, it would only make you feel cheapened. Really I've been keeping it to myself. But of late, I'm beginning to spew it out. It's almost as though I sensed my body and soul had had quite enough.

It builds and builds and builds in your guts. Near crying. I can think about it . . . (She cries softly.) 'Cause you're tired. When the night is done, you're tired. You've had so much, there's so much going . . . You had to get it done. The dread that something wouldn't be right, because you want to please. You hope everyone is satisfied. The night's done, you've done your act. The curtains close.

The next morning is pleasant again. I take out my budget book, write down how much I made, what my bills are. I'm managing. I won't give up this job as long as I'm able to do it. I feel out of contact if I just sit at home. At work they all consider me a kook. (Laughs.) That's okay. No matter where I'd be, I would make a rough road for me. It's just me, and I can't keep still. It hurts, and what hurts has to come out.

POSTSCRIPT: *"After sixteen years — that was seven years ago — I took a trip to Hawaii and the Caribbean for two weeks. Went with a lover. The kids saw it — they're all married now. (Laughs.) One of my daughters said, "Act your age." I said, "Honey, if I were acting my age, I wouldn't be walking. My bones would ache. You don't want to hear about my arthritis. Aren't you glad I'm happy?"*

Jim Grayson

A predominantly black suburb, on the outskirts of Chicago. He lives in a one-family dwelling with his wife and five-year-old son, whose finger paintings decorate a wall.

He is a spot-welder, working the third shift. His station is adjacent to Phil Stallings'.

He is also a part-time student at Roosevelt University, majoring in Business Administration. "If I had been white, I wouldn't be doing this job. It's very depressing. I can look around me and see whites with far less education who have better paying jobs with status.

"My alarm clock goes off in the mornings when I go to school. I come back home, take my shirt and tie off, put my brief case down, put on some other suitable clothing. (Laughs.) I go to Ford and spend the night there . . ." (Laughs.)

As, on this late Sunday afternoon, he half-watches the ball game on TV, turned down low, his tone is one of an amused detachment. His phrases, at times, trail off . . .

Oh, anything away from the plant is good. Being on the assembly line, my leisure time is very precious. It's something to be treasured. I don't have much time to talk to the family. I have to be a father, a student, and an assemblyline worker. It's just good to get away.

On our shift we have lunch about seven thirty. A lot of times I just read. Sometimes I just go outside to get away from . . . I don't know if you've heard of plant pollution. It's really terrible. Especially where I work, you have the sparks and smoke. You have these fans blowing on us. If you don't turn the fans down the smoke'll come right up.

They don't use battery trucks. They should. They use gasoline. Lots of times during lunch I never stay on the floor. I usually go outside to get a breath of fresh air. The further you are from the front door, the worse it is. You can cut the heat with a knife, especially when it gets up in the nineties. You get them carbon monoxide fumes, it's just hell.

Ford keeps its overhead down. If I had to go a few feet to get some stock, that would be the time I'm not working. So Ford has everything set up. If you run out, the truck'll come blowin' carbon monoxide all over your face. But it's making sure you'll never run out of work. I mean you're *really* tied down to the job. (Laughs.) You stand on your feet and you run on your feet. (Laughs.)

We get forty-eight minutes of break — thirty minutes in the morning and the other eighteen in the evening. You always go to the bathroom first. (Laughs.) It's three flights up. You come down, you walk to another part of the plant, and you walk up another three flights to get a bite to eat. On the line, you don't go the washroom when you have to go. You learn to adjust your physical . . . (Laughs.) For new workers this is quite hard. I haven't gotten used to it yet. I've been here since 1968.

The part of the automobile I work on is before it gets all the pretties. There's no paint. The basic car. There's a conveyorlike . . . Mr. Ford's given credit for inventing this little . . . (Laughs.) There is no letup, the line is always running. It's not like . . . if you lift something, carry it for a little while, lay it down, and go back — while you're going back, you're actually catching a breather. Ford has a better idea. (Laughs.) You hear the slogan: They have a better idea. They have better ideas of getting all the work possible out of your worn body for eight hours.

You can work next to a guy for months without even knowing his name. One thing, you're too busy to talk. Can't hear. (Laughs.) You have to holler in his ear. They got these little guys comin' around in white shirts and if they see you runnin' your mouth, they say, "This guy needs more work." Man, he's got no time to talk.

A lot of guys who've been in jail, they say you don't work as hard in jail. (Laughs.) They say, "Man, jail ain't never been this bad." (Laughs.) That's the way I feel. I'm serving a sentence till I graduate from college. So I got six more months in jail. Then I'll do something else, probably at a reduction in pay.

If it was up to these ignorant foremen, they'd never get a car out. But they have these professional people, engineering time study. They're always sneakin' around with their little cameras. I can smell 'em a mile away. These people stay awake nights thinking of ways to get more work out of you.

Last night I heard one of the guys say we did 391 cars. How many welds are we supposed to put in a car? They have governmental regulations for consumer protection. We just put what we think ought to be in there and then let it go. (Laughs.) There are specifications, which we pay very little attention to.

You have inspectors who are supposed to check every kind of defect. All of us know these things don't get corrected. I was saying about buying a car, not too long ago. "I hope this buggy lasts till I get out of college." I can just look at a car and see all kinds of things wrong with it. You can't do that because you didn't see how it was made. I can look at a car underneath the paint. It's like x-ray vision. They put that trim in, they call it. The paint and all those little pretties that you pay for. Whenever we make a mistake, we always say, "Don't worry about it, some dingaling'll buy it." (Laughs.)

Everyone has a station. You're supposed to get your work completed within a certain area, usually around ten, maybe fifteen feet. If you get behind, you're in the hole. When you get in the hole, you're bumping into the next worker. Man, sometimes you get in the hole and you run down. Th next worker up from you, he can't do his job until you get finished. If you're slowin' up, that starts a chain reaction all the way up the line.

Ford is a great believer in the specialization of labor, brings about more efficiency. Actually, I can be thinking about economics, politics, anything while I'm doing this work.

Lotta times my mind is on schoolwork. There's no way I could do that job and think about what I'm doin', 'cause it's just impossible for me. The work is just too boring. Especially someone like myself, who is going to school and has a lot of other things on my mind.

"I get pretty peeved off lots of times, because I know I can do other work. They have their quota of blacks and they have just enough so you can't say they're prejudiced. I'm trying to graduate from college and I'd like to go into industry, where the money is.

"I have all sorts of qualifications for the kind of work I want, but none has been offered to me. In 1969 they ran an ad in the paper wanting a junior accountant. I have a minor in accounting, so I applied. They wanted a person with good aptitude in mathematics and a high-school graduate. I had an associate arts degree from junior college and two years of accounting. They took me to the head of the department. He asked, "What makes you want this type of work?" (Laughs.)

You can compare the plant to a miniature United States. You have people from all backgrounds, all cultures. But most of your foremen are white. It seems a lot of 'em are from Alabama, Arkansas, a large percentage Southern white. They don't hide their opinions. They don't confront me, but I've seen it happen in a lot of cases. Oh sure, they holler at people. They don't curse, cursing is not permitted.

They'll do anything to get production. Foremen aren't supposed to work on the line. If he works, he's taking away a job from a union man. The union tries to enforce it, but they do anything they want. Then they complain, "Why didn't you get your people to come to work every day?"

There's quite a bit of absentees, especially on Mondays. Some guys just can't do that type of work every day. They bring phony doctors' excuses. A lot of time, they get the wife or girlfriend to call in: "Junior just broke his leg." (Laughs.) "Your mother-in-law's cousin died and you have to rush home." They don't send you home unless it's an emergency. So lotta guys, they make up their own lies. Monday's the biggest day. You'll have three days off right in a row.

The company is always hiring. They have a huge turnover. I worked at Harvester for five years before I started college. You would find guys there, fifteen years service, twenty, twenty-five. You meet an old-timer here, you ask, "How long you been here?" "About three years." (Laughs.) I'm twenty-nine and one of the oldest guys around here. (Laughs.)

Auto workers are becoming increasingly young and increasingly black. Most of the older workers are a lot more — shall we say, conservative. Most of the older men have seniority, so they don't have to do the work I do. They put 'em on something easy. Old men can't do the work I do. They had one about a year ago, and he had three heart attacks. And they finally gave him a broom. He was about forty. Yeah, forty, that's an old man around here.

I read how bad things were before the union. I was telling some of our officials, don't become complacent. There's much more work to be done, believe me. One night a guy hit his head on a welding gun. He went to his knees. He was bleeding like a pig, blood was oozing out. So I stopped the line for a second and ran over to help him. The foreman turned the line on again, he almost stepped on the guy. That's the first thing they always do. They didn't even call an ambulance. The guy walked to the medic department — that's about half a mile — he had about five stitches put in his head.

The foreman didn't say anything. He just turned the line on. You're nothing to any of them. That's why I hate the place. (Laughs.)

The Green House, that's where the difference of opinion is aired out. Ninety-nine percent of the time, the company comes out winning. If I have a problem, I go to the Green House about it. They might decide against me. They say, "This is it, period." I have to take the time off. Then I can write a grievance. It could be three weeks, three months, three years from now, they could say, "Back in 1971 you were right." So if a union doesn't want to push your particular grievance, you're at the mercy of the company.

They had a wildcat, a sit-down related to me. This particular foreman . . . I think it's jealousy more than anything. They don't like to see, you know — I'm going to school every day. I would bring my books and I'd read during the break. They'd sneak around to see what I'm reading. I seldom miss a day's work and I do my work well. But this guy's been riding me about any little thing. One night he said the wrong thing.

I was going on my break. You're supposed to wear your safety glasses all the time. They don't enforce these things. I took mine off just to wipe my forehead. He said, "Get your glasses on!" It's these nagging little things building up all the time. Always on my back. So I grabbed him, shook him up a little bit. And I went on to lunch. I came back and they were waiting for me. I was supposed to have been fired. I got the rest of the night and two days off.

These guys that worked with me, they didn't like it. So they sat down for a while. I'd already gone. They refused to work for about twenty minutes or so. Now this takes a lot of nerve for the guys to . . . good guys. But oh, I definitely have to get away from this. (Chuckles, suddenly remembering.) One night, there was something wrong with the merry-go-round. We call it that 'cause it goes round and round. They had to call maintenance right away. About six guys came, white shirt, tie, everything. You shoulda seen these guys. On their hands and knees, crawling all over this line, trying to straighten it out. They wouldn't stop it.

Now I couldn't see myself — what kind of status would I have, with my white shirt and tie, crawling on my hands and knees with a crowbar, with grease all over . . .? It was pretty funny. Some of these guys who've been on a farm all their life, they say, "This is great, the best thing ever happened to me."

Phil Stallings said his ambition is to be a utility man. More variation to the job.

Well, that's a hell of an ambition. That's like the difference between the gravedigger and the one who brings the coffin down. So (laughs), he can have it. My ambition is higher than Phil's.

There's no time for the human side in this work. I have other aims. It would be different in an office, in a bank. Any type of job where people would proceed at their own pace.

Once I get into industrial relations — I got corporate law planned — then it won't be a job any more 'cause I will enjoy what I'm doing. It's the difference between a job and a career. This is not a career.

Barbara Terwilliger

She is in her thirties. She has an independent income and is comfortably well-off. During her less affluent days she had worked as an actress, as a saleswoman, engaged in market research, and had assorted other occupations.

It can be splendid not to work for a while, because it changes the rhythm. You can reflect on what you've done. There's no feeling of being indolent. I like being by myself for long periods of time and do not need an occupation. After two months, though, it doesn't work for me. I begin to feel the need for a *raison d'être.* Unless I'm in love. If I should be in love, after months I would begin to feel parasitic and indolent.

What's love got to do with it?

Oh well, love is a woman's occupation. (Laughs.) It's a full-time occupation if you're married. Since I'm not married, I'm talking about a love affair. If you have any sort of ego, you can't make a love affair a justification for life.

About work and idleness . . .

You raise the subject of guilt.

(Slightly bewildered) I did?

I have come to some conclusions after having been free economically from the necessity of work. To be occupied is essential. One should find joy in one's occupation. A great poet can make love and idleness fructify into poetry, a beautiful occupation. He wouldn't think of calling it work. Work has a pejorative sound. It shouldn't. I can't tell you how strongly I feel about work. But so much of what we call work is dehumanizing and brutalizing.

I've done typing as a young girl. I've worked in places where the office was like a factory. A bell rang and that was time for a ten-minute coffee break. It was horrifying. Still, most people are better off — their sanity is maintained in anything that gives their life some structure. I disliked the working conditions and I disliked the regimentation, but I enjoyed the process of typing. I was a good typist. I typed very fast and very accurately. There was a rhythm and I enjoyed that. Just the process of work. It's movement. There's something enlivening . . . A blank piece of paper, your hands on the keys. You are making something exist that didn't exist before.

I tried to pay very much attention to the words I was typing down. I care about language. Some of the words were repugnant to me. If I were having to type some porno stuff or having to say, "Dry cereal is the best thing to feed one's kids night and day, they're going to flourish eating Crunchy Puffs," I wouldn't have been able to do it. But the process gave me satisfaction. There weren't very many erasures. It was neat.

I really feel work is gorgeous. It's the only thing you can depend upon in life. You can't depend on love. Oh, love is quite ephemeral. Work has a dignity you can count upon. Work has to be a game in order for it to be well done. You have to be able to play in it, to compete with yourself. You push yourself to your limits in order to enjoy it. There's quite a wonderful rhythm you can find yourself involved in in the process of any kind of work. It can be waxing a floor or washing dishes . . .

I worked for an employment agency, doing placements. They divided the girls into placeables and unplaceables. I was usually drawn to the unplaceables. These were girls who seemed to me to have some sort of — maybe, inchoate — creative gifts. They wanted jobs where they could feel as individuals. The girls whose hair was not in place, who looked untidy, who weren't going to be that easily accepted. There were some eccentricities involved. I would spend most of my time with them. I would make phone calls to — God forgive — advertising agencies, radio stations.

If you concentrated on the placeables, you made money. These were the girls who came off the production line of high schools, particularly the Catholic schools. They seemed to be tractable young girls. They went into banks as filing clerks in those days. You called the banks and you had your card file and you sent the girl over to the job. You could be a mass production worker yourself, working these girls into the system. There were no tough corners, nothing abrasive. One of my colleagues made two hundred dollars a week shoveling people into these slots. I wasn't doing what the other girls at the desks were doing. I found myself haunted at night by the unplaceable girls. The unplaceable girls were me. If I failed them, I was failing myself. I couldn't make any money. I quit in three weeks. They probably would have fired me anyway.

They were pretty intense weeks. I suffered a lot. I needed the money. I was living on practically nothing. My girls were losers. I found it unbearable to reject them. You say, "We have nothing for you," and send them away. Your time is money, you work on commission. There was a code on the application blank, so you could give the girl the brushoff and she'd never know why.

There were a couple of times I found jobs for the unkempt girls, whose stockings were baggy. And there was even some pleasure in placing those sweet naïve girls, who wanted nothing better than to work in banks, and they were grateful. Even there, the process — being part of something, making something happen — was important. That's the difference between being alive and being dead. Now I'm not making anything happen.

Everyone needs to feel they have a place in the world. It would be unbearable not to. I don't like to feel superfluous. One needs to be needed. I'm saying being idle and leisured, doing nothing, is tragic and disgraceful. Everyone must have an occupation.

Love doesn't suffice. It doesn't fill up enough hours. I don't mean work must be activity for activity's sake. I don't mean obsessive, empty moving around. I mean creating something new. But idleness is an evil. I don't think man can maintain his balance or sanity in idleness. Human beings must work to create some coherence. You do it only through work and through love. And you can only count on work.

Fred Roman

I usually say I'm an accountant. Most people think it's somebody who sits there with a green eyeshade and his sleeves rolled up with a garter, poring over books, adding things — with glasses. (Laughs.) I suppose a certified public accountant has status. It doesn't mean much to me. Do I like the job or don't I? That's important.

He is twenty-five and works for one of the largest public accounting firms in the world. It employs twelve hundred people. He has been with the company three years. During his first year, after graduating from college, he worked for a food chain, doing inventory.

The company I work for doesn't make a product. We provide a service. Our service is auditing. We are usually hired by stockholders or the board of directors. We will certify whether a company's financial statement is correct. They'll say, "This is what we did last year. We made X amount of dollars." We will come in to examine the books and say, "Yes, they did."

We're looking for things that didn't go out the door the wrong way. Our clients could say, "We have a million dollars in accounts receivable." We make sure that they do, in fact, have a million dollars and not a thousand. We ask the people who owe the money, "Do you, in fact, owe our client two thousand dollars as of this date?" We do it on a spot check basis. Some companies have five thousand individual accounts receivable. We'll maybe test a hundred.

We're also looking for things such as floating of cash. If a company writes a check one day and deposits money the next day, it tells you something of its solvency. We look for transfers between accounts to make sure they're not floating these things — a hundred thousand dollars they keep working back and forth between two banks. (Laughs.)

We work with figures, but we have to keep in mind what's behind those figures. What bugs me about people in my work is that they get too wrapped up in numbers. To them a financial statement is the end. To me, it's a tool used by management or stockholders.

We have a computer. We call it Audex. It has taken the detail drudgery out of accounting. I use things that come out of the computer in my everyday work. An accountant will prepare things for keypunching. A girl will keypunch and it will go into the monster. That's what we call it. (Laughs.) You still have to audit what comes out of the computer. I work with pencils. We all do. I think that's 'cause we make so many mistakes. (Laughs.)

You're an auditor. The term scares people. They believe you're there to see if they're stealing nickels and dimes out of petty cash. We're not concerned with that. But people have that image of us. They think we're there to spy on them. What we're really doing is making sure things are reported correctly. I don't care if somebody's stealing money as long as he reports it. (Laughs.)

People look at you with fear and suspicion. The girl who does accounts receivable never saw an auditor before. The comptroller knows why you're there and he'll cooperate. But it's the guy down the line who is not sure and worries. You ask him a lot of questions. What does he do? How does he do it? Are you after his job? Are you trying to get him fired? He's not very friendly.

We're supposed to be independent. We're supposed to certify their books are correct. We'll certify this to the Securities Exchange Commission, to the stockholders, to the banks. They'll all use our financial statements. But if we slight the company — if I find something that's going to take away five hundred thousand dollars of income this year — they may not hire us back next year.

I'm not involved in keeping clients or getting them. That's the responsibility of the manager or the partner. I'm almost at the bottom of the heap. I'm the top class of assistant. There are five levels, I'm a staff assistant. Above me is senior. Senior's in charge of the job, out in the fields with the client. The next level is manager. He has over-all responsibility for the client. He's in charge of billing. The next step is partner. That's tops. He has an interest in the company. Our owners are called partners. They have final responsibility. The partner decides whether this five hundred thousand dollars is going to go or stay on the books.

There are gray areas. Say I saw that five hundred thousand dollars as a bad debt. The client may say, "Oh, the guy's good for it. He's going to pay." You say, "He hasn't paid you anything for the past six months. He declared bankruptcy yesterday. How can you say he's gonna pay?" Your client says, "He's reorganizing and he's gonna get the money." You've got two ways of looking at this. The guy's able to pay or he's not. Somebody's gotta make a decision. Are we gonna allow you to show this receivable or are we gonna make you write it off? We usually compromise. We try to work out something in-between. The company knows more about it than we do, right? But we do have to issue an independent report. Anyway, I'm not a partner who makes those decisions. (Laughs.)

I think I'll leave before I get there. Many people in our firm don't plan on sticking around. The pressure. The constant rush to get things done. Since I've been here, two people have had nervous breakdowns. I have three bosses on any job, but I don't know who's my boss next week. I might be working for somebody else.

Our firm has a philosophy of progress, up or out. I started three years ago. If that second year I didn't move from SA–3, staff assistant, to SA–4, I'd be out. Last June I was SA–4. If I hadn't moved to SA–5, I'd be out. Next year if I don't move to senior, I'll be out. When I make senior I'll be Senior–1. The following year, Senior–2. Then Senior–3. Then manager — or out. By the time I'm thirty-four or so, I'm a partner or I'm out.

When a partner reaches fifty-five he no longer has direct client responsibility. He doesn't move out, because he's now part owner of the company. He's in an advisory capacity. They're not retired. They're just — just doing research. I'm not saying this is good or bad. This is just how it is.

It's a very young field. You have a lot of them at the bottom to do the footwork. Then it pyramids and you don't need so many up there. Most of the people they get are just out of college. I can't label them — the range is broad — but I'd guess most of them are conservative. Politics is hardly discussed.

Fifteen years ago, public accountants wore white shirts. You had to wear a hat, so you could convey a conservative image. When I was in college the big joke was : If you're going to work for a public accounting firm, make sure you buy a good supply of white shirts and a hat. They've gotten away from that since. We have guys with long hair. But they do catch more static than somebody in another business. And now we have women. There are several female assistants and seniors. There's one woman manager. We have no female partners.

If you don't advance, they'll help you find another job. They're very nice about it. They'll fire you, but they just don't throw you out in the street.(Laughs.) They'll try to find you a job with one of our clients. There's a theory behind it. Say I leave to go to XYZ Manufacturing Company. In fifteen years, I'm comptroller and I need an audit. Who am I gonna go to? Although their philosophy is up or out, they treat their employees very well.

Is my job important? It's a question I ask myself. It's important to people who use financial statements, who buy stocks. Its important to banks. (Pause.) I'm not out combatting pollution or anything like that. Whether it's important to society . . . (A long pause.) No, not too important. It's necessary in this economy, based on big business. I don't think most of the others at the firm share my views. (Laughs.)

I have a couple friends there. We get together and talk once in a while. At first you're afraid to say anything 'cause you think the guy really loves it. You don't want to say, "I hate it." But then you hear the guy say, "Boy! If it weren't for the money I'd quit right now."

I'd like to go back to college and get a master's or Ph.D. and become a college teacher. The only problem is I don't think I have the smarts for it. When I was in high school I thought I'd be an engineer. So I took math, chemistry, physics, and got my D's. I thought of being a history major. Then I said, "What will I do with a degree in history?" I thought of poli sci. I thought most about going into law. I still think about it. I chose accounting for a very poor reason. I eliminated everything else. Even after I passed my test as a CPA I was saying all along, "I don't want to be an accountant." (Laughs.) I'm young enough. After June I can look around. As for salary, I'm well ahead of my contemporaries. I'm well ahead of those in teaching and slightly ahead of those in engineering. But that isn't it . . .

When people ask what I do, I tell them I'm an accountant. It sounds better than auditor, doesn't it? (Laughs.) But it's not a very exciting business. What can you say about figures? (Laughs.) You tell people you're an accountant — (his voice deliberately assumes a dull monotone) "Oh, that's nice." They don't know quite what to say. (Laughs.) What can you say? I could say, "Wow! I saw this company yesterday and their balance sheet, wow!"

(Laughs.) Maybe I look at it wrong. (Slowly emphasizing each word) *There just isn't much to talk about.*

Alternatives to traditional careers: Resources*

Although most of the information contained in this chapter is about traditional career fields, there are other directions for those interested in them. Recent research has shown a decline in the number of students interested in social action or working for a cause. We believe that today numerous change-oriented students are finding meaningful employment in traditional settings. They are working for change either avocationally or within their respective institutions. Keeping in mind the difficulty of defining what is traditional and what is not, we approach the following section with a little caution.

Career resources as well as career directions (of the not-so-typical nature) are discussed in the context of the previous career information and exploration. Our purpose is to initiate your awareness of as many career options as possible. You should examine this material in the same manner as you did the previous career information. Evaluate your own interests, skills, and aspirations in respect to the activities and values about which you're reading. If you are interested in further exploration of this area, check your career planning and placement office or school library for copies of these or similar resources.

WorkForce is a bimonthly magazine that began "at first by offering suggestions and ideas for the creation of alternatives to traditional jobs and more recently by encouraging the attempts of people with 'straight' jobs to make their workplaces more humane." Not only are jobs, new groups, and resources to aid in directing energies and efforts listed, but also "conspiracy notes" where boycotts and causes in need of immediate support are reviewed. Each issue covers a different subject of current concern; for example, "Science for the People," "Research," "Radicals in Health," and "Gay Liberation." *WorkForce* also has a resource guide listing groups that the editors consider to be major sources of information and that can help people who want to start local social action programs.

Colleges do not have the corner on the learning market — contrary to what some people would like to think — alternatives such as workshops, institutes, community centers, and networks offer those dissatisfied with traditional sources of learning another opportunity. These are described in *Somewhere Else,* edited by the Center for Curriculum Design, which is comprised of 400 entries — people, places, networks, centers, books, and groups. Subjects range from artisan centers and spiritual centers to women's networks. Variety is the key to this resource as it includes the entire realm of learning centers — from the fairly traditional to the truly experimental — throughout the United

*Adapted from an unpublished pamphlet (1975) by JoAn Mann, Assistant Director of Career Planning and Placement, College of Sciences and Humanities, Iowa State University, Ames, Iowa. Used by permission of the author.

States and also abroad. *Somewhere Else* is an idea book that you can refer to for summers, interim terms, vacations, postgraduate years, or for any time when life becomes a mechanical routine.

Integrating one's work with life is the subject of *Working Loose*. Members of the American Friends Service Committee share their experiences of searching for and discovering work that lets them develop as individuals while aiding others. Through poems, dialogue, and essays, the message is transmitted that knowing one's own needs, aims, and talents give one the possibility of creating or finding work that is not separate from living and learning. Resources at the back of *Working Loose* can direct you to groups, books, or individuals for "information and energy" to create your own way.

Though just a beginning of what should expand into a nationwide index of local alternative centers, the San Francisco and Boston *People's Yellow Pages* directories are available for ideas of nontraditional contacts in those two cities. Community centers and services are listed as well as suggestions about where to go for recreation, volunteer work, schools, bookstores, and so forth. Each of these could hold possible employment for someone interested in such ideas or resources. Many similar centers and services are located across the country, making these two sources versatile.

Outdoor jobs are naturals for conservation careers. The kinds of jobs available in this area plus information on salaries, education requirements, and employing agencies are found in *Making a Living in Conservation*. Emphasis is placed on entry-level jobs that do not require previous experience rather than on those for the highly trained and experienced person. The nine categories covered range from forestry to oceanography to environmental health. They are supplemented by tips on job hunting and education, as well as an additional information section.

A Different Drummer describes social action opportunities, basically in the Philadelphia–Washington, D.C., area but, again, which can be applicable for all areas of the country in concept. Listings in *Different Drummer* include such areas as consumer protection, ecology, experimental and alternative schools, working for peace, and community action. Prerequisites, if any, are stated in most instances as well as insight as to abilities and talents helpful for the position. Regarding the prospects of finding a permanent job in any of the suggested agencies and organizations, *A Different Drummer* does say, "you'll have more luck job hunting in the future if you spend some of your time in a volunteer job now." Hence, this resource as well as the others suggests viable interim internships and summer jobs, which can give you the direction and experience necessary to land or create a position that will enable you to expand and share your experiences.

Another resource that could offer suggestions for gaining valuable work experience is *A Guide to Volunteer Services*. "Being a volunteer only requires a frame of mind — the desire to do something, with no financial reward, for someone else who could not receive that service unless *you* do it with him or for her." Organizations concerned with health care and welfare (such as hospitals, the Salvation Army, the Red Cross, volunteer services). Again, permanent employment is always a possible outcome of any volunteer position.

As a concluding thought, learning through experience is vital for both knowing yourself and preparing for future work directions. Thorough examination of opportunities is certainly one of the best ways to discover the direction you wish to take — be it a well-traveled path or a trail you blaze alone.

Conclusion and organization of data

Whatever the resource or method you use to gather career information, we would like to emphasize a couple of points pertinent to how you use the information. First, don't just read a career pamphlet or brochure, listen to a career tape, and so forth, and then leave it feeling you've done your bit in exploring careers. We urge you to take some notes (something new, huh?) and organize the information for easy future reference. Career information is too easily forgotten and too complex for you to rely on memory alone. We recommend something like the Career Information Organizer chart, not only to organize your comments and perceptions, but to be sure you have considered all aspects of the career that are important to you. There are many criteria to consider when exploring a career — that chart lists some of them and helps you organize them in regard to the careers ycu are exploring.

As well as being a self-help method of organizing your perceptions and comments, this kind of chart is a very helpful tool to bring to a career counselor (or anyone, really) to get some additional input as to your thinking, organizing, and approach to different careers. Complete it on your own but then get feedback from someone else — get their reactions and suggestions.

As a final point of suggestion, don't be satisfied with information from just one source. For example, we think you'll agree that it would be rather foolish to disregard a career you think you might like because one individual tells you it doesn't pay very much. Relating back to our chart as well as to the career development model, pay is just one of many things to consider in career choice. Also, the opinion of a single individual (who knows how knowledgeable he or she is anyway?) should certainly not be conclusive evidence for you.

As a second example, you would not base your decision to go to law school on a 1965 article (you'd be surprised how many are still around and used as career information) saying that there is a need for lawyers. Be aware of publication dates and remember a book or article may contain the unsubstantiated, biased opinions of uninformed individuals.

Careers	Criteria to consider in exploring careers				
	Career activities	Preparation and skills required	Work setting and location	Job outlook	Miscellaneous comments

Career information organizer

Be sure to check out your information and the reliability of its source — confirm it with a career counselor or placement person as well as other reliable resource people. A useful pamphlet "Are You an Occupational Ignoramus — Most Students Are and It's Risky Business," published by the College Placement Council, can be helpful in checking out your information. Ask your career planning personnel about it.

Career development model—Chapter 5

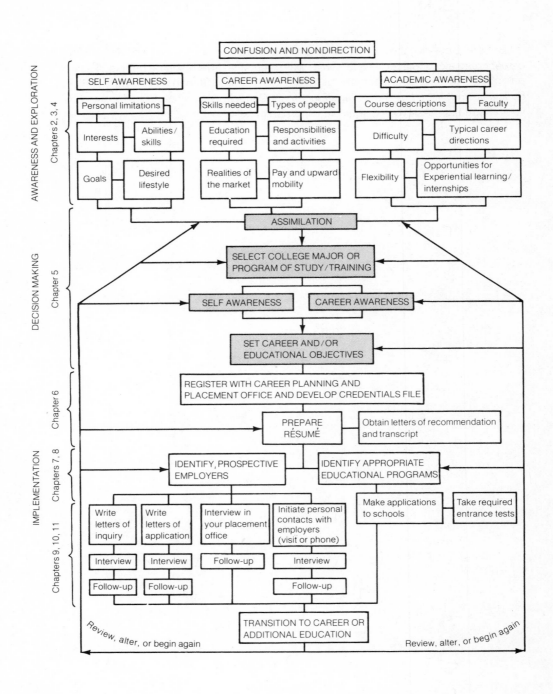

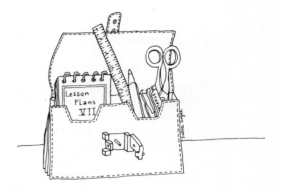

5 Setting educational and career objectives

Decision making as it regards your program of study or training or your choice of career is a critical step in our systematic model for career development. It is in this decision that everything we've accomplished in the first three sections comes together. Decision making, setting objectives, problem solving, or whatever we want to call it is basically a confrontation with one particular aspect of your own career development and your resulting concern about how you're going to resolve it. It may be as basic as wanting to know where a particular piece of career information is or as complex as how you see yourself fitting into a particular career. Whatever the problem or decision, the steps to solve it are quite similar.

To be consistent with our model, as well as to illustrate perhaps the most common (and most difficult) decisions that we all must make, we will examine the problems of choosing a career and choosing a college major or program of study or training and some ideas that may help you make your decisions. Again, looking at our model, we use the word *assimilation* to describe the process by which you put together self-awareness — knowing your likes, dislikes, skills, abilities, goals, lifestyle, limitations, and so forth — with career awareness — knowing important things about different careers like activities and responsibilities of the job, skills needed, number of jobs available, pay, challenges — as well as academic awareness — understanding the make-up and implications of programs of study or training *—and ultimately coming up with a career direction.* If you are already in a particular study or training program, then we also want to review self- and career awareness as part of your career decision-making process (look back at the appropriate chapters.) Easy, huh? Unfortunately, not for the majority of students.

In some instances, however, it is very simple and as a result of completing one or all of the previous chapters, your decision as to program of study or training and career direction will automatically result. For example, you may read something about a particular career, be turned on by it, and ultimately decide to pursue it; or maybe a scale on an interest inventory pointed to a particular career, the same career turned up several times in the questions you answered in the second chapter of this book and after a summer job in the same field, you decided it was definitely for you. If this happened to you, then you are, needless to say, feeling pretty good about having cleared this hurdle and being ready to proceed on to Chapter 7, "Identifying Appropriate Educational Programs," and Chapter 8, "Identifying Prospective Employers." If not, then read on, and we will try to help you through another important step in your career development — decision making.

A step-by-step approach

Just as our model uses a systematic approach to career development, the following approach to making a decision or solving a problem is likewise systematic.* It follows a pattern of steps that should be completed sequentially to give you the best chance for success at the finish. *A word of caution* — this approach is *not* going to startle you with its profundity or uniqueness. It is, rather, a logical procedure that is quite similar to the ideas of many other educators about this subject. It is not a panacea but a method that may offer some assistance in answering your career choice questions.

Our logical systematic approach to making a career decision or solving a career-choice problem is as follows.

Formulate the problem or decision and set your goal

Needless to say, before you can set about the task of solving a problem, a clear definition of the task and the steps necessary to accomplish it are necessary. The first step then is to get this problem clearly defined in your own mind — the clearer it is, the easier will be its

---

*Some of the ideas for this systematic approach have been incorporated from the film *Career Decision Making* by John D. Krumboltz and Don L. Sorenson (16mm sound/color film, 27 min.; produced by Counseling Films, Inc., Box 1047, Madison, WI 53701; Library of Congress catalog no. 76-710926; copyright 1974); and an unpublished "Career Exploration Program," by Dr. Thomas Irwin, President of Career Planning Consultants, Inc., Charlottesville, Va., 1973.

solution as well as the procedures you go through in attaining that solution. Writing some things down as well as talking with a career counselor or placement person can assist you in this step.

One common error in this step is to believe that you are defining the problem when actually you are talking about a symptom of the problem. For example, in some cases an inability to decide on a career direction is really a symptom of the problem. The actual problem is your own unwillingness to spend sufficient time and energy in making that decision. To solve the problem, then, you can't devote efforts to the symptoms but must attack the essence of your concern — namely, the allocation of time devoted to career decision making.

Commitment of yourself: Time, energy, and resources

As implied in the previous step, commitment on your part to do the necessary work involved in making a decision is critical to the process and ultimately to making a successful decision. So, this then is the second step in the process. As we have mentioned previously — but it bears repeating — think of all the hours you spend studying and reading, in many cases, for courses that have little practical meaning to your life. Isn't it worthwhile to devote an hour or so a day to an important decision that will definitely affect the rest of your life?

Gather information and explore alternatives

This step in the decision-making process relates very closely to what you have been doing in the preceding chapters of this book. You have been gathering or compiling information about yourself, about study or training alternatives, and about career alternatives. Another valuable area of information is the identification of your skills. The following section and accompanying exercise will give you a clearer perspective on how to identify, examine, and operationally present and demonstrate your own skills.

One further suggestion before you begin looking at your skills. We believe that you will find it helpful, when gathering information about any decision or problem, to organize it and write it down in a systematic format. The Career Information Organizer that appears in Chapter 4, "Career Awareness," will provide you with a good model for organizing the information you gather.

A detailed look at skills

During the previous discussion, we have tossed the word *skills* around quite profusely. If you have picked up on our implications, you probably realize the significance of skills to any discussion of career development. On the surface, the idea of skills — their identification as well as their application to work settings — may not appear to be a difficult one to grasp. After all, if you as a student know your skills (what you can do and to what level of excellence) and how they apply to work situations, you have half your battle won. Right? Well, maybe not.

There are varying levels of sophistications at which one can talk about skills. In fact, the area of skills can be a discipline in itself, quite complex in its own study and make-up. To avoid getting bogged down in complexity, let's take a brief look at skills from the perspective of some experts in the field.

Although we haven't talked much about a resource entitled *The Dictionary of Occupational Titles* (DOT), it is most useful regarding the application of skills to various job situations. The DOT examines just about every career field imaginable with respect to its occupational groupings and a "worker-traits" arrangement. This dual approach provides you with information on relationships among career fields and also an idea of the necessary skills, experiences, and potential for various job areas. More specifically, there are coded groupings of information for each career field that indicate knowledge, abilities, aptitudes, temperaments, and physical demands. Also, each career field is coded to indicate the amount of involvement and complexity with data, people, and things (see later paragraphs on this concept). This type of information can be extremely valuable in helping you assimilate aspects of self- and career awareness in your search for a general career direction.

Finally, each career field is discussed in terms of work performed, worker requirements, training, and methods of entry, a qualifications profile, related classifications, and a most interesting type of information — clues for relating applicants and requirements. This final category gives brief statements on interests, hobbies, areas of college activities, and skills that relate to the career being discussed. Thus, although your skill areas are significant in determining your career direction, don't forget these other considerations — your interest and enthusiasm for the activities of the career field, flexibility that allows you to change direction, types of people generally found in the field, as well as other criteria specifically important to you. All of them deserve your attention. (See Clarifying Career Values exercise later in this chapter).

It is important to remember that the DOT is a valuable tool in your approach to career awareness and career exploration (Chapter 4). It appears complicated at first, but with the assistance of a counselor and your own determination, its information can provide insights that no other resource can.

The DOT is especially important to our discussion of skills. Most of the research is credited to a Dr. Sidney Fine, who categorizes skills into three succinct areas: skills in working with *data,* with *people,* and with *things.* The diagram, "Summary chart of worker function scales," illustrates levels of sophistication from simple (at the bottom) to complex (at the top) in each category.

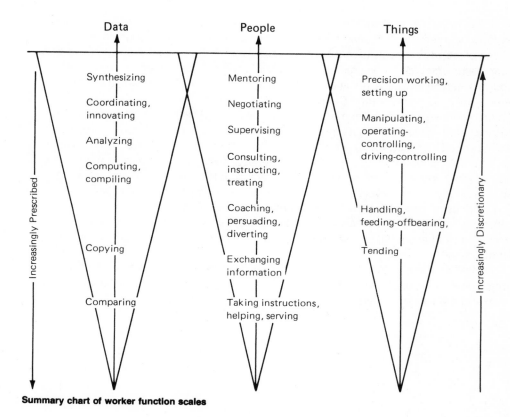

Summary chart of worker function scales

We believe this diagram can be interpreted in different ways depending on one's perspective and intentions. For our immediate purpose, most career fields deal with data, people, and things in some way, shape, or form. The distinguishing factor remains the quantity or amount of "dealing." The importance of each category varies with different jobs. As indicated by Dr. Fine's descriptive words of ascending complexity within the inverted triangles, we can take a job, look it up in a career resource, and determine its relationship to working with data, people, and things. Thus, knowing our own skills and experiences with each category, we can develop points of departure for career exploration in fields suitable to our skills.

Your own skill identification and demonstration
Reading that a college education develops skills applicable to career fields is not going to convince you that you're hireable. Also, simply talking about skills per se —

functional, adaptive, work-specific, or dealing with people, data, and things — to an employer on a résumé or in an interview will not guarantee success in your job search.

One of the key elements is your ability to base these skills in actual experiences and accomplishments (skill demonstration) and then communicate them to employers through either the traditional résumé or interview approach or the Bolles "empowerment" method, which is discussed (in Chapter 10.)

When we speak about skill demonstration, we are (and will be throughout the following exercise) dealing with skills that can be related to Dr. Fine's schema. From our point of view, however, it's not critical for you to relate each of your own skills to this schema. If you can, so much the better for your personal awareness of your own knowledge and skills and how they relate to work situations. On a practical level, if you use the following exercise simply to identify your skills, "demonstrate" them, and then take the one step we can't emphasize enough, research employment organizations or vacancies thoroughly so that you can communicate how your skills can be beneficial to work situations, you will be more than off and running in your pursuit of a career direction or a specific job within that direction.

The following exercise will assist you in identifying experiences and abilities that demonstrate your skills and, it is hoped, facilitate your communication of those experiences and skills to employers.

Directions   Check those experiences and/or abilities that were integral to your *overall* college experience. In so doing, you will have identified a skill applicable to the work world as well as marketable to employers.

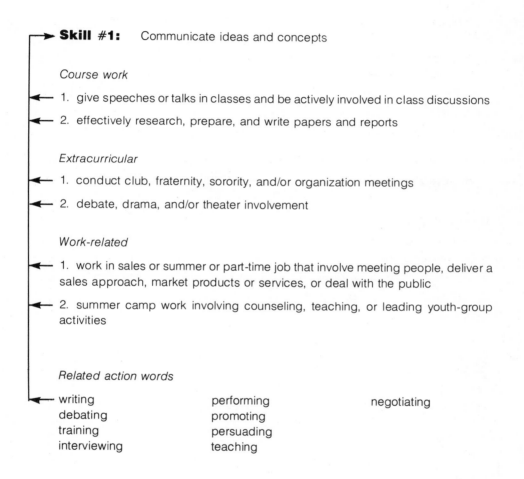

Skill #1:   Communicate ideas and concepts

Course work

1. give speeches or talks in classes and be actively involved in class discussions

2. effectively research, prepare, and write papers and reports

Extracurricular

1. conduct club, fraternity, sorority, and/or organization meetings

2. debate, drama, and/or theater involvement

Work-related

1. work in sales or summer or part-time job that involve meeting people, deliver a sales approach, market products or services, or deal with the public

2. summer camp work involving counseling, teaching, or leading youth-group activities

Related action words

writing	performing	negotiating
debating	promoting	
training	persuading	
interviewing	teaching	

Skill #2:   Think analytically, objectively, and evaluatively in solving problems and making decisions applicable to various work operations

Course work

1. analyze information, synthesize important concepts, and effectively communicate them on tests and papers

2. budget time, schedule courses, and allocate resources in planning curricular and extracurricular activities

Extracurricular

1. budget finances for clubs or groups

2. plan and administer group or club activity, policies, and directions

3. develop strategies in athletic, recreational, or contest-related endeavors

Work related

1. various work situations involving decision making, scheduling, planning strategies, and developing directions

2. sales or clerical responsibilities involving exchanging money, dealing with a product or service, as well as contact with the public

Related action words

creating   designing
planning   theorizing
researching   visualizing
inventing

Skill #3:   Think creatively and use imagination in the formulation of innovative ideas, projects, and programs

Course work

1. develop independent study, special project, or research requiring imagination and creativity

2. majoring in self-designed or interdisciplinary course of study requiring innovative planning or scheduling

3. create study techniques used in completing course assignments and preparing for examinations

Extracurricular

1. initiate new campus activities or programs or modify existing ones

2. instigate new approaches or practices as part of club, athletic, theater, or activity processes

Work related

1. Work or job situations where personal ideas were used to increase efficiency of, or expand, present operations

Related action words

perceiving
imagining
inventing

designing
developing
innovating

Skill #4: Possess working knowledge of employment organizational structure, process, operations, and systems

Work, course work, or internship

1. familiarity with the world of work (or specific employment setting) through direct or indirect involvement

Skill #5: Organizational, creative, and communicative ability in *writing*

Course work

1. develop ideas, construct outline, and communicate through course papers and projects

Extracurricular

1. write reports, summaries of meetings, and communiques to students or college regarding issues and programs

Work related

1. experience with business correspondence, office memos, or writing up programs, activities, and so forth

Related action words

correspond	type
dictate	communicate

Skill #6:   Utilize complex and sophisticated tools of quantitative analysis

Course work, extracurricular, and/or work related

1. experiences and competencies in using computer, calculating machines, accounting, and systematic approaches to problem solving

Related action words

data processing	calculating	budgeting
inventorying	figuring	financing

Skill #7:   Creative self-expression through fine arts and/or media talents

Course work

1. musical, drama, theatrical, or artistic ability expressed through course projects

Extracurricular

1. perform recitals or organize showings for creative art work

2. active in drama and theater from various perspectives, including acting, directing, or crew

Work experience

1. summer stock experience

2. recitals, concerts, performances

3. involvement in audio-visual media in the area of equipment operation, production, and editing

4. develop portfolio of personal work

Related action words

conducting	performing	dramatizing	painting
composing	drawing	acting	

Skill #8:   To work effectively with people toward a group goal

Course work

1. involvement in group discussion contributing ideas and input

2. work efficiently and cooperatively with other students in class project or assignment

Extracurricular

1. working member of college committee(s), fraternity, sorority, athletics, student government, newspaper, and so forth

2. work with group of students (individuals) in carrying out an assignment significant to a group program — voluntary, community, or college related

Work related

1. summer or part-time job with involvement in a process, program, or product — shift work, warehouses, assembly line, youth work, camping, and so forth

Related action words

listening   input
cooperating   compromising
follow-through
contribute

Skill #9:   Supervise people and/or a process in the accomplishment of a goal

Course work

1. group or discussion leader in class

2. project chairman for group study responsible for delegating duties, organizing re-search techniques, and final completion

3. student or volunteer teaching, responsible for curriculum planning, instruction, and evaluation

Extracurricular

1. fraternity, sorority, club or committee leader with responsibility for planning and conducting meetings as well as determining group direction or responsibilities

2. volunteer tutor assisting students in planning and study-skill development

Work related

1. summer job as camp counselor or park director involved in supervising and adminis-tering

2. part-time or informal teacher of arts, crafts, athletics, or recreation

3. residence hall staff or college work-study project in administering college policies and assisting students

4. laborer or construction worker at times assuming responsibility for supervising prod-uct, process, or people

Related action words

administering	evaluating
managing	teaching
supervising	instructing
delegating	problem solving

Skill #10:   Use personal traits, a commitment to helping, and knowledge of inter-personal relationships in assisting individuals to solve problems

Course work

1. tutor classmates in academic skills — studying, scheduling, assignments, preparing for tests

Extracurricular

1. informal "counselor" and listener for friends' problems in a wide range of areas

2. volunteer tutor or counselor in community or social service programs

3. involvement in youth services-related activities

Work related

1. summer camp counselor or recreational program director

2. residence hall assistant or assistant in college student services

Related action words

counseling   helping
advising   providing information
listening   assisting
referring   tutoring

A final reminder

A college education, as well as everyday life, develops usable skills. We hope that the previous exercise has evidenced some of them and, equally as important, that you have demonstrated the experiences and accomplishments on which these skills are based. Indeed, these are important insights for you. However, becoming more familiar with work settings and job situations specifically applicable to these skills is equally significant. Without your taking this step, plus creating opportunities to present these skills to people in work settings, the process is incomplete — the job is half done. It's like developing a super résumé and then leaving it in your desk drawer — where it cannot work for you.

Know yourself (gain self-awareness and identify your skills), but then be sure to use this knowledge in the other steps of the career development model to help accomplish one of two objectives — determining a career direction, or securing a position consistent with your career objective.

Evaluate each alternative through decision-making exercises

Now that you have learned about skills in general and what yours are in particular and have added this piece of information to others gathered about yourself and your alternatives, you are ready for the next step. In a sense, you have already partially completed this step if you have done a thorough job on the Career (or Academic) Information Organizer. If, when you read about different careers or study programs, listened to career information, experienced different career-related situations, and so forth, you kept asking yourself the questions, How do I fit in? Would I like it? How well would I do in it? and so forth, and more importantly, came up with some answers to these questions, then you are already well into this evaluation step.

The following exercises* can help you organize this evaluation process. Another word of caution — these exercises are not a decision-maker for you; they have no statistical basis and should be used instead as general aids that can give you important pieces of information in making your decision.

Before proceeding with the exercises "Clarifying Curricular Values" and "Clarifying Career Values," let us briefly explain their significance. Although you will obviously make many decisions during your lifetime that will affect your career development, we believe there are two primary decision points during your academic career that are of paramount importance. These are (1) the selection of an academic major or program of study and (2) the selection or, more probably, the tentative selection of a career. The two exercises that follow will help you to collect, organize, and evaluate information that you have gathered about yourself, various academic programs, and various careers. It will, thus, be easier for you to rationally evaluate the alternatives available to you.

*The concept behind these decision-making exercises comes from Dr. Michele Wilson, Counseling Psychologist, Center for Counseling, University of Delaware, Newark, Delaware.

Clarifying curricular values

Directions

1. Look at the chart titled "Curricular values clarifier." Under the heading "Criteria to consider in making an academic decision" are several aspects of college programs that many people believe are important in making such a decision. There are also blank spaces where you can fill in your own criteria — those *you* particularly value that are not included in our chart. Examples of these are

practicality
enthusiasm of faculty
types and diversity of courses
type of students in a particular area
difficulty of courses
class size
opportunities to take courses outside the department
quality of scholarship
reputation of professors

2. You will also notice that on the left side of the chart, there are spaces for you to list college programs you feel may be interesting. They may include academic disciplines that piqued your interest in the second or third chapter of this book or just areas of study that you've always liked or curiously contemplated.

3. Using information gathered from your college catalog, from Chapter 3 of this book, and from conversations with faculty, counselors, and friends, begin to assign specific values for each criterion at the top of the chart to each program. Use a number from 0 to 3 to indicate *compatibility* between you and what you know about the particular criterion and how it relates to a specific college major. Number 3 designates a high degree of compatibility; 2 average; 1 very little; and 0 shows that you could care less in terms of that criterion meeting your *needs* in any particular college program. Say, for example, you're trying to decide between an economics and a business major and an important consideration is flexibility — flexibility in time to take numerous other liberal arts courses as well as an internship to gain some practical experience. If one or the other college program has fewer course requirements, that college major would probably score a 3 on flexibility while the other major might score only 1. Another example: You're trying to decide how the practicality criterion relates to majors in history and in English. You already know that liberal arts graduates in each of the majors proceed to numerous jobs each year in business and industry, and each major is a good prerequisite for a graduate program in business (M.B.A.) or law. However, the kinds of things you see yourself doing in a job someday are very communications oriented. In this case you might place a numerical

Criteria to consider in making an academic decision

College program of study/training	major issues and activities	Interest in college	Type of courses, class size, assignments	Faculty	Opportunities for internships/experiential learning	Typical careers and job outlook		Total

College program with highest total

Next highest total

Lowest total

Curricular values clarifier

value 3 on English and only a 2 on history. While any liberal arts degree provides communications skills, an English concentration might intensify those skills and thus be more *practical* for a career direction emphasizing communications.

4. A couple of cautionary points before proceeding:

a. Leave some "academic criteria" spaces blank. Chances are, once you begin using a resource with this exercise, you'll discover new criteria that are important to you.

b. If you feel that one or two criteria are especially important or meaningful to you, double their number when you're assigning values.

c. Don't feel that this exercise is a one-shot deal. Your values may change just as your interests may change. The important thing is to choose a major that best fits your interests, abilities, and present goals, as well as allows for their development in the future. It is essential to keep in mind that the choice of a college major does *not* completely determine a future career. If you can select an area of study that incorporates ideas, issues, and concepts related to broad career goals then you will be in a good position to refine these goals through increased future exploration — both inside and outside your major.

d. No college program decision is irreversible in terms of your career direction. The list is endless of history majors becoming accountants, math majors becoming social workers, certified teachers becoming business executives. Your only limitations are your willingness (or lack thereof) to adapt and work toward a newly developed idea or career direction.

5. When you have completed all the criteria for the college majors you have listed, add up the values and check the comparative totals. You now have an *objective* comparison of different majors as they correspond to your values. *Not* that the highest total is the area for you, but rather that you have just obtained an important piece of information in helping to select a college major. Use it with other information about careers and the college programs of study or training as well as information about yourself to piece together a potential direction for you.

Clarifying career values

Directions

1. On the "Career values clarifier" chart you will find the head "Criteria to consider in making a career decision" at the top. This identifies different aspects of a career decision. There are also blank spaces where you can fill in your own criteria — those *you* particularly value that are not included on our chart. Examples of these are:

leisure time
helping people
fringe benefits
pressure

Criteria to consider in making a career decision

Careers	Interests in career activities	Abilities for doing the job	Preparation required	Job outlook, number of openings	Financial rewards, salary, benefits					Total

Career with highest total

Next highest

Lowest

Career values clarifier

prestige
location
variety of tasks
advancement possibilities
creativity
moral fulfillment
adventure

2. You will also notice that on the left side of the chart, there are spaces for you to list careers that you feel may be interesting. They might include career fields listed in Chapters 2 and 3 that looked as if they might be right for you or just careers that you've also kind of liked or been curious about.

3. Now is where the work begins. Using information gathered from the resources discussed in Chapter 3 (books, visits, work experiences, pamphlets, audio-visual information, media, etc.) begin to assign a value for each criterion (listed across the top) to the careers listed on the left. As you remember the information from previous career exploration or use a career resource (the *Occupational Outlook Handbook* or the *Job Index* discussed in Chapter 4 are excellent for this method) while you are doing this exercise, attempt to put a value on the career criteria as they relate to the careers you are exploring. Now, what exactly do we mean by value? In order to compare the careers, we need to assign a *number value* to each of the career criteria. We'll use the numbers 0, 1, 2, and 3; with 3 designating a high degree of compatibility between what you know about the career criterion for the particular career you're evaluating and how it meets your needs for a career, 2 designating an average degree of compatibility, 1 indicating a less than satisfactory degree of compatibility, and 0 meaning you could care less about the particular aspect in a career or that there is no way you can evaluate that criterion as it relates to that career.

For example, if the *Occupational Outlook Handbook* indicates that salaries for accountants are quite high and amount of money is very important to your choice of a career, then you would place a 3 under the salary criterion for the career accountant. If your grades in one accounting course were only average, you might rate the ability criterion a 1 or a 2. As another example, suppose that in your reading as well as in talking to social workers, you conclude that social workers' greatest job satisfaction is in helping people. If you're not really concerned with helping people in a job or feel that it is not very important to your happiness in a job, you will most likely rate social worker under the career criterion helping people as a 1 or even 0.

4. A couple of cautionary points before proceeding:

a. Leave some spaces for career criteria blank. Chances are, once you begin using a resource with this exercise, you'll discover new criteria that are important to you.

b. If you feel that one or two career criteria are especially important or meaningful to you, double their number when you're assigning values.

c. Don't feel that this exercise is a one-shot deal. Your values may change just as the different careers in which you are interested may change. Also, as you gather more career information and begin to know more about careers, you will probably also change the values you place on the career criteria.

5. When you have completed all the criteria for the careers you have listed, add up the values and check the comparative totals. You now have an *objective* comparison of different careers as they correspond with your values. *Not* that the career with the highest total is the career for you, but rather that you have just obtained an important piece of information, which can help you formulate a career direction. Use it with other information about careers as well as about yourself to arrive at a potential career direction for you.

Decide tentatively — consider alternative and back-up plans

In this step consider all your evaluations (look at your completed *Values Clarifiers* as well as other information). Use all the information to put together a *tentative* career direction. It is important that when you view this information, you are aware that some criteria are more important to you than others and therefore should be given more weight. You can do this by doubling or tripling the values you assign to different criteria, as explained in the previous exercise.

Also, in making this tentative decision, the career or academic direction that allows for flexibility, experiences that might tie into other careers, and those that allow possible back-up directions in case something goes awry are also important considerations. When using the exercises, too, always be sure to review your self-, career, and academic awareness while going through the decision-making process.

A good way to check on your decision is to relate it back to your problem formulation in the first step of this decision-making model, as well as to the information gathered in Chapters 3 and 4, and evaluate it for consistency. If they jibe, then you're in business — if not, then you might want to go back and do some revision.

As has been emphasized throughout this book, this is a self-help process structured to allow you to be involved in activities and accomplishments by yourself and ultimately to secure a career consistent with your abilities, interests, skills, and goals. However, and especially in relation to the fifth step in this model, it can be advantageous to discuss some of your thoughts and work in this book with a career counselor or placement advisor. Working by yourself is great and very satisfying when success is achieved — when you're in a jam, though, bouncing your thoughts off a trained "helper" can be just the thing to stimulate new thinking and problem solution.

A misconception that should be discussed in this context is the expectation that a counselor will make a decision for you. Sound decisions involve a sense of commitment. You can't be committed to a decision someone else has made. Therefore, a counselor should allow you the freedom to make your own decision. He or she can help you to weigh the alternatives, but he or she can not make the ultimate decision for you.

Review and reevaluate periodically

Your career or academic decision and direction should be the best one possible *at this point in time.* As you gather new information and weigh future experiences, however, this direction can easily change. Some people feel that a decision should only be made when they are absolutely certain they are making the right choice — once they make a decision, it is irrevocable. No choice that requires any debate consists of two alternatives — one totally black, the other all white. There are plusses and minuses to each possibility, and therefore, *complete certainty is hardly ever feasible.* You must choose the alternative that will *probably* lead to the most desirable outcome. Once you make a decision, you are usually still free to change your mind. Don't feel that once you choose a major, a program of study or training or a career, you are no longer free to change that decision. Especially in this area of career choice, you can almost always explore new directions and make new choices as you learn more about yourself and about various careers.

Also, you should not feel that there is only one career field for you and that one endeavor alone will make your life happy and successful. For all of us, there are numerous areas with the potential to bring us satisfaction and accomplishment. Therefore, determining a career decision is not the end of your career development; there is always opportunity for fulfillment in career areas before unthought of as well as the ever-present opportunity for career change. But, don't waste time worrying about that now. Changing careers is fine — once you've actually been in a career for a while and then determined that you need a change.

Presently, it is estimated that Americans change careers up to five times during their lifetimes. If these changes are the result of a carefully thought-out and planned decision-making process similar to the one stressed here, then this is certainly healthy. There is considerable comfort in knowing that you have developed a plan for career direction. Just as important, however, by following a systematic process for making career decisions, you not only have developed a rational, logical direction, but you can look back and be assured that you have sound reasons for this direction.

In quick review, the decision-making or problem-solving steps are

1. Formulate the problem or decision and set your goal.
2. Commit yourself — your time, energy, and resources.
3. Gather information and explore alternatives.
4. Evaluate each alternative.
5. Decide tentatively.
6. Review and reevaluate periodically.

Choosing a major

Before concluding this section on career decision-making there are a few other points you should keep in mind. Although every student is different in terms of exactly when he or she makes specific decisions and takes specific steps, and although every college has different requirements about when one must declare a major, the following guidelines regarding "typical" academic and career development at four-year colleges are suggestions for you to consider in your own progression.

Freshman year

In most cases, you are just starting to formulate your ideas on choosing a major and on career direction. This is to be expected, and you should not be concerned about not having made clear, definite plans regarding your future. By involving yourself in different courses and experiences during your freshman year as well as exploring your ideas with advisors, career planning and placement counselors, and other students, you will gain information and assistance in establishing a direction. Generally, your freshman year should include a diversity of courses , as well as experiences that will allow you to identify and further develop your interests, abilities, and goals.

Sophomore year

Typically, during the sophomore year, one declares his or her academic major or area of concentration. Although this decision does *not* determine your career, it is an important factor to consider when thinking about a career direction. Prior to making this decision, we recommend that you do a thorough job of gathering and evaluating information. Talk with your faculty advisor and other people on and off campus and continue to explore ideas and options. Valuable information can also be gathered by exploring off-campus activities, involving yourself in extracurricular activities, and taking courses from many diverse areas.

Junior year

By this point in your academic and career development, you should at least begin thinking about how your courses and experiences in college are contributing toward your plans beyond graduation. Is further education desirable or necessary to attain your goal? Begin now to identify the types of organizations toward which you are heading and become familiar with what you must do to apply for further education and/or employment (i.e., Graduate Record Examinations, Law School Admissions Tests, credentials files, letters of recommendation). Talk with your faculty advisor and counselors in your career planning and placement office.

Senior year

Planning for your future becomes critical as you enter your final undergraduate year. Much of this planning will involve making final decisions as to graduate school or career options and getting involved in the process that will help you make that transition. Discussion with your advisor and an early visit to your career planning and placement center will help you identify, contact, and apply to appropriate graduate or professional schools and/or employers. Be certain to set up your placement credentials file early in the fall of your senior year. Find out about interview procedures on your campus. Inquire about and attend seminars on interview preparation, résumé writing, letter writing, and other subjects, sponsored by your career planning and placement office.

Two-year colleges

Quite obviously, the previous guidelines are aimed at four-year college students and are not directly applicable to the two-year college student. However, although the time frame is severely contracted, the basic ideas and activities are relevant and adaptable. One of the primary differences is that in the two-year college, you will probably not be able to delay the decision concerning which curriculum to enter until your second year. It is, thus, even more important for you to become acquainted with and talk to advisors and counselors and to gain relevant curriculum and career information as quickly as possible.

Some final thoughts on decision making

Since every decision that you make involves compromise, the selection of one particular option or course of action, and the elimination of other courses of action, be certain that a decision is actually called for before you make it. Maintain all your options as long as possible and then, only when a final decision is inevitable, choose one option. An example may be helpful here. Bob has taken a number of employment interviews. He believes that two interviews went particularly well and that he will be offered employment by both organizations. One firm is based in Los Angeles, the other in Bangor, Maine. Bob decides that he will accept an offer from the Los Angeles organization. He, therefore, decides that he will no longer need his fur-lined winter clothes and gives them away. As you can probably guess, what actually happens is that Bob does receive two offers. One from the organization in Bangor, Maine, and the other from an organization in Nome, Alaska. He has made a premature decision and is now caught with his fur-lined pants gone. The moral of this story, and the point that we are trying to make, is *never make a decision until you have to*.

Also, in some cases, a decision is not really a deciding *between* two alternatives; in others it may not be necessary to make a decision until a later date. For example: You may combine departments in a major, formulate your own program of study, set career objectives that include more than one career field, apply to more than one type of school and see which one materializes, or not select a college major until the following semester after you have had the opportunity for additional exploration.

Students often try to make decisions before there are actually alternatives from which to choose. For example, you might attempt to decide between law school or graduate business school before there are "real" acceptances from one or both. A possible

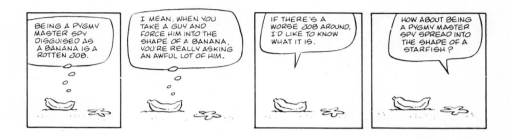

solution might include applying to both professional schools and waiting to see which one accepts you. A better solution might be to examine each type of professional study, including career directions, thoroughly and determine which is most suitable for you. This example applies to any decision where you have the advantage of declining one offer in favor of another, once all choices become evident. In selecting courses, faculty advisors, what activity to join, or who to go out with on Friday, however, this approach is probably not so workable! When a decision can wait, wait! We've talked to too many students who were sorry they limited themselves and their futures because they made a choice when they really didn't have to.

Career development model — Chapter 6

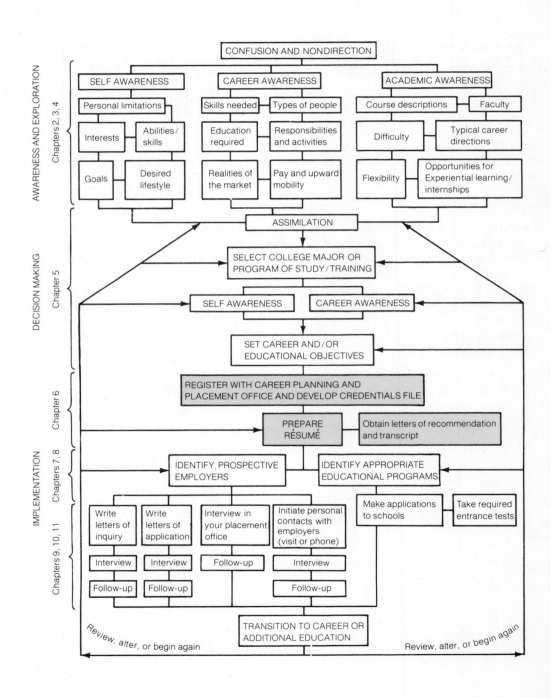

CONFUSION AND NONDIRECTION

AWARENESS AND EXPLORATION — Chapters 2, 3, 4

SELF AWARENESS
- Personal limitations
- Interests
- Abilities/skills
- Goals
- Desired lifestyle

CAREER AWARENESS
- Skills needed
- Types of people
- Education required
- Responsibilities and activities
- Realities of the market
- Pay and upward mobility

ACADEMIC AWARENESS
- Course descriptions
- Faculty
- Difficulty
- Typical career directions
- Flexibility
- Opportunities for Experiential learning/internships

ASSIMILATION

DECISION MAKING — Chapter 5

SELECT COLLEGE MAJOR OR PROGRAM OF STUDY/TRAINING

SELF AWARENESS   CAREER AWARENESS

SET CAREER AND/OR EDUCATIONAL OBJECTIVES

Chapter 6

REGISTER WITH CAREER PLANNING AND PLACEMENT OFFICE AND DEVELOP CREDENTIALS FILE

PREPARE RÉSUMÉ   Obtain letters of recommendation and transcript

IMPLEMENTATION — Chapters 7, 8

IDENTIFY PROSPECTIVE EMPLOYERS   IDENTIFY APPROPRIATE EDUCATIONAL PROGRAMS

Chapters 9, 10, 11

- Write letters of inquiry → Interview → Follow-up
- Write letters of application → Interview → Follow-up
- Interview in your placement office → Follow-up
- Initiate personal contacts with employers (visit or phone) → Interview → Follow-up
- Make applications to schools
- Take required entrance tests

TRANSITION TO CAREER OR ADDITIONAL EDUCATION

Review, alter, or begin again   Review, alter, or begin again

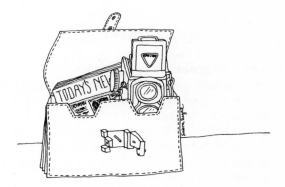

6   Developing a credentials file

Now that you have tentatively set your career and/or educational objectives, you are ready for the next major step in the career development process — developing a credentials file and registering with your office of career planning and placement.

Since the registration procedures and policies vary widely among career planning and placement offices, you should check with the office on your campus for specific instructions. Also, employers vary as to what specific types of credentials they wish applicants to submit.

Typically, however, a credentials file includes a résumé, any relevant academic transcripts, and letters of recommendation or references from previous employers and/or professors. Once you have set a career objective (general or specific) and have identified employers in organizations that are consistent with that objective, contact them by letter and résumé or by telephone. If the employers are interested in you, chances are they will want to view a set of your credentials prior to interviewing you. Because a credentials file can be updated throughout your career planning and because the process described above remains fairly consistent no matter what kind of employment you're applying for, a credentials file can be useful throughout your life.

Résumés

The most critical item in your credentials file is your résumé. It is a summary of your personal data; your educational background, training, and skills; your employment

199

experience; and your career objectives. Often, we confuse a résumé with a data sheet. They are not, however, the same thing. A data sheet is a standardized form used by many placement offices and by some employers in which you simply fill in the blanks. A résumé, while containing much of the same information, provides you with greater flexibility and can be personalized and elaborated to emphasize your own skills, abilities, interests, and experiences. One quick word on the content of a résumé regarding these skills, interests, and experiences. We have found that when many students sit down and rough out a résumé, they say they have great difficulty because "they haven't done anything that an employer would want to read." Chances are they're wrong. As we stated in our discussion of skill identification and demonstration (see Chapter 5), employers are interested in anything and everything in which you were involved during your college years that required some responsibility, creativity, organization, planning, communications, super-vision — the list is endless. And, equally as endless is the list of courses, extracurricular activities, volunteer experiences, athletics, independent studies, internships, and part-time or summer jobs in which the above list of résumé-worthy items are found. Make a list with the help of a career counselor, and we guarantee it will be longer than you think.

Your résumé is critical because it is your calling card or door opener. It represents you when you cannot be there in person. Although it cannot get you a job, a good résumé will elicit enough interest on the part of a prospective employer that she or he will wish to talk with you further. A poor résumé, on the other hand, will almost certainly eliminate you from further consideration.

Because people vary widely, résumé styles and formats vary widely. Yours should reflect you and you alone. There are some general considerations, however, that you may wish to keep in mind in preparing your résumé.

A résumé should be comprehensive, yet concise. That is, it should include all *relevant* information about you, yet not be wordy or a showplace for your prose style. Headings and dates should be highlighted or set to one side so that the reader can easily locate those items of special interest to him or her. Although there is no magic formula as to length, résumés are typically one to two pages. Remember that personnel people read hundreds of résumés each day. They don't want to wade through extraneous verbiage to find what they are looking for.

Sample résumés are included at the end of this section. They are only *samples* of styles and formats. Your office of career planning and placement probably has many more. If you decide to use one of these samples as a guide, be certain that it accurately reflects *you*.

Whatever style and format you select, it is a good idea to begin with a rough draft — a data sheet can be useful as a guide. Once the rough draft is completed, or if you have any questions, feel free to consult your career planning counselor for assistance in writing the finished résumé.

When you are ready to begin your final draft, ask yourself these questions:

1. How does my résumé look through the eyes of the employer?
2. Is there sufficient "white space" so that it doesn't look crowded on the page?
3. Have I adequately and accurately demonstrated and communicated my abilities, interests, and skills?
4. Is my résumé free of irrelevant material?
5. If I include a career objective, is it clear and accurate?
6. Are my spelling and grammar correct?
7. If I were an employer, would I be able to say, "This document stimulates my interest in discussing employment possibilities with this candidate"?

If the answer to any of these questions is no, then you need to make some changes. As the quality of your résumé is reflective of your quality, we feel that the role of the résumé cannot be emphasized enough.

The following section includes numerous samples of résumé formats — use the one that you feel most comfortable with and that best outlines your academic and work experiences. We would suggest that you write a rough draft of your résumé and take it to a career counselor for his or her suggestions, critique, and help in determining the final form of your résumé.

Sample résumés

LESLIE A. SMITH

<u>Permanent Address</u>   <u>Present Address</u>
3504 Larchwood Drive   3217 14th Avenue S. E.
Minnetonka, Minnesota 55343   Cedar Rapids, Iowa 52403

Born May 5, 1954   Single   Excellent Health

career
objective — To work in a position of responsibility within the general field of business or management. Desire especially to use and develop communication skills acquired through college education and experiences.

education — Coe College, B.A.   English   1975

1971
to 1975 — Will receive B.A. degree in English in June 1975, with strong supporting course areas in business administration and psychology. Extracurricular activities have included volunteer tutoring of elementary school children, secretary of Alpha Omicron Pi Sorority, and representative two years in the Student Senate.

Served as dormitory resident assistant during senior year with responsibilities for conducting floor meetings and advising students.

Planned and researched Cedar Rapids community services regarding their financial planning for senior seminar in Psychology.

(Emphasize the positive aspects of your academics and extracurricular activities. Describe honors, responsibilities, involvements, and practical applications of courses such as independent studies, special projects. and presentations.)

career-
related
experiences
1974
to 1975

Responsible for planning, organizing, and implementing sorority rush program resulting in largest pledge class in past five years. Activities included communicating with freshmen, contacting alumni, planning social events, and supervising the evaluation of candidates.

Conducted research project on the use of psychology in marketing household items for Marketing II course and presented study to class.

Spring
1974

Internship for three months in City of Dubuque Bureau of Parks and Recreation. Involvements included writing programs for parks' summer leaders, participating in all staff meetings, and doing odd jobs for the director.

January
1974

One month internship in Community Theatre with responsibilities for scenery, props, and staging organization.

summers
1972
to 1974

Worked in Woolworth Department Store, Minnetonka, Minnesota. Various jobs included: check out, stocking shelves, and eventually assisting in purchase of products.

(Describe work experiences in reverse chronology. Stress tasks related to the position you are currently seeking. Eliminate minor details and emphasize major responsibilities. Indicate progressive increases in responsibility where they have occurred. Include civic projects, volunteer work, practical courses, extracurricular activities, summer experiences, etc.)

skills
and
interests

Interest and ability in writing. Have written numerous articles for the college newspaper and literary magazine. Was assistant editor of yearbook during senior year and wrote introduction for each section. Have submitted an article to *The Student Journal* — "Student Rights on a 'Controlled' Campus" and am awaiting evaluation.

(This section simply continues to fill out your character. It is basically personal as opposed to professional. Something in it might strike a note of interest with a prospective employer. Skills and interests that are especially career oriented might be mentioned. This section is optional.)

references References furnished upon request by Career Counseling and Placement, Coe College, Cedar Rapids, Iowa 52402.

FRANKLIN L. BROWN

Permanent Address   Present Address
1521 Main Street   1810 Jefferson Street
Alexandria, Virginia 20308   Charlottesville, Virginia 22903
Telephone: (703) 445-2024   Telephone: (804) 962-4503

Born December 4, 1952   Single   Excellent Health

job
objective To obtain a position in the field of banking with the eventual goal of obtaining a management position in international finance.

(Describe succinctly the type of job that you want. If you are interested in a broad occupational field, state it as clearly and concisely as you can. Suggest strong alternative or related interests if you have them.)

education UNIVERSITY OF VIRGINIA, B.A.   History   1973

1969
to
1973 Candidate for the degree of Bachelor of Arts, with honors, in history, June 1973. Concentrating in Far Eastern history with emphasis on modern China and supporting field in economics. Dean's List. Have been active in the Jefferson Society, the Marketing Society, ABC Fraternity (President and Rush Chairman), and intramural athletics.

(Emphasize the positive aspects of your academic career and extracurricular activities. Describe any academic honors or financial awards you have received as well as any positions or leadership you have assumed.)

work
experience
summer
1972 Worked as a Financial Assistant for First National Bank Securities in Richmond, Virginia. Primary duties involved working with a securities analyst on overseas investments.

summers 1969 & 1970
Worked as a lifeguard for the Department of Parks and Recreation in Virginia Beach, Virginia. Served as a beach guard in 1969 and was promoted to beach captain in 1970. In latter position was responsible for all guards for a five-mile stretch of beach.

(Describe work experiences in reverse chronology. Stress tasks related to the position you are currently seeking. Eliminate minor details and emphasize major responsibilities. Indicate progressive increases in responsibility where they have occurred. Include civic projects, volunteer work, etc. Be specific and avoid vague generalities. Do not overlook periods of self-employment and include all employment experiences, summer or otherwise, if relevant.)

early background
Born and raised in Alexandria, Virginia, as the younger of two children. Father works for the Internal Revenue Service. Attended local public schools for twelve years and graduated from high school in June 1969. Member of the national honor society and varsity football and baseball teams.

(There is quite a bit of discussion surrounding the advantages and disadvantages of this section. Some prefer to omit it, which is prefectly all right. Others have found that mentioning of hometown, father's occupation, or a significant early experience has actually paved the way for fruitful employment contact. Basically it is designed to fill out your character and present you as a person as opposed to a purely academic being.)

skills and interests
Command of written and spoken French. Traveled in Europe for one summer (1971) and have camped up and down the eastern seaboard. Enjoy travel, camping, folk music, and the outdoors.

(This section simply continues to fill out your character. Like the section above, it is basically personal as opposed to professional. Something in it might strike a note of interest with a prospective employer.)

references
References furnished upon request by the Office of Career Planning and Placement, 5 Minor Hall, University of Virginia, Charlottesville, Virginia 22903.

LINDA J. SMITHSON

1245 Z Avenue N.W.
Cedar Rapids, Iowa 52410
(319) 398-9988

personal	Married (5/74) 5′10″ 130 pounds 23 years old
career objective	Advertising officer with an international business firm, utilizing my foreign language background.
	Major concentration in French language and literature, with special interest in European art history. GPA: 3.5 out of possible 4.0.
	Spent 1973–1974 academic year in Paris, studying at the University of Paris (Sorbonne).
work experience Feb. 1975 to present	Receptionist/secretary, Maxwell and Hart, Attorneys at Law, Cedar Rapids, Iowa. Handled reception, telephones, and messages for this medium-sized firm of 15 attorneys, with a staff of 10. Responsibilities included light secretarial duties, set-up of new files, and updating of old files and legal resource materials.
Aug. 1974 to Dec. 1974	Assistant Manager, Open Drawer Office Supplies, Cedar Rapids, Iowa. Responsibilities included inventory and ordering of stock, daily accounting for company reports, and supervision of part-time employees. Most work was unsupervised, the store being my responsibility during most of my working hours.
April 1973 to Aug. 1974	PBX Operator, Cedar Rapids Public Library. Operated the telephone system for administrative offices and service centers. Duties also included staffing an information desk serving the library main entrance.
office skills	Typing (60 wpm), Dictaphone, IBM Selectric Composer, Bell PBX and Call-Director telephone systems.
background and activities	Born and raised in Northeastern United States. Have traveled extensively in the United States and Western Europe. Interests include classical music, European history and literature, and sewing. Served as a summer program counselor in college and acted as Business Manager for campus coffee house.
references	References will be furnished upon request.
	June 1975

FRANK J. BROWN

<u>Permanent Address</u>   <u>Present Address</u>

6745 3rd Ave. N.W.   Box 1233
Cedar Rapids, Iowa 52404   Coe College
Telephone: (319) 362-2916   Cedar Rapids, Iowa
                                                              Telephone: (319) 364-5750

Born: September 30, 1952   Single   Excellent Health

**job
objective**
To obtain a position of responsibility in a commercial broadcasting, advertising, or public relations company, with the opportunity to use skills gained through academic and work experiences as well as to learn more about the field of communications.

education
Coe College, B.A.   Speech   1975

**1971
to
1975**
Will receive B.A. degree in Speech in May 1975. Have taken a broad range of courses providing a wide and varied educational background. Have lettered four times on the basketball team and was captain my junior year. Spent the fall of senior year in Washington, D.C., working on an independent project with NBC news. Responsibilities included covering the Rockefeller confirmation hearings, the Watergate cover-up trial, and assistance in the preparation of an edition of the NBC evening news. Dean's List junior and senior year.

**work
experience
1972
1973
1974**
Worked for the City of Cedar Rapids as a lifeguard at the public pools. During the summer of 1974 was assistant manager of Ellis pool, responsible for the daily operation, maintenance, and bookkeeping. Also served as a neighborhood basketball team coach during these summers. Worked as a Red Cross volunteer during summer 1974 teaching Junior Life Saving swimming course at Ellis pool.

**year
round
work
1971
1975**
Have worked part time at two radio stations in Cedar Rapids. KCDR from May 1971 to October 1972. Currently employed at KIOA, working year round as a part-time disc jockey, responsible for weekend operation of KIOA, some programming at KIOA and KCDR, and news preparation at KCDR.

**early
background**
Born and raised in Cedar Rapids, the youngest of five children. Father is a local postman. I have worked part-time since the seventh grade. Attended

local public schools, member of Honor Society, holder of Eagle Scout Award, and was basketball captain junior and senior year. Played trumpet since fourth grade and sat second chair in the high school band.

references   References furnished upon request by Career Counseling and Placement, Coe College, Cedar Rapids, Iowa 52402.

CAROL ANN SMITH

Permanent Address   Present Address
345 Country Club Road   Box 50
Baldwin Hills, California   Coe College
Telephone: (805) 228-2132   Cedar Rapids, Iowa
                                             (319) 364-1133

Born: September 7, 1953   Single   Excellent Health

Career objective   To teach secondary school psychology and/or social studies in a public school system. Would also like to work with students through extracurricular activities.

Education   Coe College, B.A.   Psychology (social studies concentration)
            1975

1971 to 1975   Will receive B.A. degree in psychology May 1975, which will include certification to teach grades seven through twelve in psychology and all social studies. Extracurricular activities have included volunteer tutoring of elementary school children, Chi Omega Sorority, Alpha Lambda Delta Honorary Society, and assistant editor of the year book.

Served as an assistant to Professor Cole in the Psychology Department. Responsibilities included typing, grading tests, general secretary work, and library research.

Served as student recruiter during senior year with responsibilities for welcoming prospective students, showing them around the college, and introducing them to professors and facilities of interest.

Career-related experiences	
Fall 1974	Completed student teaching experience in psychology at Central High School, Cedar Rapids, Iowa.
Summer 1974	Worked as a salaried teacher's aide for the Title I program at the Lincoln Elementary School, Baldwin Hills, California. Responsibilities in this remedial reading program included individual tutoring, assisting with group work and field trips, and supervising educational games.
Spring 1973	Tutored with the Upward Bound Program of Cedar Rapids, Iowa, under the supervision of Coe College. Responsibilities involved encouraging and assisting a seventeen-year-old remedial reading student with course work at his high school.
January 1972	Educational Internship in English at Riverway High School, Baldwin Hills, California, with responsibilities for cataloguing and filing educational materials, assisting with introductory English composition classes, and the assigning and grading of compositions.
Spring 1970	Served as counselor for an educational outdoor camp. Responsibility for supervising all activities and classes of students assigned, as well as assisting with science and art classes.
Spring 1969	Served as an aide during an outing for handicapped and mentally retarded youth.
Summer 1968	Worked as a volunteer swimming instructor for preschool through junior-high-school-age children at Baldwin Hills YMCA.
Other experiences	
Summer 1973	Worked for Mountain View Nursing Home, Montgomery, California, in a capacity of cook's helper.
Fall 1972 to Spring 1973	Worked as cook's helper for Crown Food Service, Inc., Cedar Rapids, Iowa.

Summer 1970	Participated in the Experiment in International Living in the Netherlands.
Summer 1969	Toured the USSR with a language-culture study group.
Skills and interests	Interest and ability concerning the publication of a yearbook, having served for two years as assistant editor of the yearbook. Other interests include painting, arts and crafts, camping, swimming, boating, needlework, cooking, reading, and traveling.
References	References furnished upon request by Career Counseling and Placement, Coe College, Cedar Rapids, Iowa 52402.

JAMES L. KERN

<u>Permanent Address</u>   <u>Present Address</u>
2 Crescent Street   Box 536
Chester, Pennsylvania   Coe College
                                  Cedar Rapids, Iowa

Born: June 5, 1955   Single   Good Health

Employment experience Summer 1974	*Etcher* for Midwest Nameplate Company. Involved in the etching of varying gauges of stainless steel, aluminum, and titanium plates. Became familiar with the entire name plate manufacturing process.
1973 to 1974	*Department Assistant for Language Laboratory,* Coe College, Cedar Rapids, Iowa. Worked in total operation, maintenance, and transportation of equipment; can diagnose malfunctions and make general repairs.
February 1973 to July 1973	*X-ray Librarian for Radiology Department,* City Hospital, Chester, Pa. Involved in operation of various stations of X-ray department, particularly the emergency room and central records. Responsibilities included locating, filing, charging, and transportation of X-rays and doctors' diagnoses of X-rays. Also involved in the verification of patients' identification numbers and sometimes functioned as a middleman between radiologists and doctors.

June 1970 to June 1971	*Janitorial Aide* for Chester County Public School System. Duties included general janitorial maintenance as well as providing laundry service for physical education classes.
Education	High School diploma from Chester High School, Chester, Pa. Listed in *Who's Who among American High School Students;* Vice President of Red Cross Club; PSAT letter of commendation; concert and marching band member; member of chess club, Latin club, French cooking club.

Coe College, 2 years. Courses include general liberal arts as well as a strong concentration in physical and social sciences (including basic psychology, biology, physics, chemistry, algebra, atomic theory, and plane and solid geometry). Have been involved in some simple radiation experiments using Coe's linear accelerator, beryllium-radium source, and other facilities. Also, have taken some communication-oriented classes. Member of International club; participated in Open Door Public Service, and assisted at the college radio station (KCOE).

Other skills and interests	Drafting and cabinet making: 3 years in junior and senior high schools. Familiar with hand and power tools, especially drill press, belt sander, band saw, and grinder (can also operate edge and surface planer, jig saw, and lathe).

Library Assistant in junior and senior high schools; familiar with use of card catalogs and Dewey decimal system.

Newscaster for KCOE radio station. Have basic understanding of all radio station equipment, including promotional room and master control panel.

Basic working knowledge of stereo and audio components, particularly in the areas of evaluation and matching cartridges, turntables, amplifiers, and speakers.

General knowledge of automobile construction and design, with some understanding of mechanics.

References	References furnished upon request by Career Counseling and Placement, Coe College, Cedar Rapids, Iowa 52402.

Robert P. Jones
88 Jefferson Park
Richmond, Virginia
(804) 783-9951

PERSONAL INFORMATION
Age: 28   Marital status: Married
Height: 5′ 10″   Military status: Veteran
Weight: 160 lbs.   Interests: Photography, reading, softball
Health: Excellent

OCCUPATIONAL GOAL: To obtain employment as a Service Manager in an automotive
repair business.

EDUCATION
High School: Jefferson High School, Richmond, Va.   Graduation: June, 1966
Courses of special interest: Automotive Shop, Math
Activities: Softball, Photography Club

College: Rockmont Community College, Cohens, Va.   Graduation: June, 1976
Degree: Associate in Applied Science
Major: Automotive Technology
Major Courses: Automotive Engines, Fuel Systems, Lubrication and Cooling Systems
Activities: Veterans Club

EXPERIENCE

Dates	Employer	Position
1972–Present (part-time)	Rockmont Community College	Automotive Lab Assistant
1968–1972	U.S. Army Ft. Dix, N.J.	Motor Pool
1966–1968	Casey Motor Co. Richmond, Va.	Mechanic Supervisor
1964–1966 (summers)	Jimmy's Garage Richmond, Va.	Clerk: Parts Dept.

References will be furnished upon request by:

Career Planning and Placement Office
Rockmont Community College
Cohens, Va.

John A. Doe*
Box 4322
Coe College
Cedar Rapids, Iowa 52402
Phone : (614) 587-2222

Home Address:
4322 Lewiston Road
Niagara Falls, N.Y. 14305
Phone: (715) 284-4560

OBJECTIVE: Management training program with eventual work in international banking.

SUMMARY OF CAPABILITIES:
Group Leader: Chm. Social Activities Council — coordinated all social groups on campus . . . Leader, Life Planning Workshops — led intensive five-hour sessions to help students establish long-range goals. Sr. Year, High School: Chm. Social and Finance Committee — raised $28,000 for school and charity . . . Honor Society President — instituted tutoring system and Talk Show on TV . . . VP, Forensic Society — annual three day debate tournament . . . Capt. Tennis . . . VP Explorer Post — Chm. light bulb sale and Capt. Basketball Team.

Communicator/Adviser: Student Academic Adviser — advised 12 pre-med students with professor in all phases of education . . . Corresponding Secretary for social fraternity — maintained all correspondence between the national, alumnae, and local — published year-end report . . . Senator, Student Government . . . Economics Dept. liaison — represented student views at faculty meetings — worked on development of new Economics major.

Administrator/Organizer: Executive Council for student government — restructured social budget and philosophy . . . Exec. Council fraternity — instrumental in setting House budget priorities . . . salesman for chandeliers, intercoms, industrial lighting — in addition to selling prepared orders for approval by VP . . . carpenter/craftsman — built and organized storage area for plumbing, electrical, construction supply . . . gas station attendant . . . Career Advisory Committee — reviewed career aids with selected faculty and students . . . House Council for dorm — established code of behavior — led hearings on misconduct.

*This résumé courtesy of David A. Gibbons, Associate Dean of Students, Denison University, Granville, Ohio.

EDUCATION: B.A. Economics, Coe College (1976) . . . minor History . . . Introductory Accounting . . . semester study at Oxford, focused on British economic problems . . . Senior Research, Inefficiencies in the British Labor Market.

AWARDS: Frank Gannett Newspaperboy Scholarship . . . Jaycees Niagara County Outstanding Teenage Youngman Award . . . Denison — Economics Honorary, Omicron Delta Epsilon.

PERSONAL: Age, 21 . . . Marital Status, single . . . Health, excellent.

SUMMARY OF EMPLOYMENT: *Summer '75* — Salesman for Industrial Supply Company, tutored high school algebra, jazz piano at local club, tennis instructor . . . *Summer '73 & Summer '74* — Carpenter/craftsman for same supply company, landscape work . . . *Summer '72* — gas station attendant, landscape work . . . *Coe '72, '74, & '76* — Saga Food Service as cook, waiter, dishwasher.

REFERENCES: Furnished upon request by the Center of Academic and Career Planning, Coe College, Cedar Rapids, Iowa 52402.

Jane F. Roe*
Box 492
Coe College
Cedar Rapids, Iowa 52402
(614) 587-2222
[Until 29 May 1976]

4321 Woodhill Drive
Gibsonia, Pa. 15044
(412) 123-4567

OBJECTIVES: A management position in Business or Industry that will allow me to combine my leadership and communication skills with my administrative abilities.

EDUCATION: B.A. expected, 29 May 1976, Coe College; Double Major-Psychology and Sociology; includes such courses as Industrial Psychology, International Relations, Computer Science, and Economics.

Additional Educational Experiences: Head Resident Training, Crisis Intervention Training, and Summer Travel in Europe.

*This résumé courtesy of David A. Gibbons, Associate Dean of Students, Denison University, Granville, Ohio.

SUMMARY OF CAPABILITIES:

INTERPERSONAL COMMUNICATOR
Head Resident (1975–1976): Selected as Head Resident, responsible for entire operation of one Residence Hall; facilitated communication between residents and dormitory staff, represented opinions of residents to University Administration, counseled personal and academic problems.

Lived, worked, and counseled with persons of other races and cultures; learned mutual understanding and practiced joint reponsibilities.

Crisis Intervention Center Volunteer (1974–1975): counseled callers and walk-ins regarding personal problems and crises; served as a referral source for community services, provided information regarding drug use and abuse.

Campus Tour Guide (1972–1976): showed prospective students the campus, answered questions and interpreted policies; communicated personal experience, interest, and enthusiasm.

GROUP LEADER
Head Resident: in addition to above, managed dormitory activities, responsible for reporting maintenance problems, planned and conducted dorm meetings; served as chairperson of House Council, carrying judicial and administrative responsibility.

Officer of National Sorority (1972–1975): Panhellenic Representative, represented opinions of house to representatives from other houses, aided in coordinating inter-sorority activities; Rituals Chairman (1975); planned and organized all ceremonial events; served on House Executive Board (1972–1975) and responsible for planning, scheduling, and executing all house events.

Elected Member of House Council (1972–1973, 1974–1976): determined violations and imposed disciplinary action on offenders; planned and scheduled Residence Hall activities, allocated activity funds.

Girl Scouts (1962–1972): Patrol leader and Junior Adviser for 5 years.
Elected President (1972).

4-H (1965–1971); Elected President, Vice-President, and Junior Leader.

ADMINISTRATOR
Departmental Assistant —Psychology Department (1973–1975): graded tests, tabulated

research results for professors, assisted with research, developed bibliographic resources, established occupational file, assisted with secretarial duties.

Teaching Assistant —Psychology Department (1975–1976): chosen to work closely with
one professor, assisted in constructing, monitoring, and grading tests, developed and
carried out class projects.

Manager Swimming Club Concession Stand (Summers of 1973 & 1974): ordered
supplies, scheduled and supervised three workers, worked 40–50 hours per week.

Head Resident as mentioned above, responsible for the total administration of one
Residence Hall.

PERSONAL DATA:
Born 9 April 1954
Health—Excellent
Marital Status—Single

Willing to work anywhere in the United States or Europe.

REFERENCES: Will be furnished upon request by the Center for Academic and Career
Planning, Coe College, Cedar Rapids, Iowa 52402.

JAMES E. DOE*
1000 University Avenue
Des Moines, Iowa 50310
Phone: (515) 235-2270

OBJECTIVE: A management position in the retailing field utilizing skills acquired through
my education and experience. I am willing to relocate and can travel dependent upon the
initial assignment.

QUALIFIED BY: Retailing experience in the Des Moines Area Community College Marketing curriculum. This experience includes applied on-the-job training in inventory control,
stock work, personal salesmanship, department management, scheduling of

*Special appreciation to Mr. Tom Dart, Director of Placement Services at Des Moines Area Community College, for
the use of this sample résumé.

employees, and conducting special in-store events. Through a program of inservice in suggestive selling among my departmental employees, gross sales increased 16% in the past fiscal year. Through market surveys which I initiated, merchandise was ordered which met with enthusiastic response from my clientele. Interior table-top displays, which I designed, prompted increased impulse purchases. Leadership skills were learned at the student leadership conference which I attended in the fall of 1973.

EDUCATIONAL QUALIFICATIONS:
Des Moines Area Community College   AAS Degree — May, 1975
Ankeny, Iowa   GPA — 3.12
Major: Retail Marketing

West High School   Diploma — May, 1973
Des Moines, Iowa
Core Area: Distributive Education

EMPLOYMENT EXPERIENCE:
X. Y. Zebra Stores   Department Manager
Des Moines, Iowa   June, 1974–May, 1975

PROFESSIONAL ORGANIZATIONS/INTERESTS:
Representative: College Student Senate, 1974
Treasurer: Alpha Mu Sigma, Marketing Fraternity
College Dean's List — 3 quarters — 1974–75

PERSONAL DATA:
Height: 5′11″ — Weight: 187 lbs. — Born: February 27, 1955 No dependants

REFERENCES:
Available through the College Placement Office of Des Moines Area Community College, 2006 Ankeny Blvd., Ankeny, Iowa 50021.
Phone: (515) 964-6215.

Career objectives as part of the effective résumé

As part of most résumés, the stating of a career objective is usually one of the most difficult areas (especially for liberal arts graduates) to define. In most cases, some conversation with a counselor or hard thinking and exploring on your part will enable you to set a general career objective. Usually this objective will focus more on the kinds of things you want to do and less on the particular job or setting in which they can be done. A viable alternative is simply to omit the "Career Objective" part of the résumé or when you have narrowed it down to a couple of choices, develop two résumés with different career objectives. If you know the field or position in which you want to work, simply stating the field is also acceptable. For example: To obtain a position in journalism. Or: To work for an advertising or marketing agency.

The following are sample career or job objectives. Use them as guidelines from which to create your own; do not use them verbatim for your own résumé. (They aren't that good, and you can easily develop a better one for yourself!)

General business

To obtain a position of responsibility and challenge within the field of business or management.
To utilize skills and experiences within a challenging managerial position.
To enter a management, marketing, or sales training program with the eventual goal of individual responsibility within a business function.
To work in production management following a period of formal and on-the-job training.
To work in a position of responsibility in a general business or management capacity.
To work in a bank, training in all areas of operation initially with eventual responsibility in management.

Education

To teach on the elementary school level as well as to be involved in the total educational program of a school.
To teach secondary school mathematics in a public school system. Desire also to coach athletics and take responsibility for extracurricular activities.
To take responsibility for curriculum planning, course instruction, and total student development within a program of junior high school language arts. Desire also to work with students through tutoring and individual work as well as extracurricular activities.

Social and community service

To work in a social welfare agency. Desire to be involved in and committed to helping disadvantaged individuals through development of personal skills as well as program objectives.
To work in community or social service with the eventual goal of program planning, implementation, and leadership.

To attain meaningful employment by a community services agency or educational institution utilizing a background in psychology and an intuitive understanding of children.

Sciences

To work in the area of general research, utilizing practical learning gained through classroom, laboratory, and work-setting experiences.

To work in the general area of conservation, ecology, and the environment. Desire to be involved in problem solving, program planning, and resource management within a government or state agency.

Publishing and communications

To use skills gained through academic and work experiences within the general field of communications.

To work in advertising, marketing, or public relations involving communication of product, service, or issue to the general public.

To achieve a position in a publishing organization. Desire to learn publications business "from the bottom up" utilizing and developing my written communication skills.

Letters of recommendation

What about references or statements of recommendation? Are these out of your hands? Not completely. You select the individuals whom you would like to recommend you. Choose them carefully. Don't be afraid to ask them if they feel that they can write an accurate and positive recommendation for you. One tip that you may find helpful is to supply all potential recommenders with a copy of your résumé. This may stimulate their interest in you, and it will tell them what type(s) of position(s) you are seeking so that they can respond in terms of the qualifications required.

No matter what course you take, be sure that you do not simply leave a recommendation form in someone's mailbox. Talk.with them, if at all possible, or at least write them a letter or note. When dealing with letters of recommendation that are confidential, be sure you feel certain that your recommender will write a positive reference. Some professors we know believe they must say a few negative things about you in order to give the letter validity. Our own opinion is that this can screen you out of some jobs. Again, communicate with your recommenders so that you have a good idea what they are going to write.

The question sometimes arises as to whether or not a letter of recommendation from an individual in "a high place" is of value to you. Our answer is yes, indeed — if, and only if, you have performed or accomplished things under him or her so that he or she can make meaningful statements about your work. As with all your recommenders, you want to be sure that they can write specific things about your work habits, scholarship, personal qualities, and potential. Vague letters that say nothing more than that you have a "pleasant appearance" and are a "good worker" don't carry much weight with an employer. That is why it's always best to seek out employers, professors, or people who know you and your work abilities to write your recommendations. This doesn't usually include members of the clergy, family friends, or personal acquaintances.

As a final point of discussion concerning letters of recommendation, you should be aware of a recent law — Public Law 93-380 (commonly called the Buckley Amendment) — now passed, which gives you the right to see your letters of recommendation written after January 1, 1975. In other words, when you set up a credentials file, the letters of recommendation you receive from an employer or professor are now open to your inspection. Accordingly, you can decide whether or not you wish to have a certain letter sent as part of your credentials file. Despite this recent ruling, you may want to consider the following points:

1. Some employers (especially those who hire people in education) put more credence in letters of recommendation if they are kept confidential from the student. Therefore, under Public Law 93-380, you can waive your right to see your reference. Thus, you still can maintain a confidential credentials file if you want. We don't believe that an honest and open recommender should be influenced in his or her writing based on whether or not you can see the letter, but since all recommenders are not honest and open, and some employers insist that a letter has no meaning if you have seen it, you may want to consider staying with a confidential file. Talk it over with your career planning and placement director before making this decision.

2. Very few employers today (other than those in education) even bother to read letters of recommendation as part of your job application. Therefore, if you aren't a prospective teacher, you may want to consider not having any letters of recommendation. Many career planning and placement offices have already gone this route in eliminating them for non-education students.

However, you never can tell when you will encounter an employer who wants references or a situation sometime when letters of recommendation are necessary (for example, going back to graduate school, being considered for a scholarship, etc.). They are good to have when you need them.

3. If you are a prospective teacher, whether you opt for an open file (only open to you and employers — no one else) or for a confidential one, the letter of recommendation from the teacher for whom you're practice teaching is one of the keys to your file as well as to getting a teaching position. Because of this importance, it is especially necessary to have good communications with your supervising teacher before the letter of recommendation is written as well as throughout your practice teaching experience.

As you can see, developing and knowing your paper credentials are as important as knowing yourself. They are a critical part of attaining an employment interview. Never take them for granted, as their successful development is one of the steps necessary to attain your career objective.

Transcripts

Obviously, an academic transcript is a "given" in that it already exists and there is little you can do now to change it. However, you can affect how a prospective employer will evaluate it.

Take a careful look at your transcript and make certain that it is complete and accurate. Are there significant trends in it that should be brought to the employer's attention? Are there reasons and explanations, *not excuses,* for low grades?

If you have some low grades or an average (or slightly below average grade point average), don't be alarmed or defensive. Every bit of existing research states emphatically that there is *no* correlation between high grades and success on the job. Accordingly, any employer worth his salt should know this and *should* be placing more emphasis on your part-time experiences, your communication skills, and the abilities and interests that are expressed through your other involvements.

Have you changed majors? Did your previous major(s) hurt you academically? Did you get most of your low grades during your first year or two of college? This is pretty typical for most students and largely due to getting adjusted to college life as well as taking diverse required courses. Are your better grades in your major field or interest and, likewise, your lower grades in areas in which you're not so interested? This is also usual, relates very closely to motivation. It might be a point of discussion for you to bring out with an employer or a graduate or professional school representative.

Remember, however, a prospective employer will probably only have a chance to glance at your overall grade point average. It is up to you to make him or her aware of what lies behind it and what that GPA means for you.

In some cases, a transcript does not accurately reflect your academic accomplishments (for some reason or another) and, in all cases, a transcript is difficult for anyone to read. In these regards, you may want to consider course listing forms, like those illustrated here for listing your courses as part of the credentials file.

The Center for Academic & Career Planning
Coe College
Cedar Rapids, Iowa 52402

Course Listing

Freshman	Sophomore
Junior	**Senior**

Blank course listing form

The Center for Academic & Career Planning
Coe College
Cedar Rapids, Iowa 52402

Name _____   College major _____

_____   _____

Career objective _____   Supporting areas _____
                                        (College minors)

_____   _____

Listing of courses and course experiences
pertinent to career objective

Freshman	Sophomore
Courses: Independent studies, class projects, internships, etc.	Courses: Independent studies, class projects, internships, etc.
Junior Courses: Independent studies, class projects, internships, etc.	Senior Courses: Independent studies, class projects, internships, etc.

Completed course listing form

Career development model — Chapter 7

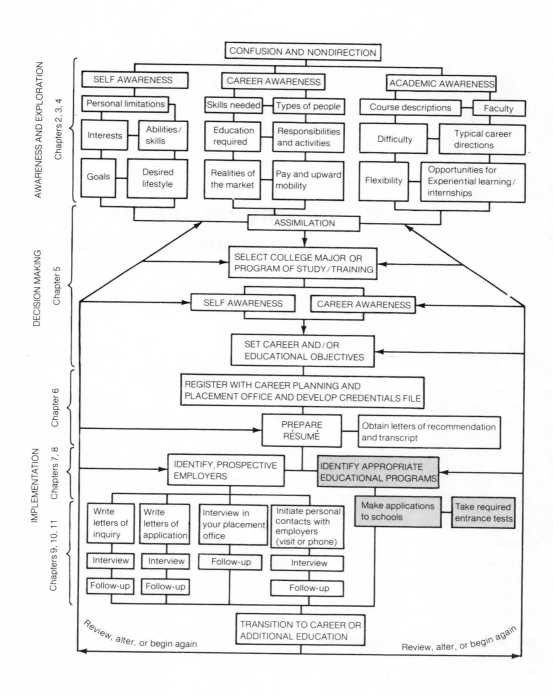

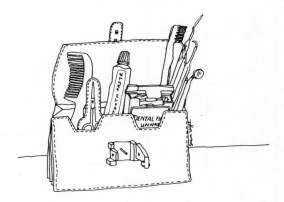

7 Identifying appropriate educational programs

Once you have decided on a career or career direction, the next step is to determine whether or not further formal education is required for you to enter and progress in the field. Keep in mind that the decision to pursue further formal education should be an active, positive decision. That is, you should know why you wish to continue your education. We believe that it is a mistake, and an expensive one at that, to continue one's education for reasons like: "All my friends are," or "I can't think of anything else to do . . . maybe I'll find the answer after a few more years in school." If these look like your reasons, you may wish to work through the previous chapters of this book again and also talk with a counselor in your career planning and placement center. He or she can help you get a better focus on your career and life goals.

Resources

If you determine that additional education is necessary, there are several excellent resources to help you identify the programs that are best suited to your skills and abilities, as well as your area of interest. Your college or university library and/or career planning and placement office will probably have most of these resources.

Two-year community college students
College catalogs Look especially for the particular institution's policies regarding transfer students. What are the preadmission requirements? What courses and credits are

transferable from your previous schooling? What will be your academic status (sophomore, junior, etc.)? How many credits, semesters, or quarter hours will you need for your baccalaureate degree? Talk with a counselor at your own school to find out what has happened to other students from your school who have applied to and attended a particular college.

College guide books These include *Lovejoy's, Baron's,* the *College Blue Book,* Cass and Birnbaum's *Comparative Guide to American Colleges.* These guides give an overview of all accredited four-year colleges, focusing on admissions requirements, enrollment figures, faculty qualifications, costs, special programs, academic opportunities, and the student body.

Lovejoy's Career and Vocational School Guide This excellent resource identifies career programs in all technical and skilled fields and describes their appropriate preparation or training. Schools are listed according to the training they provide. The career fields to which the training leads are described in detail — including listings of employers.

Four-year college students

Graduate and professional school catalogs This is probably the first resource that occurred to you, as it does to most people — it is a good one. However, there are a few problems. First of all, a graduate or professional school catalog is designed to attract potential students to that particular institution. Therefore, its approach may be somewhat biased in favor of that institution and its programs. Secondly, unless you are certain which institutions offer the program(s) that interest you, you are probably going to waste a lot of time searching through catalogs.

Of course, you will want to read the catalogs eventually. However, for the reasons just stated, we believe that it would be preferable to look at some more general resources first. Among the most useful are the following.

The Annual Guides to Graduate Study (Peterson's Guides Incorporated, Princeton, New Jersey) These guides attempt to cover, field by field, every institution in the United States and Canada that offers graduate programs leading to a degree in each of the fields considered. At the very least, the names and addresses of institutions offering the degrees will be listed. For many institutions, there will be a brief, one-page description of the program, research facilities, financial aid, cost of study, cost of living, student body, application procedures, and whom to contact for further information.

Graduate Programs and Admissions Manuals (Educational Testing Service) This is a reasonably comprehensive source of information, provided in tabular rather than narrative form, about graduate schools in the United States.

Guide to American Graduate Schools (The Viking Press)   "This volume is designed to provide the kind of basic information students need to reach sound decisions in the selection of appropriate institutions at which to continue their education."

An Assessment of Quality in Graduate Education (American Council on Education)   A comparative study of graduate departments in twenty-nine academic disciplines.

Graduate Study in Management (Graduate Business Admissions Council)   This book provides an overview of management and the role of the manager, information about graduate management (business) education, discussing such matters as curricula and teaching approaches, preparation for graduate education in management, including such factors as academic background and work experience. Also, information on admissions procedures and the factors that shape admission decisions, financial aid, and information for special student groups are presented.

Prelaw Handbook (Association of American Law Schools and the Law School Admission Council)   In addition to descriptions of individual law schools and a sample Law School Admissions Test, this handbook includes information about the legal profession, prelaw curricula, the study of law, and admission to law school.

All students

Along with carefully studying the information in these books and individual catalogs, there are a number of other steps you might take to help narrow the range of individual choices. If possible, talk with alumni of the schools you are considering. Remember that the requirements and atmosphere of many have changed and that alumni may be biased about their alma mater.

Talk with department faculty and advisors in your own institution. They often have special insight into various schools. If possible, visit the schools and get your own feel for the place.

In talking with these people, there are a number of questions you may wish to have answered. The answers to these questions will help you to do a better job of choosing the right institution for you.

1. What are the students like? Are their views and lifestyles compatible with your own? The school newspaper and other publications can provide some feel for this.
2. What are the admissions requirements? Can you realistically meet them?
3. Where is the school located? Are the geographic area, climate, and community suitable for you?
4. What does it cost to attend? Is housing provided and/or available and at what cost? What are the financial aid resources and required qualifications?

5. What is the school's reputation with alumni, students, other educators, and employers?

6. What are the specific graduation requirements for your prospective major field of study or program of training?

7. What is the student/teacher ratio and the typical class size in your area?

8. What counseling services are available, and how well are they regarded?

9. What career planning and placement services are available, and what has happened to recent graduates?

10. Are the courses you wish to take taught primarily by faculty members or teaching assistants (graduate students)?

11. What is the rate of graduation compared with the flunk-out and drop-out rates?

Make applications to schools and take required entrance tests

Once you have determined that further formal education in a graduate or professional school is desirable and/or necessary for you to pursue the career of your choice, you are ready to begin the application process. You will need to determine what, if any, tests or examinations are required, secure and complete the necessary application forms, secure letters of recommendation, and, in some instances, take interviews.

Tests and examinations

Most graduate or professional schools require at least one test as a part of their admissions process. Generally, graduate schools of arts and sciences require the aptitude (or morning) part of the Graduate Record Examination (GRE) or the Miller's Analogy Test (MAT). Some schools also require the advanced section of the GRE, which is an achievement test focused upon a specific discipline such as history, education, or psychology. One of the publications cited earlier in this chapter — the *Graduate Programs and Admissions Manuals,* for example — can usually give you an idea of which tests are required by particular institutions. Of course, the most reliable sources for this information are the schools' catalogs and admissions forms.

Virtually all law schools require the Law School Admission Test (LSAT). Graduate business schools require the Advanced Test for Graduate Schools of Business (ATGSB). Medical schools require the Medical College Admission Test (MCAT). Dental schools require the Dental Admission Test (DAT).

To transfer to a four-year college or university from a two-year community college, ACT (American College Test) or SAT (Standardized Aptitude Test) scores are required as part of the application. Information on time and place of testing should be available from the college to which you hope to transfer or from your community college counselor.

In all instances, you are advised to refer to the graduate or professional school or college catalogs for specific test requirements. Also, talk with your academic advisor, any pre-professional school advisors on your campus (prelaw, premedical, etc.), and your office of career planning and placement for more complete information about test application forms, test dates, and the best time for you to take a particular test. Regarding this last question, the general advice is to take the test as early as possible in your senior year. This way, your applications will be completed as soon as possible. Also, if you are sick and cannot take the test or do unusually poorly on the test, you will be able to take it later in the year. A brief word about retaking a test on which you do poorly. Usually, all scores for a particular test will be sent to the institutions to which you are applying. As a general rule of thumb, your scores on the second test must be at least 100 points higher than those on the first test for them to have any positive effect on an admissions committee.

Preparing for the test

A frequently asked question is, How can I prepare for a particular test? All of the test application forms contain sample questions. It is wise for you to complete these carefully and to be familiar with the test items and format. Although you really cannot study for an aptitude test, it should be remembered that most of these tests are speed or time tests. Thus, it is wise for you to be familiar with the test format and types of questions so that you will not waste valuable test time trying to figure out the test directions. This same advice holds true for test review books put out by independent publishers. If you feel that going over the questions and answers in one of these books will make you more relaxed during the actual administration of the test, by all means do it. Just keep in mind that probably the most important key to doing your best on a standardized admissions test is for you to be as relaxed as possible. So, trite as it may sound, do be sure that you get a good night's sleep before the test and that you allow plenty of time in the morning so that you do not have to rush to get to the test on time.

We do not advise that you take crash courses in test preparation. If you have any questions about the advisability of a particular preparation procedure, check with your advisor or career counselor.

Applications

There is not an awful lot that we can say about specific applications other than to read them carefully and complete all the required information as completely and honestly as possible. Failure to follow directions properly on an application form will be looked on unfavorably by an admissions committee and could seriously jeopardize your chances of being accepted. Also, inaccurate or false information will probably catch up with you and could well end your career before it begins. Again, if you have any questions about how to complete parts of an application, do not hesitate to ask your advisor or counselor.

Letters of recommendation

This is a potentially tricky area. As we said earlier, you are the one who selects the individuals who write your recommendations. Choose them carefully. Obviously, you want to select those individuals who can best speak to your potential as a graduate or professional school or college student. Not quite so obviously, these are not necessarily the people from whom you got the best grades. All of us have taken courses where little was required or performed, and yet we made good grades. We have also taken courses where we worked hard, demonstrated initiative and intelligence, and received a lower grade. Try to be sensitive to this when you select prospective recommenders. Most of us have also taken courses where there were a great many students in the class and the professor never got to know us very well. In this situation you might give the professor copies of work you have done in his or her class to refresh his or her memory of you. As we said earlier, be sure that you give a prospective recommender the courtesy of personally handing the recommendation form to him or her.

Finally, check with your preprofessional advisor and/or career planning and place-ment office to see what recommendation services are available to you. Often, these services will save a good deal of time for you and your recommenders in terms of maintaining, reproducing, and transmitting letters of recommendation to prospective graduate or professional schools. Review the section in Chapter 6 on obtaining letters of recommendation as part of developing your credentials file.

Interviews

Some graduate and professional schools, especially medical schools, require an inter-view as part of the admission process. Some schools strongly recommend an interview for all applicants. Others suggest it for marginal applicants. Still others, due to the number of applicants, discourage formal interviews although applicants are still encouraged to visit the school. It is important for you to determine from the catalogs and applications the category into which you fall.

If you are going to have interviews for admission to graduate or professional schools, most of the rules and suggestions contained in Chapter 11, "The Employment Interview Process," will be applicable. Read the chapter carefully.

A few basic tips may help you. Read the catalog and know as much as you can about the school. Know why you wish to pursue that particular program and go to that particular school. Be on time for the interview (this cannot be stressed too strongly). Know the interviewer's name and how to pronounce it. Know and use his or her title. Treat everyone with respect and courtesy — remember, secretaries and receptionists are people, important people who can and often do affect the tone of an interview situation. Above all, even though you will be understandably nervous, keep your cool and be yourself. Chances are, being yourself will allow you to be your own best salesperson.

Career development model — Chapter 8

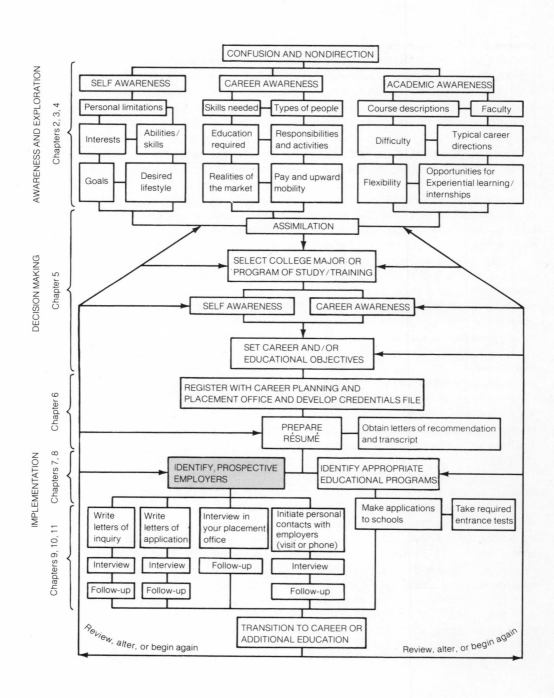

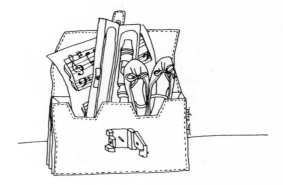

8 Identifying prospective employers

If you determine that you do not need, at least at this time, further formal education in order to pursue your chosen career, you will need to identify employment resources and begin to get them working for you.

Try to keep an open mind. Don't reject any resource because of generalizations and prejudices you may have developed. It's important to look at, explore, understand, and utilize all the resources available to you. Once you have reviewed all of them, you can determine which ones appear to be getting you the best results. Then you can begin to order your career priorities, select the resources most useful to you, and concentrate your efforts on them.

Above all, do not sit passively and wait for resources for career opportunities to come to you. Seek them out. A resource will only be useful if you are aware of it and use it.

The resources that follow are not listed in any particular order. Every individual's circumstances are different, and the utility of a specific resource will depend on each person's particular needs and interests.

Friends and associates

Who do you know, or know of, who is presently, or has been, employed in your field of interest? Make a list. It's probably longer than you think. Don't be bashful, shy, or afraid. Contact as many of these people as possible. Don't ask them for a job, but do ask them about their job and how they got into it. Most people are more than happy to talk about what they do and how they got where they are.

This approach will serve several purposes. First, you will learn some approaches to entering the field. Second, you will learn more what the job or career actually entails. Third, your friends and associates may identify some job leads for you. And fourth, these people will become aware of what you are seeking and may keep you in mind should they hear of any available positions.

Professors, teachers, and advisors

Most of these people will have excellent contacts both within and outside academic circles. They, too, are usually more than happy to share these contacts and leads with you. However, they cannot share these leads unless you make them aware of your interest.

Career planning and placement offices

The career planning and placement office of your college is a source of many employment leads. You probably think first of the organizations that visit your campus and conduct employment interviews there. Check with the office on your campus and find out what organizations will be visiting, what they are looking for, and the procedure for scheduling interviews with the organizations that interest you. You are probably also aware that your career planning and placement office posts many notices of available positions or vacancies. In other chapters of this book we have discussed how you can put together a credentials file that will present you in the best manner, and we will discuss how to conduct a letter-writing campaign — two follow-up activities that allow you to use these employment resources to your best advantage.

A third valuable resource in your career planning and placement office is the staff itself. Never assume that they know what careers you are looking for. Sit down and talk with the placement counselors. Let them know as explicitly as possible what your abilities, qualifications, interests, and goals are. They can give you many helpful suggestions and can also keep you in mind should they hear of an opening in your field.

Also available in the career planning and placement library are many of the other resources that we discuss in this chapter. Do not hesitate to ask if you can't find a resource.

College Placement Annual

This book, which is distributed without charge to students and alumni by college and university placement offices and by the armed forces, contains much information of value to you. Along with several helpful articles, it lists over 2,000 organizations alphabetically, with a summary of the types of employees they are seeking. Employers are also cross-referenced by types of college majors and geographical location.

Advertisements

Don't let your prejudices and misconceptions dissuade you from using this source. There are many good employment leads here.

The classified section of your local newspaper or a newspaper in an area where you would like to work can be a good source of openings if properly utilized. Richard Bolles discusses many important points concerning newspaper want ads in his job hunter's manual, *What Color Is Your Parachute?* Check your placement office for it.

Position wanted ads in journals and newspapers for the industry, discipline, or profession of your choice are also quite useful.

Before responding to any ads, be sure that you read them carefully, preferably several times, to figure out what they are really looking for and follow the instructions closely. Many employers screen out candidates according to how well they follow the directions.

Employment agencies

Although there is disagreement about the value of employment agencies, we believe they can be a worthwhile source of employment leads. However, we also believe that you should not have to pay a fee for doing what you can do just as well, or better, yourself — finding a job.

Therefore, we suggest that you only work with those agencies that will agree, in writing, that you will only accept fee-paid jobs. In a fee-paid job, the hiring organization pays the agency's fee.

Above all, be certain that you read any contract completely and carefully and check out anything you do not understand *before* signing.

Job clearing-houses

Many industrial and professional societies and associations compile listings of employment opportunities, which they supply to members. There is usually a nominal fee (ranging from $5 to $50) for receiving these listings. You can write to the national or regional headquarters of the association or inquire at your placement office for more information on the clearing-house most useful to you. Most placement offices subscribe to many of these clearing-house publications.

Professional directories

Many professions publish directories and/or journals. These publications often provide the names, titles, and addresses of people in the profession as well as job vacancies. These people can be invaluable sources of information about the profession, as well as possible sources of employment. Many professional directories are available in your career planning and placement office, college or community library, or through professional associations.

State employment services

The office of your local state employment service can often provide you with employment leads. Usually, the job leads available through state employment offices run the gamut from unskilled labor, to skilled labor, to professional positions. Some state employment offices will make available employment vacancies (either typed or on microfiche) to your career planning and placement office. As these lists can be quite comprehensive, they can be a good resource for you. Don't confuse this office with employment through your state government (civil service) — mentioned below. State employment services deal with all jobs, not just those in state agencies, departments, and offices.

Government employment resources

All states and the federal government have civil service commissions. Each of these commissions provides manuals or guides to employment opportunities, qualifications, and requirements with that particular governmental body. Before you can be considered for possible employment with the state or federal government, you must usually get a civil service rating or classification. Requirements differ, depending on the academic degrees you possess and your field of specialization. Some ratings are based on civil service examinations scores, while others depend on area of training or advanced degrees. For more information on employment with state government, contact your state civil service commission and/or your office of career planning and placement.

Along with the regional federal civil service office in your particular area of the country, another valuable source of information concerning employment with the federal government is the *Federal Career Directory: A Guide for College Students*. This book relates specific academic majors to career opportunities with the federal government and gives valuable information concerning entry requirements. Your career planning and placement office probably has a copy of this directory. It is also available through your regional civil service commission area office.

A final word about employment with the government — state and/or federal. Once you have received your civil service rating, your name will be placed on a state or federal register. Agencies having vacancies for persons in your area of expertise will turn to these registers for the names of "eligible employees." This does not mean that you should not continue to seek government employment on your own initiative. Do *not* wait to be contacted or notified of an opening. Find out from your career planning and placement office and specific agencies where the jobs are that appeal to you and for which you are eligible. Then contact the appropriate agencies by letter or, if possible, in person. In a cover letter give your civil service rating, explain your interest in the position, and ask the agency to tell you what you should do next to be considered further.

Seeking further assistance

These are some of the main resources available to you in your employment search. Use many of them at first. Then narrow your scope to those most relevant to you. If you think, or hear of, other resources, by all means use them. But first, check them out thoroughly for accuracy, up-to-dateness, and relevancy of information before spending additional time on follow-up activities.

If you feel confused by the number of resources available to you that identify possible employment, seek out a counselor's assistance to organize a plan for using them. Basically, these resources are divided into those that identify actual job vacancies (or openings) and those that identify organizations that typically hire people in different fields. Both types of resources can help in your job search and, of course, require different approaches on your part. Again, talking with a career counselor can help you get off to a good start in this phase of your career development.

Career development model — Chapter 9

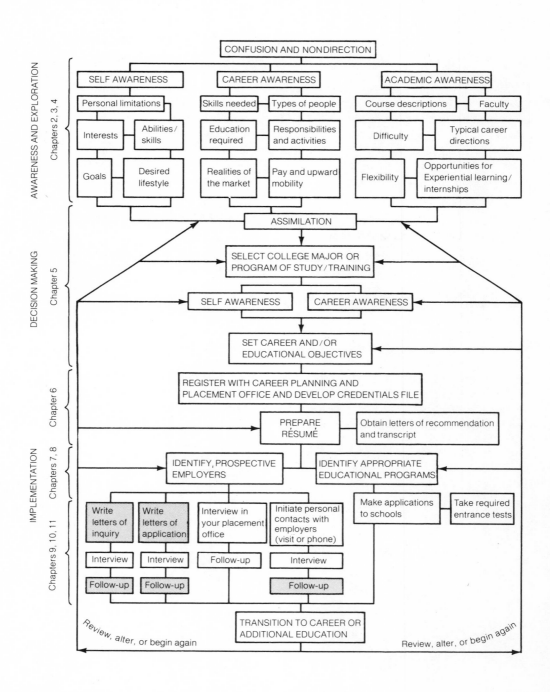

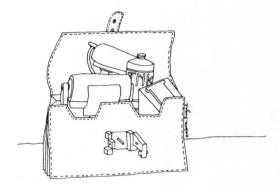

9   Letters of inquiry, application, and follow-up

Most literature on job campaigns emphasizes the conduct of the job interview. As this is the crucial step when you, as the prospective employee, must sell yourself to the employer, this is probably justified. Ultimately, the decision to hire or not to hire an individual will be based on a successful or unsuccessful interview.

Despite this emphasis, many important strategies must be successfully completed prior to the interview stage if you are to attain that job. One such preliminary strategy is letter writing. Because a letter is often the initial contact between you and an employer, its content will make an important first impression. Therefore, before you can sell yourself in an interview, it is of paramount importance that your letters also contain selling qualities. This chapter contains information and examples that can assist you in your letter writing as one of the beginning steps in your job search.

Different strategies

Most employers attach considerable importance to the quality of the letters they receive from candidates. Therefore, your ability to communicate effectively in a letter is a prerequisite for further consideration in securing employment. Careful attention to the preparation of letters with special emphasis on *effective communication* is an important aspect of this step of the job-hunting sequence.

Just as in résumé writing and interview techniques, there is more than one school of thought as to correctness in letter writing. There are some advocates who favor a "hot" promotional letter that amplifies your assets and, by withholding the résumé, sparks additional interest. Though a particular type of employer may look favorably on such an approach, it is generally considered in poor taste as well as ineffective.

Another approach advocates that a letter summarize the facts of the enclosed résumé in such a way that the employer will be interested enough to read the résumé. This approach is based on two main assumptions: (1) the purpose of an employment letter is to make the employer read the résumé, and (2) an employer is not likely to carefully read a résumé unless the cover letter brings it to his or her attention. Again, these tactics are successful in some cases. It is important to remember that different employers react differently to different approaches. Since in most cases you will not be familiar with your prospective employer, it is your task to find an approach or style that is acceptable and attractive to a majority of employers.

The right approach

"An employment seeking letter should be a simple communication which is business-like but not overly formal, respectful without being shy, and personal but at the same time dignified."* This type of letter allows the résumé to speak for itself and is the most generally acceptable as well as the most effective means of presenting yourself to an employer.

At this point, you are probably saying to yourself, "This all sounds fine and good but *how* do I write a letter that will make this favorable impression?" The information and examples that follow will help you. A final and important consideration, however, is that the letters you write are "communicative extensions" of yourself and, accordingly, should be consistent with your personality. This means that you should feel comfortable with what you say in a letter. Except in cases where formal phrases are necessary, your written expressions can be very similar to those you would use when speaking to an individual employer. This is not to say that informality should be a part of a business correspondence; only that being yourself in a letter is important. Using an impressive vocabulary that consists of "ten dollar" words whose meanings you have to look up is an example of not being yourself. This will create a superficial impression that can be seen through by the average college interviewer or personnel manager. By utilizing some of the principles and examples in this book and practicing the art of being yourself through written correspondence, you can find the right combination of sincerity, confidence, and selling to create that favorable first impression in a prospective employer.

*Allen Rood, *Job Strategy for Effective Placement in Business and Industry*, McGraw-Hill Book Company, New York, 1961.

General principles

In general, you can write three kinds of letters when you are pursuing an employment opportunity: letters of inquiry or cover letters; letters of application; and follow-up letters. Though their purposes are different, the content and points to be aware of are, in many cases, similar. Each of these types will be discussed separately. However, the following points are applicable to all employment-related correspondence.

1. Use plain white paper and matching envelope of substantial quality and of the usual business-letter size, 8½ by 11 inches. Personal stationery is undesirable.

2. Always type a letter. No matter how legible and neat your penmanship, handwritten correspondence is not considered acceptable. Your name (signature) should *always* be written in longhand.

3. The letter should be neat and free of errors. You should proofread it carefully for correct format, spelling, grammar, and punctuation. With employers getting more applications for each position than ever before, they are using (sometimes out of desperation) neatness and clarity as discriminating items in sorting through applications.

4. Keep letters brief and to the point — a one-page letter is the accepted standard. Employers lose interest if they must read irrelevant information.

5. In all letters avoid negative approaches, boastfulness, apologies, exaggeration, insincerity, and inconsistency. Do not waste the employer's time by telling him or her things he or she already knows or that appear on your enclosed résumé.

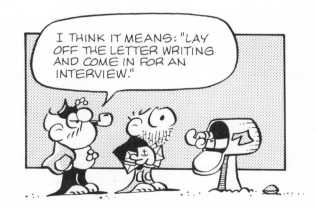

Where to find prospective employers

Employment area	Resource
Higher education	*Higher Education Directory* *Patterson's American Education*
Elementary and secondary education	*Patterson's American Education* State education directories
Business and industry	*The College Placement Annual* Business and industry publications Yellow Pages of telephone directories State manufacturing directories
Government	Federal and state employment directories *United States Government Manual*
Individual career fields	Individual career directories: *American* *Bank Directory, Directory of Advertisers*, etc.

Letters of inquiry (cover letters)

Letters of inquiry or cover letters are written to prospective employers to learn of possible vacancies and to request further information about these vacancies. Essentially, you are asking an employer if he or she has any employment openings in your field and that you be considered as a potential applicant for such openings. These letters should be addressed to a specific individual in a specific "hiring" position within the company, school, or agency — the superintendent of schools, dean of instruction, personnel manager, or director of personnel and employee relations, for example. Names of specific individuals in hiring positions can be found in some of the resources in the accompanying table, "Where to find prospective employers," which your career planning and placement office should have. When you use these resources, it is especially important to be aware of publication dates. If you are absolutely unable to locate a current listing, address the letter to a specific title rather than use the wrong name. Before resorting to this, however, we suggest you telephone the organization and request the individual's name and title from his or her secretary or the switchboard operator.

You might give serious consideration to the following points when writing an effective cover letter or letter of inquiry:

1. Always enclose a résumé with a cover letter. Your purpose is to interest the employer in hiring you, granting you an interview, or giving you additional consideration.
2. Address your letter to a specific person. Be certain that the name and title of the addressee are correct and from a reliable, current source.

3. The first twenty words are important; they should attract the employer's interest.

4. The letter should "sell" you in terms of the contribution you can make to the employer or past accomplishments that indicate potential success. If possible, include some challenging thoughts that will cause employers to feel it will be worth their while to talk with you — even if they really had not planned to hire at this time.

5. With local employers, take the initiative and telephone for an interview.

6. Refer the employer to the enclosed résumé for additional facts and details.

7. Use simple and direct language. Allow your letter to reflect your individuality but *avoid* cute, humorous, or *overly* aggressive phraseology.

8. Keep your letter short. You don't need to repeat things that are included in your résumé. Whenever possible, use the letter to raise questions, to ask for a commitment on the part of the employer, or to emphasize and expand on some item in the résumé.

It is not necessary that you follow each of these points exactly. They are guidelines that you should consider, but you can deviate from them or add to them depending on the individual situation. The following examples of cover letters utilize these guidelines in this manner.

Letter of inquiry or cover letter *Guide**

Return Address
City, State, Zip Code
Date

Full name of "employing" individual
Title of "employing" individual
Organization
City, State, Zip Code

Salutation:

Purpose of letter — inquire as to positions in your field which may be open in that organization, school or agency.

Point out significant experience or accomplishments in your field which make you a desirable employee for that organization.

Refer to the attached resume for additional details not covered in your letter and inform the employer where and how he/she can obtain your credentials.

Restate your interest in the organization and thank the employer for his consideration and interest. Have an appropriate closing to pave the way for the interview by asking for an appointment, giving your telephone number or by offering similar suggestions to facilitate a favorable reply.

Complimentary closing,

Full name *signature*

Full name *typed*

---

*Adapted by permission from *Educators' Placement Guide*, National Center for Information on Careers in Education, Washington, D.C. 1972.

Letter of inquiry*

216 No. Madison Street
Charlottesville, Va. 22903
July 24, 1975

Martha Johnson Community Center
927 E. Main Street
Charlottesville, Va. 22902

Attention: Director of Personnel

Dear Sir:

Through Mrs. Bettie Watson, who worked in your center until last May, I have learned that you are hiring a number of Social Service Technicians with AAS degrees.

I recently completed my Associate of Applied Science degree with a major in Community and Social Service at Piedmont Virginia Community College. In addition, I earned a certificate as a Child Care Specialist.

I am especially interested in a full-time position working with pre-school children. I can be reached during the day between 9:00 a.m. and 6:00 p.m. at 296-8701 or by letter at the address above. I look forward to hearing from you.

Yours truly,

Roxanne Slade

Roxanne Slade

*Courtesy of Dr. Jacquelyn Tulloch, Counselor, Piedmont Virginia Community College.

Letter of inquiry*

234 Sixth Avenue
Minneapolis, Minnesota 34972
January 5, 1973

Mr. Robert E. Taylor
Director of Marketing and Planning
Department of Health Products
State Office Building
Des Moines, Iowa 52400

Dear Mr. Taylor:

I am writing to inquire about job opportunities in your department for a college graduate with a B.A. degree in mathematics, strong course areas in psychology and business, and three years of active duty as a Transportation Officer in the U.S. Army.

You will see from my enclosed resume that I am interested in Marketing and Advertising. However, I would be equally interested in an opportunity in an area of administration for the purpose of experience. My major interest presently is gaining experience by being exposed to modern business practices as well as making a comprehensive contribution to your department.

As I will be traveling in your area in February, I will call your secretary to arrange a meeting convenient to your schedule. I look forward to meeting you and gaining more information about your department. Thank you for your consideration.

Respectfully yours,

Ross W. Smith

Ross W. Smith

*Adapted from *Job Strategy for Effective Placement in Business and Industry* by Allen Rood. Copyright © 1961 by McGraw-Hill, Inc. Used with permission of McGraw-Hill Book Company.

Letter of inquiry

Phi Delta Theta
Oshkosh State University
Oshkosh, Wisconsin 34576
May 23, 1973

Mr. Harold E. Miller
Superintendent of Schools
Fifth School District
Winnebago County
Neenah, Wisconsin 54956

Dear Mr. Miller:

This June 23, I expect to complete my Bachelor of Arts degree at Oshkosh State University and am interested in opportunities that you may have for history-social studies teachers next year.

My major area of study has been in World History with a minor in Sociology. In addition, I have completed the education courses necessary for state certification and did my practice teaching at Oshkosh High School during the past fall semester. While at Oshkosh, I also had the opportunity to assist in the coaching of the varsity football team and I would like to pursue this activity in my teaching career.

I am especially interested in vacancies in the high school history department but would also like to be considered for positions in the general curriculum areas on the junior high school level.

If you anticipate vacancies in these fields, I would sincerely appreciate your consideration. If convenient to your schedule, I will call your secretary the first of this month in order to arrange an appointment. Thank you for your assistance pertaining to this matter.

Sincerely yours,

Paul L. Collins

Paul L. Collins

Letter of inquiry

2763 Spring Road
Des Moines, Iowa 50312
April 1, 1976

Mr. B. R. Customer
Coordinator of Executive Development
General Mills Inc.
P.O. Box 1113
Minneapolis, Minnesota 55440

Dear Mr. Customer:

I am writing to inquire about career opportunities in your organization for a college graduate with a degree and a background in business administration and economics.

You will see from my enclosed resume that I am interested in general management as a career objective. My major ambition is to apply my college and work experiences to the challenge of management in your company.

May I please call on you for an interview in the near future. I would be pleased to complete your application for employment if you will forward it to me. Thank you for your time and consideration.

Sincerely yours,

John Edward Roberts

John Edward Roberts

Letters of application

Letters of application are sent in response to actual notices of vacancies received through your office of career planning and placement, replies to your letters of inquiry, newspaper ads, trade journals, and other official sources (see Chapter 6). Hearsay or conversation with people who are not working in the employment area are not considered official sources. You should not apply for a specific position within an organization unless you have official verification that an opening exists. If you are in doubt or are unable to receive confirmation, it is always best to write a letter of inquiry (cover letter).

As in all job-hunting correspondence, letters of application should be prepared according to the highest standards of business correspondence. They should be written clearly, succinctly, and in a courteous tone; be typed; and cover not more than one page in length. Details concerning punctuation, spelling, grammar, and sentence structure should be carefully considered. It's also advisable to make a copy of the letter for your own personal reference. Finally, the letter should be addressed to a specific individual including first name, middle name or initials, last name, and title. This information can be found on the written notification of the employment opening or in the sources previously listed under "Letters of Inquiry."

A letter of application should consist of three or four paragraphs. Some recommended information and ideas to be included in each of the paragraphs follow.

1. The first paragraph should establish a point of contact — either how you became aware of the opening or a similar association. It should also contain an introduction of you, the applicant, the exact job title for which you are applying, and your degree or the date on which you expect it to be conferred. It can also include your major and minor fields and, in the case of education students, certification status.
2. The second paragraph is designed to demonstrate how your education and experiences fit the requirements of the position that you are seeking. This is considered the selling aspect of the letter, and it should focus on how your skills and accomplishments fit the needs of the employer. Also, if you have a genuine rationale for your interest in this particular organization, you may wish to state it in this part of the letter. If these reasons include criteria that influenced your decision to apply, it would probably be to your advantage to state them. However, it is important to avoid reasoning that is general in nature and comes off as flattery.
3. Toward the end of the letter you can refer the employer to your enclosed résumé for information that is not included in the letter and indicate that your full credentials (transcripts, letters of recommendation) can be obtained through your office of career planning and placement. Give the employer the option of deciding whether he or she will request your placement office to forward the credentials or whether you should do it.
4. The final paragraph should stimulate action toward an interview. "May I call on you at your convenience for an interview?" "Please inform me when you can arrange an

interview," or "I will telephone your secretary to arrange an appointment convenient to your schedule" are much better statements than, say, "Please tell me about the possibilities of work in your organization." The answer to the latter is too easy. The key point here is to let the employer know that you want to be considered for the vacancy and that you are willing and committed to seeing him or her. Assuming that the vacancy needs to be filled in a short time, it is to your advantage to *initiate an interview* as soon as possible. Don't wait to be called in for an interview by the employer. Be aggressive and call for an interview on your own. Even if the vacancy is filled when you call, a persistent effort to see the employer (just to learn more about the organization) can be beneficial and may lead to other contacts.

All the letters and résumés in the world won't get you a job unless you interview. Use the telephone to follow up your letters and initiate the interview yourself — don't wait for the employer. How about ending each of your letters with: "Even if you do not have any vacancies, I am still very interested in Sears and would like to find out more about your opportunities. If convenient for you, I will call your secretary (I will stop by your office) and arrange an appointment."

Despite the availability of some on-campus interviews, we advise you to state in your letter that an interview can be arranged at the employer's convenience. Many times, however, it is not possible to travel long distances for an interview, nor is an employer always going to be able to cover your travel expenses. In such cases, interviews on your campus (if a representative is scheduled), at some other college, at a convention, or at some central meeting place may be possible. In these situations, it is of special importance to phrase the request with emphasis on employer convenience.

5. A final point that you may want to consider concerning the content of a letter of application is articulated by Richard A. Bolles in his job hunter's handbook, *What Color Is Your Parachute?* When answering a specific ad for a job vacancy, Bolles advises that you tailor your letter and/or résumé exactly to the stated job specifications and omit all else from your response — there is no excuse, therefore, for screening you out. The catch, of course, is to be able to successfully explain your tailored response if confronted in an interview situation. Also, if the ad requests salary requirements, it is suggested that you either ignore the request or state a range between $3,000 and $10,000 and add the phrase "depending on the nature and scope of responsibilities." If the ad does not mention salary requirements, you shouldn't either. It will just be an excuse for screening you out.

6. Always include a résumé with the letter of application. It permits you to keep your letter short as well as giving the employer valuable information that may cause him or her to pursue additional steps leading up to hiring. As in letter writing, résumé preparation is an important factor in obtaining an interview and should be accomplished with care and precision. Utilizing the guides provided by your office of career planning and placement and outlined in this book, as well as conferring with the counselors in the office, are steps you can take to improve your preparation of résumés and letters.

The following examples of letters of application use many of the previously mentioned principles in their format and content. These examples, as well as the principles we have discussed, can be used as guidelines in the preparation of your own letters of application. Again, and it is a point that cannot get enough emphasis, you should make additions and/or deletions according to the situations. Anything you incorporate into your letters should be consistent with your own style.

Letter of application *Guide**

Return Address
City, State, Zip Code
Date

Full name of "employing" individual
Title of "employing" individual
Organization
City, State, Zip Code

Salutation:

State why you are writing, name the position for which you are applying and how you became aware of the opening.

Explain why you are interested in this particular position and your qualifications-accomplishments in this field that would make you a desirable employee. This is the "sell" portion of your letter and it is here where you must distinguish yourself from other candidates.

Refer the employer to the attached application blank or resume which details your experiences, accomplishments, and ambitions.

Have an appropriate closing that initiates the interview by asking if you may call for an appointment, leaving your telephone number, or offering other suggestions to facilitate an immediate and favorable reply. Thank the employer for his or her consideration.

Complimentary closing,

Full name *signature*

Full name *typed*

*Adapted by permission from *Educators' Placement Guide,* National Center for Information on Careers in Education, Washington, D.C., 1972.

Letter of application *Example**

February 15, 1972

Mr. John E. Edwards
Director of Personnel
American Can Company
Greenwich, Connecticut 06437

Dear Mr. Edwards:

I wish to be considered for full time employment in your biological or chemical research department. Mr. Johnson, an employee in your Paper Chemistry Department, has advised me of an impending vacancy.

My resume is submitted for your review. I will be graduating with a B.S. degree in chemistry from Maryland Institute of Science and will be available for employment after June 7, 1973.

Any consideration given me will be greatly appreciated. May I please contact your secretary for an interview? I look forward to hearing from you.

Very truly yours,

Richard M. Morris

*Adapted from *Pathway to Your Future,* by Kenneth Adler (Bellman Publishing Company, P.O. Box 164, Arlington, MA, 1971). Used by permission of Bellman Publishing Company.

Letter of application

Box 234, Hallaway Dormitory
University of North Carolina
Chapel Hill, North Carolina 34567
March 12, 1974

Mr. Thomas D. Burke
Superintendent of Schools
Durham, North Carolina 34762

Dear Mr. Burke:

The Office of Career Plans and Placement, University of North Carolina, has notified me of a vacancy in your high school English Department and I would appreciate. being considered an applicant for this teaching opportunity. To support my candidacy, I am enclosing a resume of my experiences and the Office of Career Plans and Placement is forwarding you my credentials.

I have completed my student teaching requirements in the Chapel Hill public schools and will graduate in June from the University of North Carolina with a major in English and a minor in Speech. I will be receiving state teacher certification upon graduation.

Your consideration will be appreciated and I look forward to hearing from you about the position. An interview can be arranged any time at your convenience. As I will be in Durham the week of April 3–7, I will call your secretary to arrange an appointment suitable for your schedule. Thank you very much for your assistance.

Sincerely,

Mary L. Roberts

Mary L. Roberts

Letter of application

2763 Spring Road
Des Moines, Iowa 50312
April 1, 1976

Mr. B. R. Customer
Coordinator of Executive Development
General Mills Inc.
P.O. Box 1113
Minneapolis, Minnesota 55440

Dear Mr. Customer:

I wish to be considered for full time employment in your executive development department. Mr. Parker, Vice-President of General Mills, has advised me of an opening in your
department and suggested that I apply.

OR

I am writing in regard to a recently announced vacancy for management trainees that
appeared in the Des Moines Register of March 28, 1976. I feel that my qualifications and
ambitions are consistent with those necessary for success in this field and would sincerely appreciate being considered as an applicant.

My resume is submitted for your review and my credentials may be obtained upon your
request. I will be graduating with a B.A. degree in business administration and economics
from Coe College in Cedar Rapids, Iowa, and will be available for employment after June
1, 1976.

Thank you for your consideration. May I please contact your secretary so we could set up
an interview? I look forward to hearing from you.

Sincerely yours,

John Edward Roberts

John Edward Roberts

Letter of application*

715 No. High Street
Charlottesville, Va. 22901
March 13, 1975

Mrs. Helen J. White
Director
Learning Resource Center
Bloomwood Community College
Bloomwood, Va. 22907

Dear Mrs. White:

I am writing in response to your advertisement for an Audio Visual Technician in the *Positions Open Bulletin* (State of Virginia, February, 1975). I will complete my Associate in Applied Science degree with a major in Electrical/Electronics in June of this year and am interested in full-time work with audio visual equipment.

While a student here at Phieffer Community College, I have worked 20 hours per week in our Media Services department. I have experience in both the maintenance and repair of tape recorders, cameras, receivers, and other equipment. I am enclosing a resume with more specific information.

I am very interested in working at your Community College. May I come to Bloomwood during April for an interview? Since our spring break is April 5–15, I can come any day during that period. Other times are possible if I know in advance. I can be reached at Phieffer during the day between 8:00 a.m. and 6:00 p.m. (703-828-4099).

I look forward to hearing from you.

Sincerely,

Joseph P. Stoney

Joseph P. Stoney

*Courtesy of Dr. Jacquelyn Tulloch, Counselor, Piedmont Virginia Community College.

Follow-up letters

Several types of letters may be written following letters of application or inquiry. Letters acknowledging offers or rejections, seeking additional information, or inquiring about the status of an application are examples of follow-up letters. When you are corresponding with a prospective employer after an initial letter, the general principles we have already discussed are in many instances applicable. In addition to these, the following suggestions may be helpful:

1. You, as a candidate for employment, need to acknowledge receipt of all offers of acceptance or rejection notices. Appreciation for the consideration given as well as arrangements for future negotiations or a request for additional job leads, depending on the employer's decision, can be included in this acknowledgment.

2. When you decline an offer, you should do it as soon as possible and with courtesy. Again, an expression of appreciation is expected.

3. When you need to know the status of your application, it is permissible to write the employer and request the information. In doing so, you can review briefly the history of your job application and clarify your reason for needing the information.

4. In some cases, you may desire further information concerning the employer, specific position, previous interview, or related aspects of your job search. Being straightforward and asking for the specific information along with an expression of continued interest in the organization should elicit the desired response.

The following letters are examples of follow-up correspondence. Like the previous examples, they should be utilized only as guides.

Follow-up letter

703 Mitchell Street
Neenah, Wisconsin 54838
October 30, 1973

Dr. Alice C. Murphey
Chairman
Department of Mathematics
University of Virginia
Charlottesville, Virginia 22903

Dear Dr. Murphey:

Thank you for your letter of October 23, offering me the position of Assistant Professor in your department. I accept with pleasure the offer and look forward to working with you, your associates and staff in furthering the development of your instructional programs in mathematics.

Regarding the June or August starting date, if it is acceptable to you, I would like to begin my teaching duties in June. I look forward to meeting with you next week to discuss the specific responsibilities of the position.

Thank you for this opportunity for professional learning and contribution in the education-mathematics field.

Respectfully yours,

William C. Reed

William C. Reed

Follow-up letter

> 3504 Larchwood Drive
> Minnetonka, Minnesota 54783
> June 23, 1973
>
> Ms. Leslie A. Smith
> Director of Personnel
> Fielder Associates
> 234 Main Street
> Appleton, Wisconsin 54683
>
> Dear Ms. Smith:
>
> I am writing to say how much I enjoyed our conversation on Monday afternoon. The Corporate Planning Position which you described sounded both challenging and interesting to me.
>
> As I had mentioned to you, my previous experience in the corporate planning area included work for both General Motors and the Singer Company. While at Singer, I had been the primary force behind the corporation's first five year plan. If you are interested in more details concerning this accomplishment, I would be happy to get together with you at a future date.
>
> In conclusion, I am very interested in the Corporate Planning Position and feel confident about the contribution that I could make to your firm. I look forward to exploring this opportunity further with you at your convenience.
>
> Thank you for your time and consideration. I hope to hear from you soon.
>
> Respectfully,
>
> *Leonard S. Goodyear*
>
> Leonard S. Goodyear

Follow-up letter*

8459 Richfield Place
Cohens, Virginia 22759
June 25, 1975

Mr. Harold Hipple
General Manager
Koontz Automotive Clinic
998 E. Main Street
Richmond, Virginia 28759

Dear Mr. Hipple:

On May 20, I sent my application for the job of Service Manager along with a request for an interview to Mrs. Marks at the above address.

Since I continue to be very interested in working for your company but have received no reply, I am writing to check on the status of my application.

I look forward to hearing from you and to interviewing for the Service Manager position.

Sincerely,

Robert P. Delaney

Robert P. Delaney

---

*Courtesy of Dr. Jacquelyn Tulloch, Counselor, Piedmont Virginia Community College.

Conclusion

As emphasized throughout this chapter, the informational guidelines and examples of employment-seeking letters can help you in your job campaign. However, as with any self-help materials where examples or illustrations are given, there is a danger in following them too closely. Just as pat responses to frequently asked interview questions can make an interview stilted, using the examples verbatim can lead to the same impersonal structure in your letters.

Our examples are meant to be used as general guidelines for your own letter writing. Do not use word-for-word copies with your own insertions. Many of the examples, as well as the principles behind them, overlap in content and format and can be used flexibly according to your needs. You may, for example, get a useful idea for a letter of application to a business company from an example of a cover letter concerning employment in education.

In conclusion, letter writing is an important aspect in searching for and securing an employment position. By utilizing the suggestions and examples provided here as guidelines and by communicating your uniqueness in writing, employment correspondence can work to your benefit. Successful accomplishment of this strategy can bring you one step closer to finding the right job.

Career development model — Chapter 10

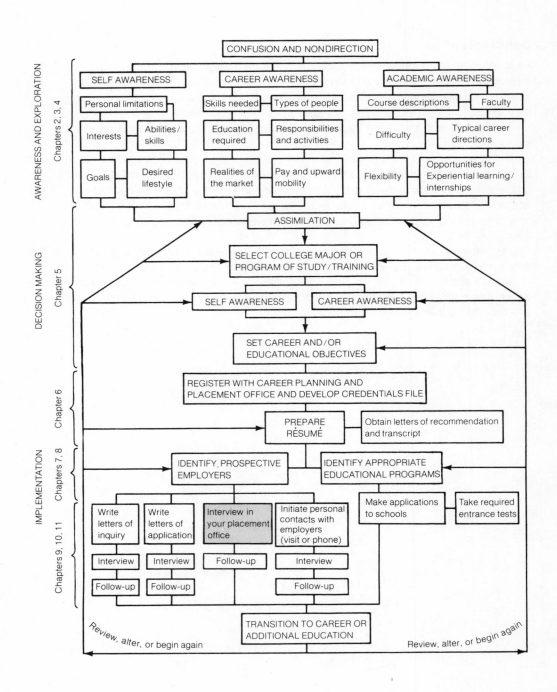

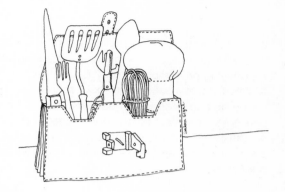

10 Initiating personal contact with employers

Interview in your placement office

Placement Office, Career Counseling Center, Office of Career Planning and Placement, or whatever the title on your campus, this service can provide you with perhaps the easiest way to make contact with employers. In almost every college or university, the career planning or counseling and placement office is very much involved in organizing on-campus employment interviews between you and varied employers from business, industry, government, and education. Because this interview process differs with each placement office, you are advised to contact your own office and discuss the exact procedures. In many cases, when you register with the office (see Chapter 5), this process will be explained to you.

You should be aware of the following general points regarding the employers that come to your campus to interview:

1. The majority of employers that visit a campus to interview students are from general business or industrial organizations. For the most part, they are seeking students to fill traditional career openings in accounting, marketing, sales, management, and general business areas. With today's demand for engineers and other technically and scientifically skilled people, engineering firms, data processing agencies, and, in some cases, scientific laboratories also send representatives to the campus.

2. School systems, both public and private, are cutting down on college recruiting because of the large oversupply of educators in today's market. A limited number are still interviewing on campus.

3. If you are interested in the social services as a career direction, chances are you will not be able to interview on campus. You will have to use other strategies outlined in *Directions* to contact social service agencies and obtain an in-house interview.

4. Banks and financial organizations still recruit quite regularly on college and university campuses. They are mainly looking for economics and business majors and liberal arts graduates.

If you are interested in some other career field, don't be discouraged. Check the listing of employers that are coming to your campus — just because we didn't mention them doesn't mean they aren't actively seeking students. Also, depending upon your part-time work experience as well as your motivation, liberal arts graduates can pursue and succeed in many of the above-mentioned fields. Research has shown that it's the specialized individual who has the better chance of obtaining an entry position in business today — but it's the liberal arts graduates who more easily climb the corporate ladder.

The on-campus interview is only one way to enter a career (the easiest for you because it cuts down your work and hassles). Other strategies in this book can help you find alternative approaches to getting the all-important interview that leads to a job in your chosen field.

Make your own contacts with employers by visit or by phone

The *direct* approach to seeking employment may not, in effect, have to be so direct. You may even have completed this step already if you've had the opportunity to visit the right employers as suggested in Chapter 3. You may recall the point that when you seek career information about a particular field from a resource (person, visit, tour, "interview," etc.) in that area, you may be able to make a favorable impression. In some cases, then, this subtle approach can stimulate employer interest, lead to an interview and, with some skill and luck, result in an employment offer.

Another strategy in using a direct approach is to know the title and area of responsibility of the individual with whom you are seeking an interview. By carefully researching the organization, you can find out the individual who is responsible for hiring in the area to which your contribution of skills, interests, experiences, and so forth, would be greatest. This is the individual with whom you want to make an appointment.

In almost all cases, experts in job seeking say, this individual will *not* be located in the typical personnel department: "The personnel department in most companies, they say, is at the bottom of the social and executive totem pole; it rarely hears of middle-high level vacancies; it rarely has power to hire; it can only screen out applicants, and refer those who survive, on up to higher executives.*

Our assessment of the personnel department is not so negative. In many cases, because you are seeking an entry-level position or because the job application process requires it, you will have no choice but to deal directly with the personnel department. This can be as beneficial for some students as it is detrimental for others. There are just too many human variables involved to make a flat statement like *do* or *do not* deal with the personnel department. For example, you might be exactly the person a company wants but because you appear overly aggressive by going around the personnel department, you don't get the job. This aggressive approach could work, however, for a different organization and with different people.

As we emphasize in our discussions of letter writing and interviewing, you are dealing with a diverse array of employers and hirers — what turns one off will just as certainly turn another on. Your task then is either to risk a bold strategy that will impress some and "depress" others or to take a middle-of-the-road approach that is not likely to affect anyone one way or the other.

Seeing the "right" person

Except for the conventional employment process where you deal with a personnel department, your task is to identify the individual who has the power to hire you and to show him or her how your skills can increase the efficiency of that organization. This may begin with the subtle approach to gathering career information that we discussed in Chapter 3, or if you have skills and experiences (we all have), it may just be a matter of getting the confidence to see the head man or woman. You might say that you would appreciate the opportunity to find out what the responsibilities and activities of his or her position are or to discuss organizational problems, or telling the employer that you have been doing some studies on the company might be one approach to a lead in. Your questions can center on traditional professional problems (planning, quality control, turnover, management, etc.), or, if you have seriously researched the organization (business publications, reports, community and company literature, surveys, *Business Week,* the *Wall Street Journal,* etc.), they may be specific to that organization. One word of warning — be sure you've got some good answers once you get in the front door. If you lack experience here, you will need to work long and hard for some sound answers (or questions) or risk serious embarrassment and the certainty that you will not receive an eventual employment offer. Practice with a friend or counselor through role playing or rehearsal techniques. We believe all that work and research is well worth it.

*From Richard Bolles, *What Color Is Your Parachute?* (Ten Speed Press, P.O. Box 7123, Berkeley, CA. 94707), 1977 edition, p. 141. Used by permission of Richard Bolles.

Who is the "right" person

Okay, now — how do we find out who this important man or woman is that we must see? Unfortunately, it's back to doing some research again — research on the companies or employers you've identified (see Chapter 8) in an effort to determine organizational areas where your education, skills, and experiences best fit and the names of individuals in these areas. It's also crucial to have done research on yourself — know where your contribution can be the greatest and most helpful for an organization. We hope the exercises and questions you answered in Chapter 2, "Self-Awareness," and the résumé you wrote in Chapter 6 will enable you to get a handle on this. Using resources like *Poors Register, Who's Who in Commerce and Industry,* and company literature as well as having some good personal contacts can help you determine the right area for you and discover the individual who has the hiring power there.

If possible, get to know a little about this individual. It can work to your benefit. Remember what we said about things you do and say turning on some employers while turning off others? By using personal contacts to learn about an employer's idiosyncrasies, you can increase your chances of turning him or her on rather than off.

What, where, how? The Crystal/Bolles approach to the job search

Essentially, any and all of these efforts are focused on *one* result — getting you together with an employer (the person with the hiring power) in a *nonstressful* meeting. Most executives are under a lot of pressure to hire successful employees and, therefore, when they are using employment interviews to actually hire someone, this anxiety cannot help but be detrimental to the way a candidate appears. Therefore, enabling him or her to view and evaluate you indirectly as a "career information gatherer" or as a potential source of help to his organization, rather than as one of a hundred job applicants, has to increase your chances of making a good impression. With follow-up and some ability on your part, you can increase the chances of an employment offer and a potential career. There's no way we can guarantee success using this approach, but we think it is a unique method that may bring you the job you're striving for. Richard Bolles, a very innovative educator in the area of getting a job, strongly supports this approach. His book *What Color Is Your Parachute? A Practical Guide for Job-Hunters and Career-Changers* (1972, 1977), can give you more detailed information concerning this step in your career development. The following section is specifically devoted to his methods.

For any discussion of the job search (or career development, for that matter), especially where the focus is on personal, direct contact with an employer, failure to elaborate on Richard N. Bolles's work based on the pioneering ideas of John C. Crystal would be a major omission. We have already spoken of Bolles's book *What Color Is Your Parachute? A Practical Guide for Job-Hunters and Career-Changers* and again encourage you to consult it for valuable input for your own job hunt. Some of his major ideas are contained in that book — they were described in the previous section of *Directions*. His recent emphasis, however, seems to stress the idea of skill identification and interviewing for information.

Dick Bolles uses the three-word structure of *what, where,* and *how* to outline this approach.* "What" designates your skills — what you can do; "where" indicates where you can use your skills (including knowing for which employing organizations your skills are applicable); "How" — how do you identify those places, and then how do you get hired there? We have already dealt extensively with the "what" and the "where" of getting a job in "Self-Awareness," "Academic Awareness," and "Career Awareness." Dick Bolles's emphasis on the "how" is simple and subtle, yet requires confidence and courage on your part. It is based on the premise that only 20 percent of the employment opportunities are ever advertised. The other 80 percent are there for those who have the initiative to seek them out. A sketch of this approach follows.†

After identifying your skills and the kind of organization that can use your skills, you can initiate a meeting with someone in one of those organizations who has the power to hire. The Yellow Pages, the local Chamber of Commerce, and professional directories can give you the right names; a letter followed by a phone call can result in a meeting. The key point lies in the reason for the meeting. Employment is *not even mentioned.* You are there to seek out information about the organization — specifically about the area of operation in which you're interested. Needless to say, you'll want to be well rehearsed and have your approach well phrased if you are arranging a meeting by telephone. Once you are in the meeting, your questions should be numerous, well-informed, and based on solid research of the organization's operating procedures. Believe it or not, people love to talk about what they do in a job and are usually more than happy to talk to you in this context.

From this point, you can seek out other organizations and resource people mentioned in your interview, or you can go back and seek out another organization on your own. Remember, *employment is not even mentioned.* Through this procedure, you are becoming more visible to employing organizations in which your interests and skills are applicable.

A return visit to your favorite (or most efficient, interesting, etc.) organization, further explanation of your interest, and an introduction of your skills and their applicability to the discussions will begin to bring an employment perspective into view. Discussing specific

---

*The material in this section is paraphrased by permission of the author from Richard Bolles, *What Color Is Your Parachute?* Ten Speed Press, Berkeley, 1972, 1977; and Richard Bolles, *The Quick Job Hunting Map,* Ten Speed Press, Berkeley, 1975.

†Invented by John Crystal, interpreted and refined by Richard Bolles. See their joint work: *Where Do I Go From Here With My Life?* (Seabury Press, New York, 1974).

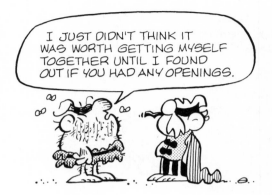

job activities and responsibilities, as well as taking the more traditional job-hunting steps (like leaving your résumé), are now appropriate. Dick Bolles refers to these two aspects of the job search as "Part I" and "Part II"; let's take a look at how he frames it:

> Beyond mechanics, it is essential for you to remember who you are, as you are going about this whole business of researching and interviewing *for information only*. The whole process will divide into two parts. Let us make clear what they are:
>
> Part I. You are the screener. The employers and organizations are the *screenees*. You are looking them over, trying to decide which of these pleases YOU. This is for information, building of contacts, and tracking down places that interest you *only*. During Part I, you can even take others with you (especially if you are in high school or college and this is all new to you, or if you are a housewife coming into the marketplace for the first time). After all, you are going out only to find information. You are not yet job-hunting, in this Part of the Process. Therefore, it's perfectly okay to take someone with you, if you want to.
>
> Part II. Having narrowed down the possibilities to four or five that really fascinate you, you now return to them . . . to seek an actual job there (doing the thing you have decided you would most like to do). At that point *and only at that point,* you now become the Screenee, and the employers or organizations, or funding-sources, or whatever, become the Screeners. Though, of course, you are still keeping your eyes and ears open in case you see something dreadful that will put you abruptly back into the role of Screener and cause you to say, to yourself at least, I have just learned this place really isn't for me.
>
> In any event, this first part of the research is Part I — where you are the Screener; and is not to be confused with Part II where you become the Screenee. If you *feel* as though you are the Screenee in this first part of the research . . . you're doing something wrong —

even if you have all the mechanics down pat. You've got rights: to go look at places and decide whether or not they interest you, and whether or not you could do your most effective work there, because you like what they're doing.*

Granted, this is a time-consuming process that takes courage and confidence, but it is, indeed, workable and capable of bringing you success. If you're shy, practice first — use your hobby and go visit people who are well-established in that area, write out a list of questions, or take a friend with you (after all, it's not a job interview . . . yet!). The more you do it, the more you will feel comfortable in your increased competency.

Our recommendations are 100 percent behind this approach to securing a job. Its emphasis on knowing yourself, knowing the work world, as well as meeting people who can potentially offer you jobs, is compatible with our idea to career development as we describe them in *Directions*. Use Dick Bolles's (and his colleague John C. Crystal's) approach, *along with* traditional methods in job search and securement. It's difficult to argue against a philosophy that urges you to use as many means as possible (within your own commitment and schedule) to secure a job. Remember, it's totally up to you — how much effort and hassle you wish to put into attaining that initial position. It is a decision that you alone must make.

*From Richard Bolles, *What Color Is Your Parachute?* Ten Speed Press, Berkeley, 1972, 1977, p. 124. Used by permission of the author.

Career development model — Chapter 11

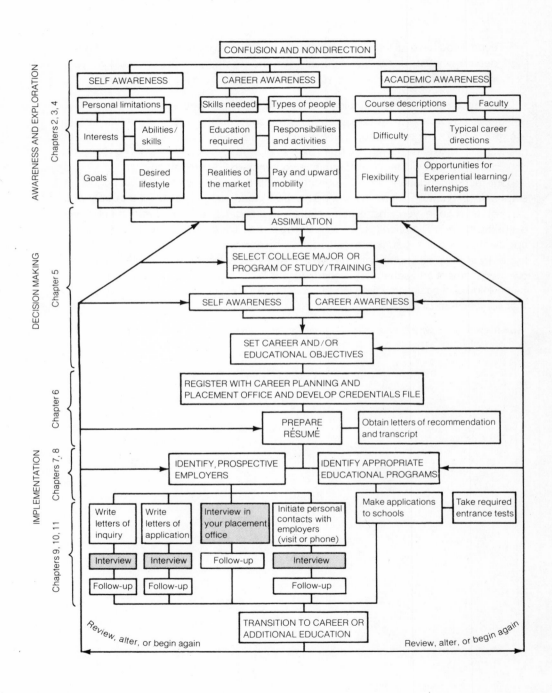

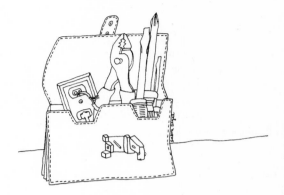

11   The employment interview process

Introduction and review

Now that you have gone through the previous steps in our career development model (self-awareness, career awareness, academic awareness, setting career and/or educational objectives, developing a credentials file, identifying prospective employers and/or educational programs, and making employment contacts) you are ready to plan and participate in the employment interview. If, after reading this chapter of *Directions,* you feel that further preparations are in order, your career planning and placement office has other resources that may prove valuable to you. Some of these are audio-visual materials that offer a number of insights, suggestions, and examples of what transpires in the employment interview. One of the most informative audio cassettes that we have discovered is "The College Interview," produced by the College Placement Council. Check with your own career planning and placement office to find out what specific materials they have and for assistance in locating and viewing or listening to these materials.

You are also encouraged to practice (audio and/or video tape, if possible) simulated employment interviews with a "placement person" acting as the interviewer. This activity will help you to develop a feeling for the interview situation. By viewing and listening to these tapes and critiquing them with a counselor, you will be able to identify your strengths and weaknesses and work toward improving your interview skills.

Before getting into the actual interview process, let's take a quick review of some of the basic steps we have followed up to this point. We are not going to review the entire career development process, but rather selected areas that tie in *directly* to success in your interviewing. We emphasize *direct* because certainly there is neither time nor space to review all the previous steps discussed in this book and, just as importantly, if you're now ready for interview preparation, it would not be practical to review all previous sections. With this in mind, the following information is crucial in the preliminary steps leading to a successful interview.

1. Understand yourself and focus on a general career field that is consistent with your interests, abilities, experiences and, if possible, your academic training.

What to do:

Read the chapters on self-awareness, career awareness, academic awareness, and
     decision-making in *Directions*.
Participate in individual or group counseling.
Take interest inventories.
Explore possible career directions by reading information materials in your college
     career planning office and/or talking to people who are in various jobs.

2. Register with your career planning and placement office.

What to do:

Pick up registration materials.
Decide whether you want open or confidential file.
Develop your résumé using guides, resources, individual or group sessions as assis-
     tance.
Carefully select recommenders and distribute letter-of-recommendation forms.

3. Identify those organizations that employ people to do the things you have identified in step 1.

What to do:

Use resources and directories in your career planning and placement office.
Pick up free copy of *College Placement Annual* that lists employment opportunities by
     major companies.
Use phone directories and professional directories in your library reference room or
     career planning office.
Become aware of those organizations, companies, and graduate or professional schools
     that come to your campus to interview.
Identify job openings and vacancies in vacancy-listings binders and resources in your
     career planning and placment office.

4. Contact employers by letter, telephone, and/or personal visit.

What to do:

Use guides and resources in *Directions*.
Write letters to specific individuals who have the power to hire and initiate an interview —
   follow letter with a phone call.
Arrange to visit employing organizations during Christmas vacation.
Use the Crystal/Bolles approach to visit employers as an information seeker.

5. Interview with employers.

What to do:

Sign up in your career planning and placement office for *on-campus* interviews.
Prepare for interviews by reading this Chapter of *Directions* and other guides and
   resources, listening to aduio-cassette tapes, viewing video tapes, or role playing
   interview sessions with your placement counselor.

6. Follow up with thank you letter or phone call.

What to do:

Initiate another meeting or interview, if necessary.

Easing into the interview

"This all sounds fine," you may say, "I'm now ready for interviewing, but what can I expect in a real-life interview? What is going to happen during that thirty minutes and what can I do to affect the outcome?"

Each interview will, of course, be unique because you will meet with different recruiters from different organizations. Some interviews will be highly structured, following a prescribed format, and some will be flexible within certain prescribed limits. Still others will be totally unstructured. Some interviewers will feed you rapid-fire questions, while others will expect you to do most of the talking.

With all these differences, however, there will be certain similarities among your interviews, and the basic evaluative criteria utilized by most recruiters will be the same. Most interviews can be broken down into four stages:

1. the introductory stage
2. a review of your background and interests
3. a discussion of the employer's opportunities and how you might fit in
4. the conclusion, in which points are clarified and the recruiter explains how and when the next contact will be made if there is to be one

Another way of dividing the interview is as follows:

1. The interviewer opens with a few casual questions to put you at ease.
2. Next, the interviewer asks you for some information about yourself or perhaps describes something about the firm he or she represents.
3. Eventually, you have the opportunity to take the initiative and point out some of your training and past experiences that could be of benefit to the employer.
4. Finally, the interviewer says what you should expect in the way of future contact from the organization.

Typically, the first part of the interview sets the stage for the entire interview. Research has indicated that the first impressions formed by the interviewer, in the initial minutes, are critical to the eventual decision as to whether or not you will receive further consideration for employment. During the remainder of the interview, the recruiter will consciously or unconsciously try to substantiate these early impressions.

Key points to keep in mind

Since the early impression is so crucial, it is important that you put your best foot forward. A few basic points should be remembered.

1. Be sure you know the exact place and time of the interview. This may sound too trite, but we've talked to unfortunate applicants who assumed that an interview was in a certain place because "all the others were."
2. Be sure you have the full name of the organization and the name of your interviewer correctly identified, spelled, and pronounced.
3. Plan to arrive at the site of your interview at least ten minutes beforehand. You can use this time to get yourself together, and there's always the possibility that the interviewer will be early.
4. Check your personal appearance again.
5. Greet the interviewer by name and in a friendly but businesslike manner. Introduce yourself in a firm voice. Shake hands firmly if the interviewer extends his or her hand in greeting.
6. Remain standing until offered a seat. Sit erect and look interested, but try not to appear rigid.
7. Be sure that you have done your homework and are prepared to answer questions about yourself and ask questions about the organization with whom you are interviewing.
8. When in an actual employment interview (not information seeking), avoid giving the impression that you have come in to look over the possibilities, and that you are not yet sure what you want. Don't say, "I'll do anything if I'm given the chance," or "I don't know

what I want to do — whatever you suggest," or "I want to work with people." Focus on a job opening or career field or be verbal and specific about your skills.

9. Be ready for at least one surprise question right at the start — some interviewers begin with the following:

a. What can I do for you?

b. Tell me about yourself.

c. Why are you interested in this organization?

d. What do you think you can do for this organization?

Maintain good eye contact during the conversation. This is significant and all interviewers are concerned with it. Remember to smile at times — during applicable situations.

10. If the interviewer does most of the talking, it's important for you to interject leading questions that will allow you to sell yourself. A question like, "Would you like to hear about my law office internship?" or "Can I share some information about my summer job with you?" will get you started.

11. Some interviewers don't like to do much talking, and in these situations you are expected to carry the ball, leading the discussion and ultimately selling yourself. Be sure you don't lecture or go on and on and on. Bring the interviewer into the conversation through good questions of your own.

12. Be sure you are communicating your positive, marketable points to him or her through the interview. We all have marketable characteristics or experiences, and before the interview ends the interviewer should hear about them.

Questions and answers to have together

Once you have been seated, the interviewer will probably begin asking you questions. The following list represents some of the questions most frequently asked by recruiters.* It will be beneficial for you to review each of these questions and prepare a brief response to them before the interview. (Not that you should memorize the answers, but rather that your preparation will allow you to quickly call to mind points once the question is asked. You won't have time to flounder once you are in an interview.) In formulating your reponses, try to put yourself in the place of the recruiter and answer the question, "If I were in the recruiter's place, working for this company, what would I want to know about me?"

1. What are your long-range and short-range goals and objectives, when and why did you establish these goals, and how are you preparing yourself to achieve them?

2. Why did you choose the career for which you are preparing?

3. What have you learned from participation in extracurricular activities?

4. What college subjects did you like best? Why?

*From "Fifty Questions Asked by Employers during the Interview with College Seniors," in *The Endicott Report,* by Frank S. Endicott, Northwestern University. Copyright © 1975 by Northwestern University. Used by permission.

5. What led you to choose your field of major study?

6. What do you know about our company?

7. Why did you decide to seek a position with this company?

8. What qualifications do you have that make you think you will be successful in business?

9. If you could do so, how would you plan your academic study differently? Why?

10. In what part-time or summer jobs have you been most interested? Why?

11. Why did you select your college or university?

12. Do you have a geographical preference? Why?

13. Will you relocate? Does relocation bother you?

14. Do you have plans for continued study? An advanced degree?

15. Are you willing to travel?

16. What specific goals, other than those related to your occupation, have you established for yourself for the next ten years?

17. In what kind of a work environment are you most comfortable?

18. What do you consider to be your greatest strengths and weaknesses?

19. Describe the relationship that should exist between a supervisor and those reporting to him or her.

20. Do you think that your grades are a good indication of your academic achievement?

21. What major problem have you encountered and how did you deal with it?

22. Describe your most rewarding college experience.

23. In what ways do you think you can make a contribution to our company?

24. Are you seeking employment in a company of a certain size? Why?

25. Why should I hire you?

In answering these questions and others do not respond with a simple yes or no, but don't be too wordy either. Phrase your answers positively and do not criticize past employers, teachers, fellow students, or fellow workers. Above all, be yourself. You must be discreetly candid and as relaxed and unaffected as possible. If you are faking your personality, an experienced recruiter will see right through you. Even if you could successfully fake your personality and secure employment, it is very unlikely that the job would be appropriate for you or that you would be happy in the job.

Be sure that by the close of the discussion the interviewer can answer these questions:

1. Why are you interested in my organization?

2. For which position(s) or career fields are you applying?

3. What are your qualifications, skills, and experiences?

4. How do you compare with other candidates? What makes you different and distinct?

If you have answered these questions, you have fulfilled a major part of your task in the interview. If, near the end of the interview, you feel that the interview is not going well and that you have already been turned down, don't let your discouragement show. You have nothing to lose by continuing to be confident and appearing positive. The last few minutes can often change the outcome as sometimes an interviewer who is interested in you may purposely discourage you in order to test your response. If you remain confident and optimistic, you will further your chances of success in the interview.

If an offer of employment is made to you following the interview, you are not obligated to give a firm answer immediately. If you are 100 percent sure that the job is the one for you, then accept it graciously. If not, tactfully state that you are flattered by the offer and would appreciate the opportunity of getting back to them in a day, a few days, a week — depending on the situation. Reassure the recruiter that you are very serious about the offer and definitely don't give the impression that you are playing one organization against another.

Some suggestions for responses

The following questions represent some more samples of what could arise in an interview. Again, don't memorize answers but decide the *major points* that you would like to make during the interview and evaluate how you would respond to these questions. The suggested approaches following each question are also for your assistance. They may or may not be applicable depending on you and your interview situation.*

1. *What do you know about our company?*
Better know something about what they do, product lines, types of services and programs, size, income, and image.
2. *What are your personal five-year goals?*
"I would like to be a project manager, head of marketing, V.P. for public relations, principal, etc." Relate answer to employer and his or her organization rather than giving a self-serving reply.
3. *With your background, we believe that you are overqualified for this position.*
This is the time to really sell yourself. Show that your so-called overqualifications can be a plus for the employer. Note that this may be a ploy by the employer to suggest a low salary. If you are interested in the position, continue to show how you can be of value to the employer.

*Questions and answer approaches from *American Institute of Aeronautics and Astronautics Employment Workshop* (New York, 1975). Used by permission of the American Institute of Aeronautics Employment Workshops.

4. *We feel that your past experiences (volunteer work, extracurricular activities, etc.) were not career oriented.*
Point out the similarities between your past experiences and the employer's requirements. Show how your past experience can be of great value to the employer as well as how your skills are applicable to his or her organization.

5. *Our experience with* _____ *(fill in the blank with liberal arts education, young, etc.) people has not been good.*
Demonstrate that what you have been doing previously can help this organization solve its problems. Show how you differ from the stereotype.

6. *What did you like least about your previous job?*
Employer wants to *see* how you react. Don't say anything negative about people. Constructively criticize or reply in a positive way by talking about things you liked about the job.

7. *What are three of your strong points?*
Know more than three.

8. *What are three of your weak points?*
Turn weaknesses 180 degrees to be positive — for example, "When schedules are pressing, I sometimes get in there myself," or "I am intolerant of sloppy work (laziness, etc.)."

9. *What do you feel this position should pay?*
You don't know; ask what range they have. Pay should be competitive with other organizations.

10. *How much do you expect (want) if we offer you this position?*
Be very careful in replying to this. Employer should have already assigned a money value to the job. Marketplace value of the job may be the key to the answer — check information in your career planning and placement office. Competitive with what other companies are paying. "I would feel good about a salary in the range of _____ to _____ ." (Again, check career information for going rates.)

11. *What is your philosophy of life?*
There is obviously no single, right answer. Be brief, concise, and don't try to overwhelm him or her with your humanity or desire to change the world.

12. *Any objections to a psychological interview and tests?*
Answer might be, "No, I don't mind as long as it's related to being a success in the job."

13. *How much do you expect to be making in five years?*
You never know what the value of money is going to be like five years from now. Talk in terms of being more interested in satisfaction to be derived from the work to be done and assuming that the financial rewards will follow.

14. *Tell me about yourself.*
Don't spend much time answering this. Tell something about yourself that relates to the job opening and let it come out in the form of a helpful experience — what you can do for the employer.

15. *Why do you want to work for us?*
Know why in your mind and answer in terms of what will interest the employer. Concentrate on organization's strengths and distinctive points. Be sure you research the organization.

If you had difficulty with these questions, you may want to role play with a friend or a career counselor. Have your friend or counselor be the employer and you the job hunter; then reverse roles and see the interview from the employer's side.

Interviewing for teaching positions*

Although the interview for prospective teachers can follow lines similar to those discussed above, there are important differences. The following typical questions asked and comments relevant to the interview are taken directly from a research study of Iowa school superintendents conducted by William J. Sloss for his masters thesis at the University of Northern Iowa. We feel it contains a wealth of information for the prospective teacher interviewing for that initial teaching position.

The following comments made by superintendents in this study are relevant to the interview process.

1. I try to determine if the candidate is willing to fit into the community. (Recognizing some communities are more permissive than others.)

2. Will he or she be good for the system? We don't want a radical element on our faculty. This does not mean that long hair and a beard will eliminate a person, but I feel they should be dressed in a respectful manner.

3. It takes time to train a good teacher. I want someone who will stay if he or she works out well.

4. I am expected to run many activities. I can't do this without people. I need people who are interested in kids and will try to avoid strict "eight-to-four" teachers.

5. Sometimes I propose a controversial viewpoint to see how well and vigorously a candidate will defend his or her convictions.

6. Does the candidate sell the interviewer the idea that she or he is well prepared to handle his subject and present it effectively to a classroom of children?

7. I try to determine what the candidate can contribute to the total school.

8. I am interested in having the applicants answer most any questions. Their ability to communicate is very important. It shows confidence in themselves or a lack of the same.

*Comments and questions from William J. Sloss, "Obtaining Teacher Employment in Iowa Public Schools as a First Year Teacher," Masters thesis for University of Northern Iowa, 1974. Used by permission.

9. I try to approach the interview using the stress technique.

10. I use a simulation of a teaching position or program to assess response of the candidates.

11. Most teachers know the subject matter, but can they handle discipline and work effectively with students and faculty?

12. I try to say something that should make him or her angry to see how he or she will react.

13. I definitely look for a neat, well-groomed individual. It's easy to get fooled if the candidate just gets shaped up for the interview.

14. I try to determine what a candidate's reaction to constructive criticism will be.

15. I seek a candidate's views toward young people who find school difficult. What will they do to help this young person?

16. I have told several teachers, "I am not so much concerned about what you can do as I am in what you can get students to do."

17. The applicant should feel that the student is all important and that she or he has something exciting to offer the student.

18. I try to determine if the applicant understands the small school setting with its many shortcomings as well as its benefits.

Here are some of the questions most frequently asked by employing personnel:

1. Do you really want to teach school or is it a stopgap toward something else?

2. How long would you plan to stay in our system?

3. How do you propose to handle first-year discipline problems?

4. What would you do differently than the way you were taught?

5. What is the building principal's role?

6. Do you perceive this job as a possible permanent location?

7. What can you do to meet the needs of individual students in your classroom?

8. What does the term *professional teacher* mean?

9. What makes you think you would be successful in this position?

10. What do you consider your greatest asset to offer teaching and our district?

11. What would you consider your greatest limitation to be regarding this position?

12. If there were one thing about your personality you could change, what would it be?

13. Are you interested in extracurricular activities?

14. What do you have to offer the students of this school that the next person waiting to interview might not have?

15. What provided you the most satisfaction in pursuing your college studies?

16. How do you as a young teacher gain the respect of the students?

17. If our program is lacking in your teaching area, how do you plan to upgrade the program and attract students to your classes?

18. Do you like to work with other teachers on a team, group, etc.?

19. Why did you select teaching as a career?

20. Coaches: What will be your reaction at contract time when the board remarks, "You should have won more games"?

21. Do you have standard levels of performance you expect from everyone? (We are looking for people that realize that each child is different.)

22. Looking back at your student teaching, what were some ways you had fun with students during this time?

23. When did you first think about becoming a teacher?

24. What do you feel is your major responsibility as a teacher?

25. Why do you want to teach in our school?

26. What is your philosophy toward kids and education?

27. Would you rather work with the above average, average, below average, or all range groups of children?

28. What ideas do you have for teaching your specific subject area? (Classroom approaches, subject approaches, classroom arrangement, etc.)

29. Will you be willing to take part in community affairs?

30. How can a teacher help children be better citizens?

31. What is your goal for yourself in education?

32. What salary would you expect to receive?

33. What rationale will you use when grading?

34. What do you expect to accomplish in the teaching profession?

35. What would you do in a certain discipline case?

36. What do you consider the most important traits for working in an educational setting?

37. How would you construct a class of whatever teaching assignment if you were to begin tomorrow?

38. What experience have you had in working with children?

39. What current literature have you read regarding your field of study?

40. What are the trends or innovative practices in education today?

41. Which group of students do you feel you will have problems relating to?

42. Do you have any ideas that you would like to try in the classroom?

43. How would you handle the student who continues to be disruptive after you have told him or her to settle down?

44. What are some essential ingredients in a successful pupil-teacher or parent-teacher conference?

45. What commitments would you make toward the improvement of our school system if we hired you?

46. What kind of things give you the most trouble?

47. What in your opinion is the most important single thing teachers need to get done?

48. Would you be happy living in a small rural town after being in a rather large town for at least the last four years?

Ending the interview

When you feel that the interview is coming to a close, do not prolong it. Without pressing, attempt to learn what follow-up action you can expect and what further action is expected of you. Also, at the close of the interview, chances are you will be asked if you have any questions. *Be sure you do.* Be prepared to ask *intelligent questions* about the organization and the position for which you are being considered. Sometimes people reveal more about themselves when they ask questions than when they provide answers. *Write* some of these questions down and go over them in your mind *before* the interview. Don't bring the written questions with you to the interview; having once familiarized yourself with them, you won't be at a loss when the interviewer asks you if you have any questions. You should have three to five questions and they should relate to the position for which you're interviewing. Sample questions can include:

Could you tell me about the training program for sales representatives — length, type of
    training, and amount of on-the-job learning?
In what ways do social worker assistants cooperate and work with other community
    agencies in Cedar Rapids?
How much opportunity is available for involvement with students in ways other than the
    classroom? Will I have opportunities for student activity advising?
What are the opportunities for furthering my education within your organization's benefit
    plan?
What are some typical career directions that are open to an individual who, say, does well
    for five years in this particular job?

Close by thanking the interviewer for the opportunity to talk with him or her and leave confidently with a smile.

Summing up the interview process

As stressed throughout this section, we strongly advise that you engage in some serious research before the actual interview. You should be very familiar with the organization — you can learn about it by reading (more than just once, five minutes before the interview) the organization's literature and descriptive brochures. Also, you should be prepared to answer the previously listed questions — don't have answers memorized but do have specific points in mind when that question is asked. In essense, you have some skills and experiences that are critical to your salability, and it is your task to communicate these qualities to the interviewer.

The more confidence you have in your ability regarding the interview process, the better your chances of coming across successfully, being offered a follow-up interview, and eventually attaining that much-valued career objective.

Why you didn't get the job

We conclude this section with a few more points for you to consider. The first is a list of reasons why students get rejected for jobs, and the final paragraph is a reprint from the *Graduate Magazine* article "Job Hunting Made Easier." We hope to assure you that lots of factors can prevent you from getting a job. Many of them you have control over, while others you don't. By controlling those you can and thinking reasonably about those you can't, your chances of taking a healthy perspective toward this whole job-search issue are better. Rejections are part of the process; however, by keeping your self-esteem and *not rejecting yourself,* your opportunity for success in the next interview is that much greater.

Why do you as an applicant sometimes receive only a thundering silence from prospective employers after your interview has been completed? A Northwestern University survey of 405 well-known firms found these reasons:*

1. Poor personality and manner, lack of poise, poor presentation of self, lack of self-confidence, timid, hesitant approach, arrogance, and conceit.
2. Lack of goals and ambition, does not show interest, uncertain and indecision about the job in question.
3. Lack of enthusiasm and interest, no evidence of initiative.
4. Poor personal appearance and careless dress.
5. Unrealistic salary demands, more interest in salary than opportunity, unrealistic about promotion to top jobs.
6. Poor scholastic record without reasonable explanation for low grades.
7. Inability to express yourself well, poor speech habits.
8. Lack of maturity, no leadership potential.
9. Lack of preparation for the interview — failure to get information about the company and therefore unable to ask intelligent questions.
10. Lack of interest in the company and the type of job they have to offer.
11. Lack of extracurricular activities without good reason.

*From "Trends in Employment of College and University Graduates," in Frank S. Endicott, *The Endicott Report,* Northwestern University. Copyright © 1973 by Northwestern University. Used by permission.

12. Attitude of what can you do for me, and so forth.

13. Objection to travel, unwilling to relocate to branch offices or plants.

14. Immediate or prolonged military obligation.

15. No vacation jobs or other work experience, and did not help finance her or his own education.

The final point: Don't reject yourself!

Your ego is going to be on the line, and it will get battered. Even if you get a great job on the very first try, there will be the night(s) before that phone call or letter comes. Nights when your stomach knots up anticipating THE REJECTION. And should THE REJECTION actually come, that pain in your stomach will become temporarily chronic. Self-esteem is highly vulnerable to rejection.

You must remember, though, that employers reject people for all sorts of reasons, few of which have anything to do with you. Perhaps they found somebody else earlier, but politely went through with the interview anyway. Maybe the budget is tight right now, but they want to conduct interviews to have names on file. Or perhaps they liked you, but your skills weren't polished enough for them yet. Economic factors may mean there are more graduates in your field than there are jobs. Or maybe they see what you don't: that the job isn't right for you, that you wouldn't be comfortable in the company.

None of this implies that you're worthless, although it may be hard to fight that feeling after a few rejections. You must keep your self-esteem up or the job hunt will get you down. And the danger of getting down, besides aggravating the knot in your stomach, is that you might start acting desperate before you really have to. You might jump for a job that is way beneath your abilities simply because you're scared. So for your own economic well-being, hang on to your ego. Job hunting is tough, chancy and time-consuming. Your belief in yourself is necessary to get you through it.*

*From "Job Hunting Made Easier" in *The Graduate: A Handbook for Leaving School* (Approach 13–30 Corporation, 1975), p. 60. Used by permission.

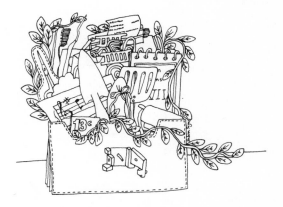

Conclusion: Where do you go from here?

Well, here you are. You have, we hope, gained some information about yourself, programs of study and training, and careers. You know the decision-making process and how and when to make decisions. You have learned about registering with career planning and placement offices, identifying employers and educational programs, the graduate and professional school application process, contacting employers, writing letters, and the interview process. You have, it is hoped, learned this career development process and now have the potential to put this knowledge to work for you in attaining a career direction or career position.

Now, you may ask yourself: "Is that it? Am I finished? Do I close *Directions* and put it on a shelf somewhere?" *No. Emphatically, no!*

You are not finished because your life goes on and with it your development and your career. Things will change. Your skills, interests, and values will change. Your desired lifestyle may change. The world of work and careers will certainly change. You will change jobs and maybe even career directions. However, the things you have learned about yourself, about decision-making, and about the entire career development process will stay with you and help you through these changes.

Career planning and development is a continuous process — a significant part of life planning and development. As the need arises, refer back to the steps you have just completed. Rework the exercises periodically so that the conclusions drawn are consis-

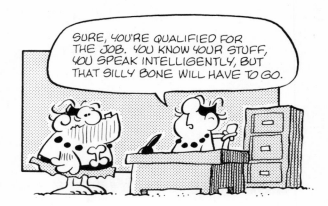

tent with where you are at that time and stage of your life and career development. Also, you can transfer your career decision-making and employment interview skills to other situations where you have to make decisions, solve problems, and communicate with others.

Career development and planning — we hope you'll agree it's more than just getting a job. The tasks accomplished and skills developed through the process of career planning are applicable to a lot of life's involvements. Don't get us wrong. We're not trying to force all this career discussion as *the* most important consideration in everyone's life — we only want to say that happiness in your daily work is a significant contributor to happiness in your life. Statements by workers like, "I think most of us are looking for a calling," "I consider myself lucky because I really enjoy what I do," and, on the other side; "You want quitting time so bad," and "Oh, my God, I've got to go to work," help to support this posture.

This book is not a universal remedy — no argument there; but when you use it to complement trained career counselors and your own personal commitment, you have the potential for attaining a meaningful career direction and influencing your future — a worthwhile accomplishment that can result in some peace of mind, satisfaction, and a happy beginning. Who could ask for more?

Index